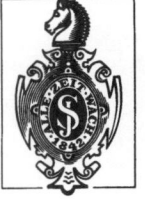

A. Cuschieri · G. Buess · J. Périssat (Eds.)

Operative Manual of Endoscopic Surgery 2

With 273 Figures in 432 Separate Illustrations, Mostly in Color

Springer-Verlag Berlin Heidelberg GmbH

A. Cuschieri, MD
Ninewells Hospital and Medical School, Dept. of Surgery
University of Dundee
Dundee DD1 9SY, Scotland, UK

G. Buess, MD
Sektion für Minimal Invasive Chirurgie
Abt. für Allgemeinchirurgie
Klinikum Schnarrenberg, Eberhard-Karls-Universität
Hoppe-Seyler-Str. 3, 72076 Tübingen, FRG

J. Périssat, MD
Cliniques Chirurgicales, 311 Boulevard du Président Wilson
33200 Bordeaux, France

Cover picture: Fig. 12.15 b, p. 233
Drawings created by M. Wosczyna, Rheinbreitbach, FRG

ISBN 978-3-662-01568-1   ISBN 978-3-662-01566-7 (eBook)
DOI 10.1007/978-3-662-01566-7

CIP data applied for

© Springer-Verlag Berlin Heidelberg 1994
Originally published by Springer-Verlag Berlin Heidelberg New York 1994
Softcover reprint of the hardcover 1st edition 1994

Reproduction of the figures: Gustav Dreher GmbH, Stuttgart, Germany
Typesetting: K+V Fotosatz GmbH, Beerfelden, Germany

SPIN: 10096524   24/3130-5 4 3 2 1 0 – Printed on acid-free paper

Preface

The second volume of *Operative Manual of Endoscopic Surgery* covers some of the operative endoscopic procedures which have been introduced into clinical practice since the publication of Vol. 1. In the general section, we have included an updated chapter on instrumentation and new chapters on anaesthetic management of patients undergoing endoscopic surgery and on video image and recording. Both topics are of importance to the practice of endoscopic surgery and have not been adequately covered in the reported literature.

Volume 2 deals with endoscopic procedures in the chest and abdomen. There have been significant advances in thoracoscopic surgery during the past 2 years; particular reference is made to anatomical pulmonary resections and oesophageal resections. As far as the gastrointestinal tract is concerned, we have included gastric and allied operations but have not covered the colorectal region as we believe that more evaluation is needed before definitive accounts can be written on endoscopic colorectal resections, especially for cancer. For this reason, we have decided to defer this important topic to Vol. 3, which is in preparation. The same applies to laparoscopic repair of abdominal hernias.

The same layout has been adopted as in Vol. 1 of the series, with heavy emphasis on illustrative representation of the operative steps and techniques. In the diagrams on sites of trocar/cannulae, we have indicated not only the site and size but also the functional role of each port.

As on the previous occasion, we are very grateful to the contributing authors for the high quality of their submissions and in this respect, our editorial task has been a light one. We also would like to acknowledge the constant support and encouragement from the staff at Springer-Verlag, especially Ms. B. Wehner, in the preparation of this volume.

A. CUSCHIERI   G. BUESS   J. PÉRISSAT

Contents

List of Contributors

G. BUESS, MD, FRCS Ed
Sektion für Minimal Invasive
Chirurgie
Abt. für Allgemeinchirurgie
Klinikum Schnarrenberg
Eberhard-Karls-Universität
Hoppe-Seyler-Str. 3
72076 Tübingen
FRG

A. CUSCHIERI, MD, ChM, FRCS Ed
Ninewells Hospital
and Medical School
University of Dundee
Department of Surgery
Dundee DD1 9SY
Scotland, UK

B.M. KOTTLER, MD
Abt. für Anaesthesiologie
Klinikum Schnarrenberg
Eberhard-Karls-Universität
Hoppe-Seyler-Str. 3
72076 Tübingen
FRG

T. LANGE, MD
Sektion für Minimal Invasive
Chirurgie
Abt. für Allgemeinchirurgie
Klinikum Schnarrenberg
Eberhard-Karls-Universität
Hoppe-Seyler-Str. 3
72076 Tübingen
FRG

G. LENZ, MD
Abt. für Anaesthesiologie
Klinikum Schnarrenberg
Eberhard-Karls-Universität
Hoppe-Seyler-Str. 3
72076 Tübingen
FRG

M. MACIOCCO, MD
C. REBUFFAT, MD
S.M. SCALAMBRA, MD
F. VAROLI, MD
C. VERGANI, MD
Università di Milano
Via S. Vittore 12
20100 Milano
Italy

K. MANNCKE, MD
Abt. für Allgemeinchirurgie
Klinikum Schnarrenberg
Eberhard-Karls-Universität
Hoppe-Seyler-Str. 3
72076 Tübingen
FRG

A. MELZER
Sektion für Minimal Invasive Chirurgie
Abt. für Allgemeinchirurgie
Klinikum Schnarrenberg
Eberhard-Karls-Universität
Hoppe-Seyler-Str. 3
72076 Tübingen
FRG

G. ROVIARO, MD
Università di Milano
Via S. Vittore 12
20100 Milano
Italy

1 Instrumentation and Allied Technology for Endoscopic Surgery

A. Melzer, G. Buess, and A. Cuschieri

Introduction

The instrumentation for endoscopic surgery has increased substantially since 1989 when the first laparoscopic cholecystectomy was performed; however, the instruments and the technology have not advanced significantly from the original devices designed and developed by Jakobeus [1], Wittmoser and Pfau [2], Semm [3] and our teams [4, 5]. Although trocars, cannulae, needle holders, scissors, forceps, and clip and stapler systems have been refined the basic technical problems of endoscopic surgery have not been overcome [6]. Sutures, ligatures and difficult organ dissections have to be executed with rigid needle holders, external slip knots and unergonomic handles across a two-dimensional operative field. Thus, complicated endoscopic operations can only be conducted safely by experienced surgeons. These procedures will be facilitated if the present disadvantages and limitations of endoscopic surgery technology due to restricted handling of tissue, lack of tactile sensation and force control are resolved [7] and three-dimensional vision is established routinely [8]. More complex and exacting procedures require even more intricate and delicate instrumentation. It is important that the surgeon become familiar with engineering and technological principles because he is the one who has to address the technical operative problems. Aside from the need for instrument development, certain basic medical and surgical principles must be followed. These include adequate operating times, completely sterile equipment, minimum malfunction and uncompromised patient safety. In this respect it is important that we encourage the industry and engineering departments to co-operate with surgeons in order to produce the instrumentation which meets the needs of endoscopic surgery.

Developmental Principles

Historically, physicians and technicians have worked closely to develop surgical instruments. Although these instruments were relatively primitive, they incorporated the necessary design features for good function using the manufacturing processes available at that time. Over the past centuries numerous instruments have been made [9]. Some were modified and then discarded, according to the progress in surgical science and current knowledge [10]. The conventional instruments of open surgery have obviously stood the test of time and over the years have been perfectly adapted to their purpose. But this tradition of instrument development and processing amongst surgeons and technicians has been interrupted and in past years the initiative has been taken over by industry.

New Area of Surgery: Old Principles of Development

Endoscopic surgery reveals the limitations and fundamental problems of current instrumentation. In this respect, the close co-operation between the engineer and the surgeon is assuming more importance, and so, as in the past, they must join effort to utilize all the available technological advances to produce the instrumentation which is best suited for the operations. Endoscopic surgery requires new instrumentation, e.g. instruments which are steerable, multifunctional, with automatic suturing, etc. Our goal has been to create the required tools by appropriate design [11]. As in former times, the instruments are designed by both the surgeon and the technician. This interdisciplinary linkage has revealed an important advantage; while

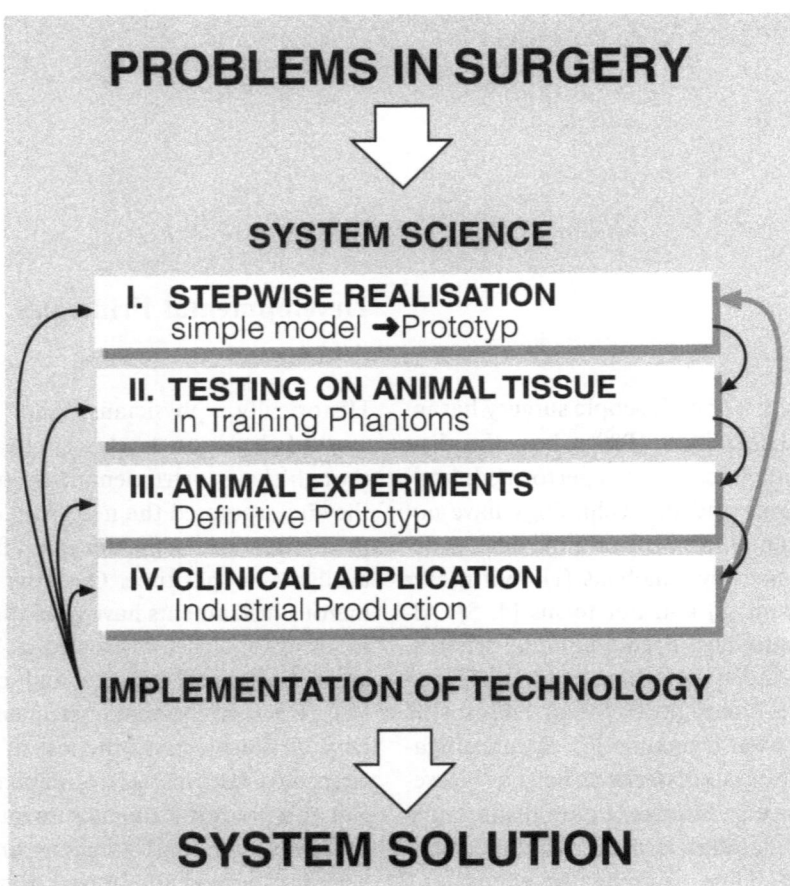

PROBLEMS IN SURGERY

SYSTEM SCIENCE

I. STEPWISE REALISATION
simple model ➜ Prototyp

II. TESTING ON ANIMAL TISSUE
in Training Phantoms

III. ANIMAL EXPERIMENTS
Definitive Prototyp

IV. CLINICAL APPLICATION
Industrial Production

IMPLEMENTATION OF TECHNOLOGY

SYSTEM SOLUTION

the surgeon is learning some important rules of design and principles of construction, the technician is acquiring knowledge concerning basic surgical and medical principles [12, 13].

Interdisciplinary Co-operation

We have established an interdisciplinary team concerned with the development of endoscopic surgical technology. This team always operates with a specific goal according to the principles of the co-operative model, which is divided into two levels:

- Level 1 entails the development of simple instruments and devices in consideration of practical surgical requirements for endoscopic operations.
- Level 2 includes system research [14] of endoscopic surgery as the cornerstone of the development of advanced, intelligent instrumentation and operating systems.

Fig. 1.1. Innovation level 1 in technology development for endoscopic surgery.
The developmental process is subdivided in four phases: first phase (*I*): theoretical solutions and simple models; second phase (*II*): practical approval of ideas in phantom experiments on animal tissue; third phase (*III*): animal experiments and professional manufacturing of prototypes; fourth phase (*IV*): clinical tests and industrial production. All sections of the development are interconnected and thus influenced and controlled by each other, not necessarily proceeding from phase 1 to phase 4. Ideas can be realized in all phases depending on their technological complexity or the medical approach

The development in level 1 is governed by the surgical problem and consists of four phases (Fig. 1.1). These phases are interconnected and influenced by current technologies as well as system analysis and techniques.

In *phase one* the surgeon and the technician discuss and outline a number of theoretical solutions regarding the instrument with sketches, drawings and simple wire or wooden models.

Phase two includes the crafting of simple prototypes, for example by modifying conventional instruments and creating test phantoms using animal tissue. At this stage the options are reduced to those which appear promising at the initial testing and only these are processed in the next phase. Whether engineers are involved in the theoretical calculation and design depends on the devices which are planned. The industry has to be involved early to consider processing, serial production and marketing.

In *phase three* the prototype is designed, manufactured and tested, first in phantoms and then in animals. Further modifications can be made in a workshop close to the animal lab. The practical experience gained by the use of the instrument in animals often requires that an instrument be redesigned.

In *phase four* a real prototype of the final instrument is manufactured by a medical instruments manufacturer. Only a device which has been successfully tested in human surgical procedures should reach the market for routine clinical application. However, reliability and clinical value of the solution only becomes apparent after an instrument has been used routinely. Not seldom, medical progress in other fields competes with or outmodes the operation itself.

This model is flexible; there are no fixed demarcations between the phases. The very first prototype of a simple instrument, for instance, can reach the routine usage phase and, by contrast, more complex developments such as manipulators or multifunctional instruments [7] may require processing through all the phases plus extensive testing and modification.

Level 2 entails systems research [14] and the development of intelligent instrument systems. The next generation of instruments will be intelligent steerable instruments equipped with microsensors, actuators [7, 15] and complex electronic controlling systems. The development of such instrumentation is, indeed, difficult and specific research must be conducted e.g. on qualification of tactile and proprioceptive impulse transmission [16, 17] or microsensor and actuator systems to achieve appropriate remote handling under three-dimensional endoscopic vision. Such delicate developments require the whole spectrum of scientific engineering. Therefore we are collaborating with research teams from the Nuclear Research Centre, Karlsruhe (KfK) Germany, the Fraunhofer Society, St. Ingbert, Germany, and the German Aerospace (DASA), Munich, Germany. The design and testing may be enhanced by simulating and modelling tools. In current microsystem engineering, computerized check of the design is indispensable [15]. The engineer proves and tests his development repeatedly to eliminate instrument failures. Such quality assurance and error analysis in endoscopic surgery will provide more reliable instrumentation. Even so, there is still the need for final experimental and clinical evaluation, because in surgical practice, instrument performance during actual operations is what ultimately determines its usefulness. It is important that the surgeon become more familiar with engineering principles and technological science, because he is the one who has to address the technical problems and to indicate the ways of resolving them. Hence, one of our most important aims is to create useful interdisciplinary co-operation in the future which requires that both groups be able to understand a certain basic language[1].

Technological and Medical Considerations Governing Safe Endoscopic Instrumentation

Reliability

Spatial restrictions put limitations on the design and construction of reliable and safe endoscopic instrumentation. Multifunctional devices are especially delicate and susceptible to breakage, and so cleaning and sterilization can damage instruments [18]. Besides the financial aspect, breakage and loss of a jaw, for instance, while clamping a vessel, is unacceptable and can cause complications. The paramount problem in technical design, though, is the narrow calibre and the length of the instruments. Critical constructions with hinges and small

---

[1] A new journal, *Endoscopic Surgery and Allied Technologies*, has been established to provide a forum for interdisciplinary communication, for example.

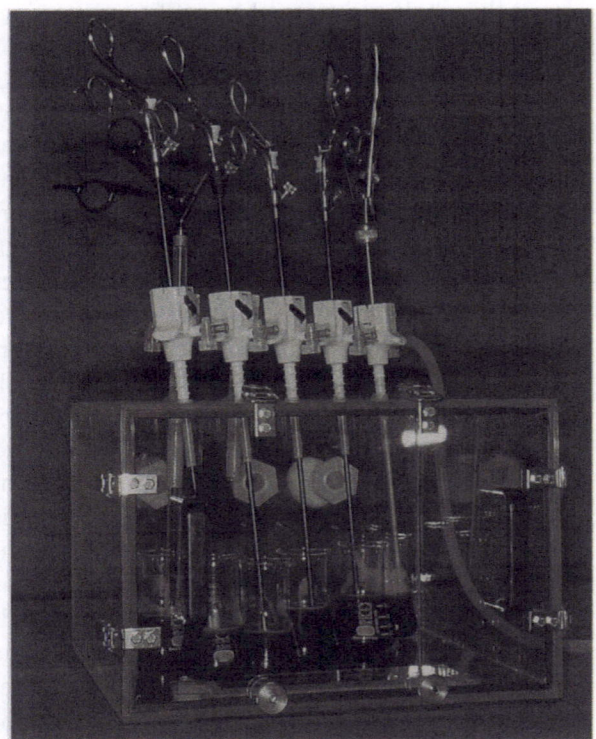

a

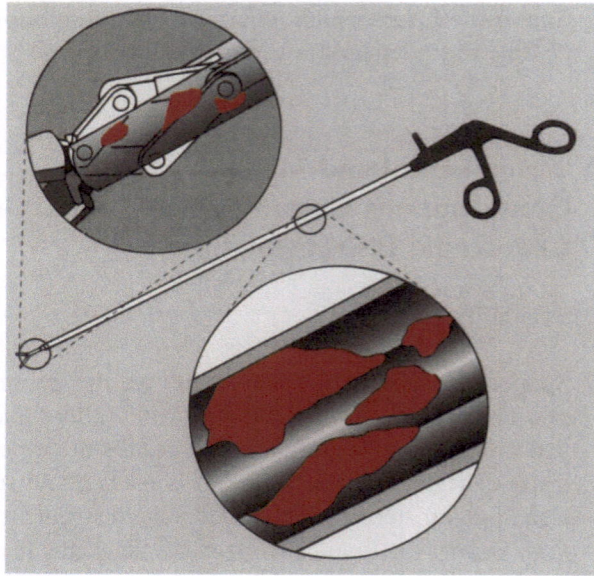

b

Fig. 1.2 a, b. Problems in cleaning endoscopic instruments.
a Samples of standard instruments were placed in a simulator box in order to examine their cleanability (Tübingen).
b Because of the tube character of the long instruments, the capillary gaps at the jaws and handle in conjunction with the intra-abdominal pressure become considerably stained with blood, which remains after routine work

bolts (Fig. 1.2) must be re-designed in order to achieve a simple and reliable action system which is simple and safe to use. Disposable instruments may solve some of the problems. They are completely sterile and the minimal lifetime requirement ensures in part appropriate function, e.g., scissors are sharp. However, the functions are often not as precise and optimal as required. Grasping forceps are sometimes unsuitable and the precise action of the jaws reduced because of instability and hysteresis of grip and hinges. Various considerations may require reduction of production costs, especially the desired low sales price. Thus either the design or the variety of construction material may affect instrument function and reliability.

In order to reduce the costs incurred in endoscopic surgery by disposables "re-posables" or semi-reusable instrumentation should be designed which meets the requirements for both endoscopic surgery and hygiene [19]. The functions should be controlled as easily as possible so that surgical procedures can be performed precisely and quickly. In addition, easy and fast sterilization and reprocessing must be possible without significant less in reliable function and lifetime of the instrument.

The parts which are subject to excessive wear and tear or which are too delicate to undergo the work-up can be disposed of, and the function of reusable parts frequently and regularly checked, preferably by specialized staff.

Applicability

Disinfection and Sterilization of Endoscopic Equipment

Hygienic requirements for instruments and equipment depend on the likelihood of contamination and subsequent infection in the patient. There are three risk levels [20]: Highly critical are those instruments exposed to the patient's blood or tissue, semi-critical are those exposed to mucous membranes, and noncritical are those only in contact with the skin. For these different levels, different reduction rates of micro-organisms are mandatory. For high-risk instrumentation a microbe reduction of 10^6, including spores, is necessary and for semi-critical equipment 10^5, excluding spores.

If an instrument is exposed to the organs and possibly to the blood in endoscopic surgery it must be treated as a highly critical item. Cross-contamination and subsequent infection must be avoided by completely cleaning and subsequently sterilizing the instruments. The optimal sterilization process is autoclaving. However, 121 °C – 134 °C pressurized and saturated water steam can severely damage heat-sensitive instruments made of plastics or optics and electronic devices. The explosive and toxic, ethylene oxide (EO) is used for low-temperature sterilization of heat-sensitive materials. The EO process requires delicate machinery and safety considerations and is less effective than steam processing. Prior to use the instrument has be to exposed to air to reduce the gas content. This airing time is up to 1 week for plastic and 24 h for metal. Thus the minimal time for an EO cycle is 1 day [21].

The low-temperature "sterilization" of the instruments using Sidex or other solutions such as glutaraldehyde, formaldehyde or peracetic acid is suitable for disinfection for semi-critical instruments but of limited value for instruments exposed to tissue and blood and cannot be recommended. There have been a few cases of proven transmission of HBV infection caused by endoscopic systems [20]. However, it is hardly possible to follow such infection pathways, and absence of evidence of infection does not mean there is no risk of infection. Hence, instruments must always be sterilized.

Newly developed methods of low-temperature sterilization can completely sterilize even delicate and temperature-sensitive systems [22]. The Sterrad System (Johnson&Johnson, Norderstedt, Germany) is a H_2O_2 low-temperature plasma process which allows nontoxic, rapid sterilization at temperatures not above 50 °C [23].

The process proceeds in the following manner: The instruments are sealed in a special package and placed in the plasma chamber of the device and a vacuum created. Approximately 1.8 ml H_2O_2 are injected into the chamber. The H_2O_2 immediately vaporizes due to the vacuum and all instruments are contacted. A radio-frequency, high-voltage field is generated and breaks down the H_2O_2 molecules into free radicals. These react with organic materials and thereby destroy micro-organisms. The whole cycle (ca. 75 min) is completed by refilling the chamber with filtered air.

Low-temperature plasma sterilization is limited primarily to surface sterilization; however, electronic equipment, in particular, synthetic materials can be sterilized and no airing is required. In addition, no special building or construction work is required in the clinic because the system is only the size of a large cleaning machine.

Basic Rules of Disinfection,
Cleaning and Sterilization

The principle rule of work-up is disinfection, cleaning and subsequent sterilization. Cleaning and disinfection is usually a combined process. It must be possible to wet all surfaces of the instrument to adequately flush and rinse it [19]. Frequent tests of sealing are mandatory since the instrument cannot be disassembled after it has been sealed.

Preliminary results of our investigations in Tübingen indicate that cleaning facilities for standard-design, rigid, reusable endoscopic forceps and scissors are inadequate (Fig. 1.2 b). Therefore, we have developed in co-operation with Netzsch Newamatic (Waldkraiburg, Germany) and Jakoubek (Liptingen, Germany) the Tübingen container (Fig. 1.3 a). After surgery the nurse places the instrument, disassembled if required, in this container and connects all tubes to special interfaces. The contents of the container are automatically cleaned and thermally disinfected, as usual. All internal surfaces of the instrument are reached by measuring the irrigation flow through all channels. The same container is then returned to the operating theatre and the scrub nurse can reassemble the instrument for the next operation. Thus, direct contact with contaminated instruments which are usually inadequately cleaned and scrubbed by hand can be minimized. Not only in consideration of recent identification of HIV virus in blood aerosols during surgical procedures [24] hand cleaning should be abolished totally.

Cleaning and disinfection depend more on the design of the instrument than on the washing machines because those have stood the test of time and their cleaning properties have been confirmed and are reliable for existing traditional instruments. Although the Association of Operating Room Nurses (AORN) strongly recommends the disas-

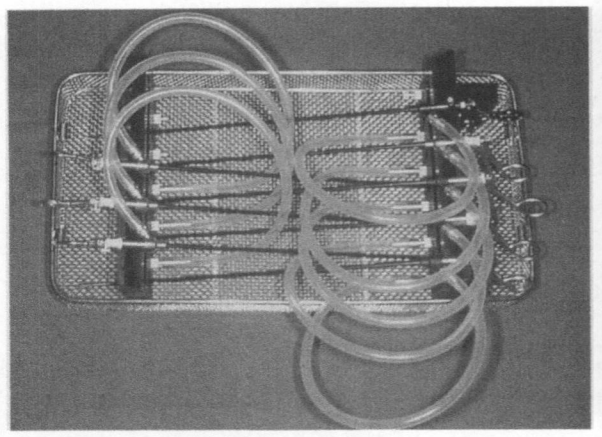

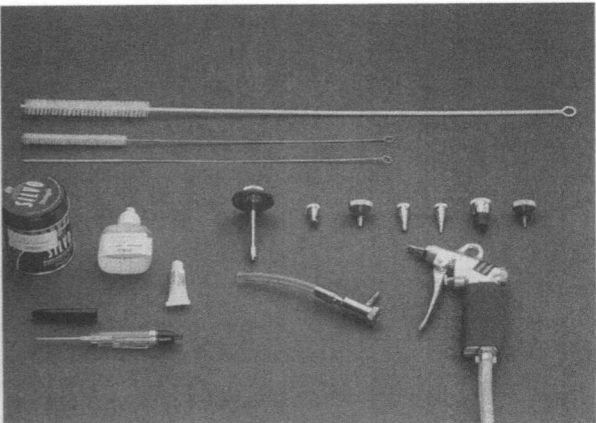

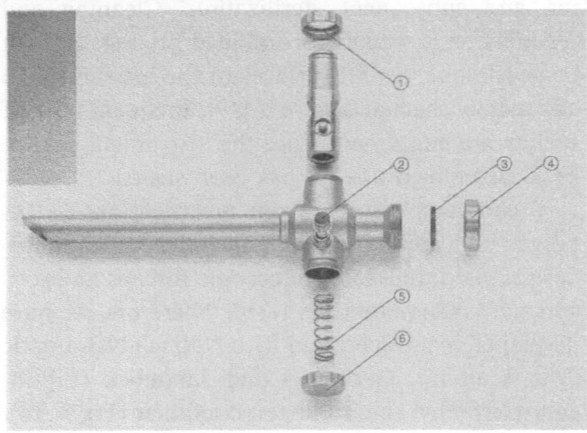

Fig. 1.3. a In the Tübingen container (Netzsch Newamatic and Jakoubek) irrigation of endoscopic instruments is automatically controlled; thus cleaning and disinfection is facilitated. **b** Cleaning usually requires considerable manual work and sophisticated equipment such as brushes, injection connectors and other tools. This adds significant risk to the person doing the cleaning of becoming contaminated and to the instrument of becoming damaged. **c** Conventional trocars and cannulae consist of several parts which are difficult to take apart and to assemble

sembling of all surgical equipment for sterilization [25, 26], endoscopic instruments can only rarely be efficiently and easily disassembled. Disassembled instruments are easier to clean and to sterilize [27]; however, the cleaning requires a considerable amount of work by hand and equipment (Fig. 1.3 b). Conventional cannulae, for example, consist of several parts which are difficult to take apart and to assemble (Fig. 1.3 c). We have attempted to develop instruments which can be easily dis- and re-assembled while maintaining appropriate and reliable functions. The first prototypes of hingeless modular instruments designed and constructed in collaboration with PCI/Jakoubek (Liptingen, Germany) and Nitinol Devices and Components NDC (Fremont, CA, USA) are promising (Fig. 1.4a). Other manufacturers such as Storz (Tuttlingen, Germany) or Wolf (Knittlingen, Germany) are marketing instruments which can be disassembled (Fig. 1.4b).

The industry should be encouraged to supply the surgeon with suitable, practical equipment which also meets the requirements for hygiene and work-up. Therefore, norms and standards must be established for endoscopic instruments[1].

The solution to these problems may be to replace reusables with disposables, but this would be of unacceptable expense. In our view the use of disposables should be restricted to certain instruments, such as staplers and other delicate ones. The shaft, handle and other simple parts should be reusable. The use of disposables leads to another important problem, that is reprocessing and reuse of disposable instruments, which seems to be practised in a number of hospitals. This policy is critical, because the manufacturers guarantee the function of their devices for the first use only. If the in-

[1] A comittee to develop DIN standards for endoscopic surgery was founded in September 1993.

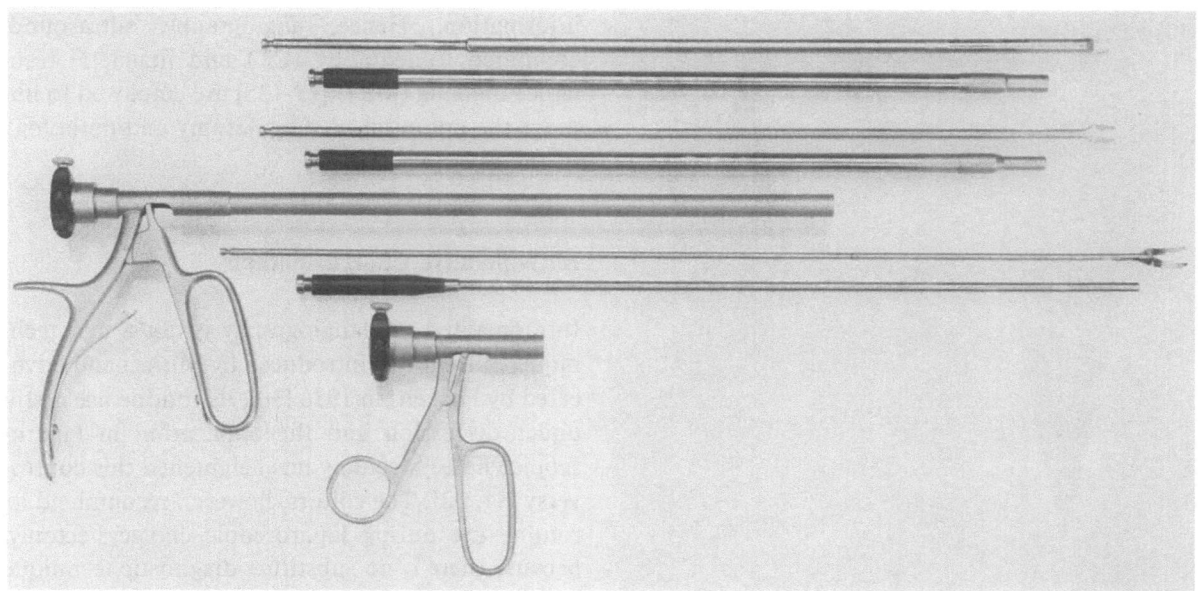

a

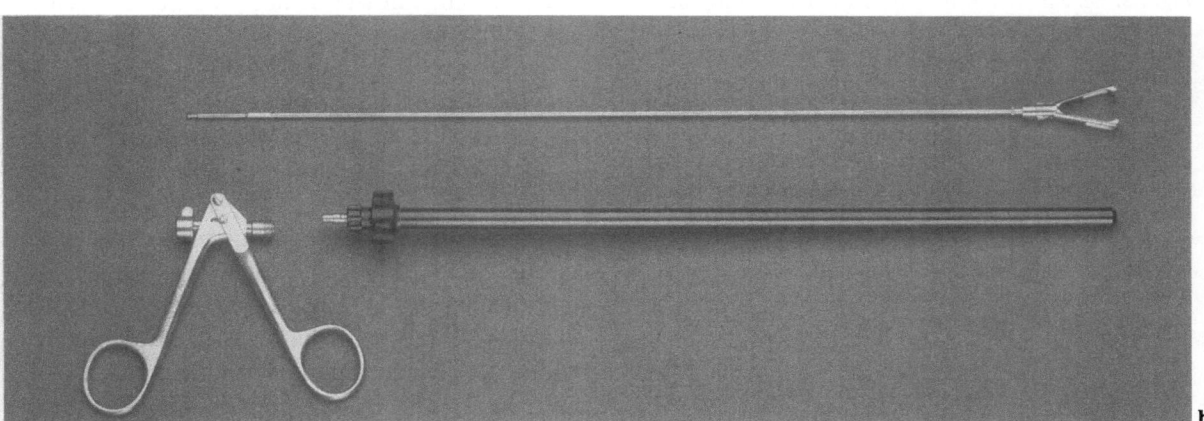

b

Fig. 1.4. a A new generation of hingeless modular instruments designed and constructed together with PCI/Jakoubek and Nitinol Devices & Components NDC can be easily disassembled and cleaned. **b** Storz, Wolf and other manufacturers are marketing standard hinge instruments which can be "taken apart" to facilitate cleaning

such as waste, energy, material and labour also need to be intensively investigated in order to find the optimal endoscopic instruments.

Biocompatibility

Biocompatibility is an important restriction in the design of endoscopic instruments as regards construction material, sealing grease and oil. The material has to meet certain requirements: no toxic effects to tissue, minimal tissue reaction, maximum chemical resistance to chemical influence, etc. [28]. The materials suitable for instruments must be of high mechanical quality. However, mechanical stability is inversely proportional to biocompatibility.

strument breaks subsequent to reprocessing, the surgeon is fully responsible for any resulting hazards [19]. We have only used reprocessed disposables in experimental surgery in animals and according to our experience the life-time of such instruments is often reduced after work-up and sterilization. However, cost-efficiency studies must be performed. Economical and ecological principles

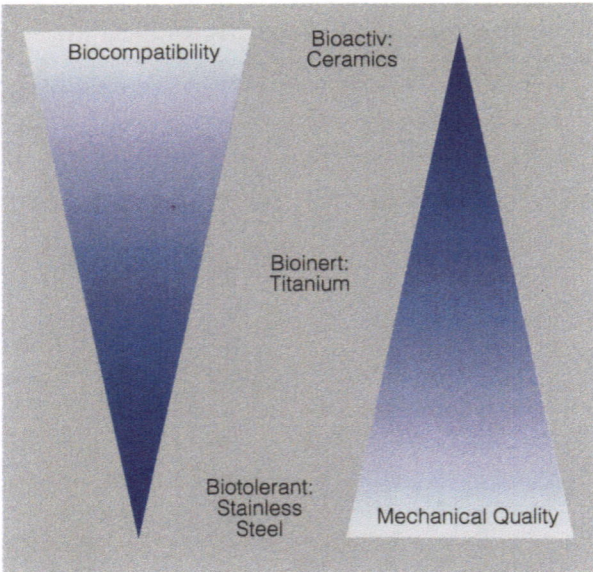

Fig. 1.5. Schematic illustration of the relationship between biocompatibility and mechanical quality of materials. The higher the level of biocompatibility of the material the lower the mechanical stability. For example, ceramics are bioactive materials, which means that the surface of the ceramic is either covered by a layer of protein molecules or it is actively integrated within tissue formation (calcium hydroxy dissolution apatite in bone). But their elasticity and mechanical stability is low. The bioinert materials such as titanium form passive oxide layers that protect within the human body. The biotolerable materials, such as tantalum and stainless steel, provide high stability, minimal tissue reaction and acceptable rate of dissolution of contents

Synthetic materials must be processed under clean conditions, e.g. the content of heavy metal must be kept to a minimum. Biodegradable plastics are preferable for clips and other implanted materials; however, their spectrum of processing is limited, there are fewer manufacturing facilities available and the mechanical stability is reduced compared to metal. Figure 1.5 illustrates the level of biocompatibility of common materials used in medical equipment.

Imaging Principles

Due to reduced sensory input such as loss of tactile feedback and the two-dimensional video image, the endoscopic surgeon requires additional anatomical information. Hence, angiography, ultrasound, computed tomography (CT) and magnetic resonance imaging (MRI) [29–35] are employed to improve the appraisal of the anatomy and pathology of the operative field.

Intraoperative Cholangiography

Intraoperative cholangiography is not a new technique. Since it was introduced by Mirizzi and advocated by Hickens in 1936 [30], its routine use is still under discussion and the application in laparoscopic cholecystectomy has heightened this controversy [31, 32]. The editors, however, recommend its routine use during laparoscopic cholecystectomy, because there is no substitute diagnostic technique which yields comparable anatomical detail. Moreover, the surgeon who is not practised in performing routine intraoperative cholangiography will not progress to more complicated procedures. The quality of cholangiography depends on the radiological equipment and its competent use [30].

Mobile X-ray machines with three blind exposures during and after the injection of different amounts of contrast are unsuitable and yield poor results. In addition, the important filling phase during contrast injection is missed. Due to such mishaps the procedure has to be repeated frequently and is time consuming. With the modern C-arm imaging systems (Fig. 1.6) with digital enhancement software such as real-time subtraction, road mapping modes and image storage provide excellent high resolutions exposures [33] (OEC Diasonics, Salt Lake City, UT, USA; Philips Medical Systems, London UK; Siemens, Erlangen, Germany). Using digital real-time subtraction angiography (DSA) with intravenous contrast injection, arteries can be visualized, obviating the need for direct arterial puncture. Unwanted background information is "subtracted", leaving only an image of the contrast-filled vessels, which is the difference between the "mask image" obtained at the start of subtraction and the contrasted exposure. When employed during intraoperative cholangiography, DSA is of particular benefit because it reveals additional anatomical details which can be obscured by overlapping structures. All the state-of-the-art C-arm machines support the subtraction technique.

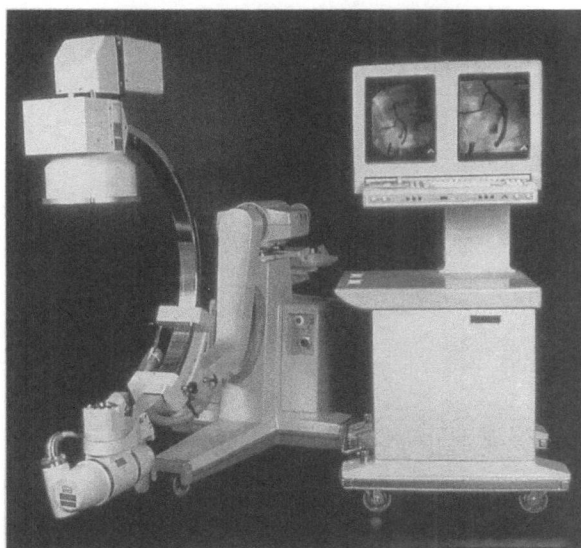

Fig. 1.6. Digital C-arm imaging systems provide superb exposures owing to new functions such as real-time subtraction, road mapping modes and image storage (OEC Diasonics, Philips Medical System, and Siemens)

The zoom, activated on the trackball panel, allows two- or four-fold magnification of a selected area of interest. "Peak opacification" compares the darkness of all pixels subsequently and replaces previous pixels by the darkest pixels acquired during the imaging process. By means of an automatic equalization of the contrast the "autohisto" takes a sampling of grey-scale values of the image and determines the correct level of an optimized and sharp exposure. The resulting image shows an optimum of contrast and quality for post-processing and image storage. The "road mapping" function obtains a sequence of subtracted images of a preselected original mask which is particularly useful for interventional cholangiography. With "real-time imaging" a selected stored image can be displayed on the left monitor and the active screening process on the right monitor. The running image can be enhanced by keeping an average of pixel values over several frames and a special feature reduces motion artefacts. It provides an average of the "noise" caused by small movements, allowing these to be viewed without undue lag. The images are stored on a hard disc, and so the surgeon can select images as they appear on the screen by means of a foot switch. These files can than be recalled and post-processed by transmitting the data on X-ray film cassettes of a mulfiformat camera or as video signals in SVHS quality on tapes or if desired as video prints by means of a laser video imager.

Ultrasound

The biliary tract and abdomen can be viewed using laparoscopic ultrasound [34, 35]. In contrast to radiological imaging, ultrasound operates on high-frequency longitudinal sound waves, which by reflection emanate an echogram of the biological tissue. The appropriate diagnostic range of the frequency (3.5 – 10 MHz) is obtained by a piezoelectric transducer. The size, shape and resonance frequency of the emitting silicon crystals determine the course of the sound beam within the examined tissue. To create a two-dimensional scanning field, the transducer crystal can be alternately moved within a sector of 60° up to 120°, or numerous transducer crystals linearly connected in a row are sequentially activated. The latter yields excellent resolution and a rectangular image which obviates the visual distortion of the triangular sector. The sound beam passes through the different cell layers that have different acoustic impedance which leads to attenuation of the sound beam. Attenuation is due to the loss of energy caused by reflection, refraction, divergence and absorption. The more attenuation caused by the sound through the tissue, the lower is the resultant signal intensity. The reflected sound signals detected by the receiver produce the image of the tissue texture according to the different signal intensities produced by the tissue impedance. The ultrasound image effects are "shadowing" and "enhancement". A sound shadow occurs when the intensity of tissue (fibrous, calcification or gas) is higher than an average attenuation according to the depth of tissue, which is balanced by means of the electronic controlling unit of the imager, whereas enhancement is caused by tissue which has lower attenuation (e.g. fluid) than that of the underlying structure.

The degree of the resolution of the image in respect of the depth of the examined tissue is determined by the frequency of the ultrasound transducers. The lower the frequency, the deeper is the exposure, but the degree of resolution decreases. By contrast, the higher the frequency (up to 20 MHz in intravascular scanning) the greater is the resolution, but the depth of the field is reduced [36]. For endoscopic purposes a range of 5–10 MHz seems to be appropriate. The ultrasound imaging systems are digitally enhanced and the pulse echo is converted into real-time, two-dimensional and even three-dimensional images. The contrast agents used are different from those used in radiology. Gas microbubbles in a fluid matrix provide the enhancement. However, the routine application of ultrasound contrast agents requires further research and evaluation.

Laparoscopic Ultrasound Probes

The ultrasound probes currently available for laparoscopy are the sector scanner made by Endomedix (Irvine, CA, USA) and the Aloka linear probe (Keymed; Southend-on-Sea, UK). However Endomedix is no longer trading. The 7.5 MHz LaproScan (Endomedix) (Fig. 1.7 a, b) employs a sector of 90°, one probe in side view and one in transverse view. Although the scanning can be controlled by the handpiece, its resolution and image qualities need further refinement.

The Aloka probe (Keymed) has a linear array which consists of aligned transducer elements. Its image is of high quality and comparable to that of hand scanners. However, the array beams in a rectangular direction, which decreases its applicability [34]. A convex surface of the transducer would represent a considerable improvement. Also a deflectable and adjustable scanning position of the distal tip is adequate [35]. The paramount problem of a deflectable probe (IV–E 1, Olympus Optical; Tokyo, Japan) is steam sterilization, because the technology employed is comparable to that of the flexible endoscope scanners (see Fig. 1.7 b).

Duplex Scanning

The Doppler effect – a reflected sound wave from an object moving away from the acoustic source has an enlarged wavelength, whereas the reflected wave from an object moving towards the source has

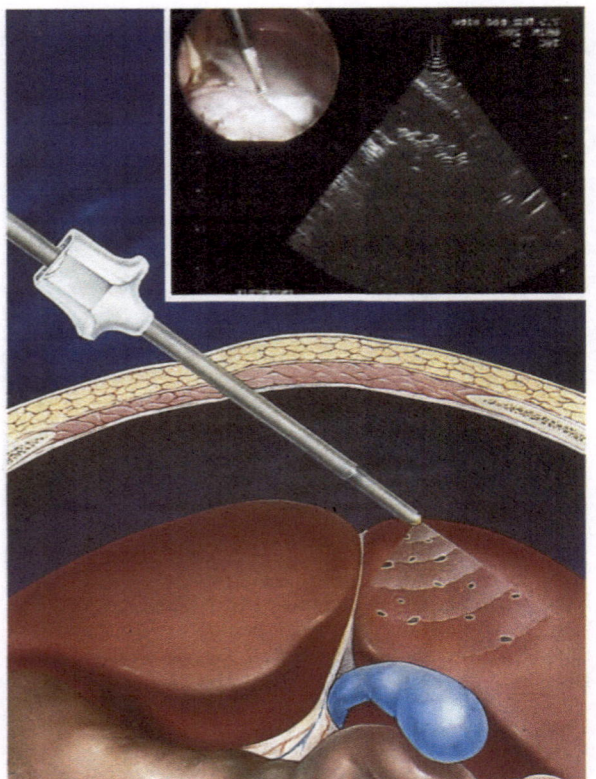

a

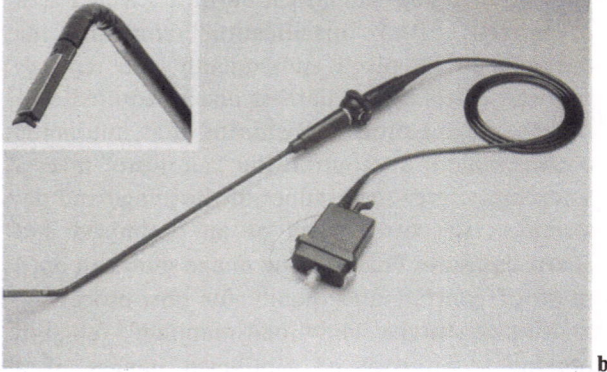

b

Fig. 1.7. a Endomedix (Irvine, CA, USA) used to market an ultrasound sector scanner which can be applied laparoscopically. Although sector scanning leads to image distortion, the scanning image can be gained from one single point. **b** A deflectable, linear sector scanner is available from Olympus Optical. The linear scanning requires a relatively large contact square to the organ; however, it produces superb images

a shortened wave length – is the principle which allows blood flow and direction to be detected and venous flow to be distinguished from arterial flow. The duplex scanning system facilitates endoscopic dissection of structures containing large vessels in difficult anatomical regions [37, 38]. Doppler probes are available from Medasonics (Fremont, CA, USA) and Meadox Surgimed (Oakland, NJ, USA).

Optical Systems

From the technological point of view the rod lens systems of rigid endoscopes are nearly optimized and further considerable improvement is physically limited. The resolution and colour quality of the current endoscopes corresponds to that which the human eye is able to perceive. Although distortion-free telescopes are available, distortion correction is still under discussion for monocular endoscopy. Distortion facilitates depth perception but the corrected optical system gives a better image (see Vol. 1, Chap. 2).

Disposable Endoscopes

The latest development in rigid endoscopes is the disposable laparoscope by USSC (Norwalk, CT, USA). Although light weight, not heat conductive and equipped with a lens cleaner, the image quality is not fully adequate for endoscopic surgery. The compromise in quality is due to the cheap production required to make the price affordable. From the technological point of view, plastic lenses made of polymethylmethacrylate can yield superb image quality (Minolta photo lenses). Especially the coating with metal oxides and nanometre-size silicate particles gives plastic both excellent dereflection and scratch resistance properties which are comparable to those of glass.

However, these lenses are larger than endoscopic ones and the correction of chromatic and spheric aberrations of lenses requires different sorts of glass with different light defraction indices. Currently, plastic lenses have approximately the same light defraction index.

In future, the plasma sterilization method will make it possible to sterilize temperature-sensitive material such as plastic lenses made of polymethylacrylate routinely. In this respect the advantages of plastic lenses – light weight, reduced heat conduc-

tion and reduced risk of damage – should be considered for high-quality reusable endoscopes.

Video Equipment

The paramount element of the image quality is the video equipment used for the operation [39]. The superb imaging quality of the telescopes are reduced by the resolution and colour quality of the cameras. The heart of the camera is the charge-coupled device (CCD) chip which is extensively described in Vol. 1, Chap. 2. The chips currently employed in endoscopic cameras are 1/2 inches diagonally. There are about 333 000 pixels and 400×400 lines; ca. 1000×1000 lines and 1 million pixels are desirable. Preliminary experience with endoscopic HDTV in Tübingen has revealed considerable advantages and enhancement of endoscopic surgical procedures due to the superb resolution 1250×920 lines and 2.2 million pixels. HDTV endoscopy will be commercialized by BTS (Eindhoven, The Netherlands) and Wolf. The minimal size of the rod lens system suitable for HDTV resolution is that of a 10-mm endoscope.

Digital video processing and recording is currently available (e.g. Canon, Sony, etc.) and holds great potential as the pictures are indefinitely stored on optic discs but current costs are prohibitively high. However, in combination with HDTV endoscopy digital video would fulfil all requirements regarding colour trueness and resolution that are necessary for adequate visualization in endoscopic surgery.

Rigid Chip Endoscopes

The integration of the CCD chip within the tip of the endoscope seems to be of considerable advantage compared to the classic endoscope and camera system. It is light weight and easy to handle and the camera does not need to be adapted. The complete set can be sterilized so that no cover is required and the loss of light through the rod lenses and above through the connection between light cable endoscope and ocular camera can be avoided. However, resolution and colour reproduction of current CCDs are inferior to that of rigid rod lens systems.

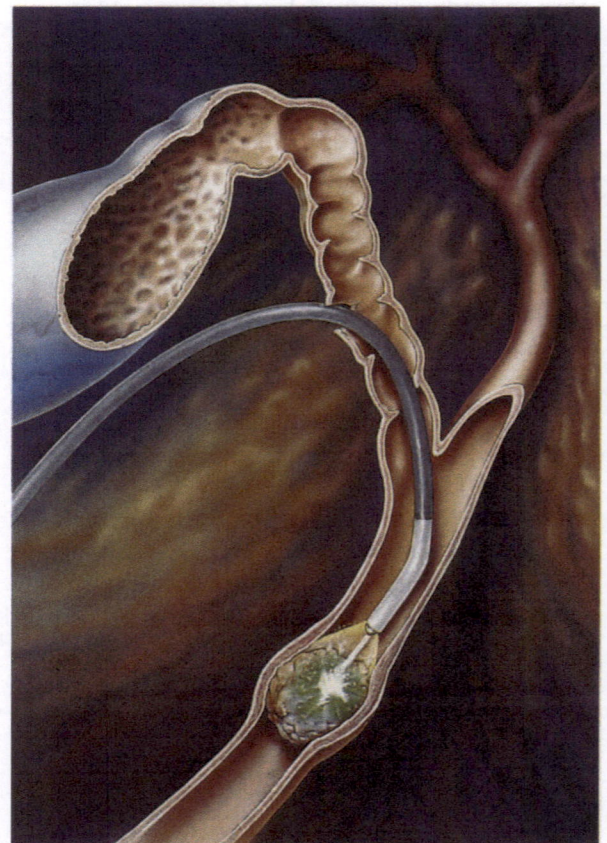

a

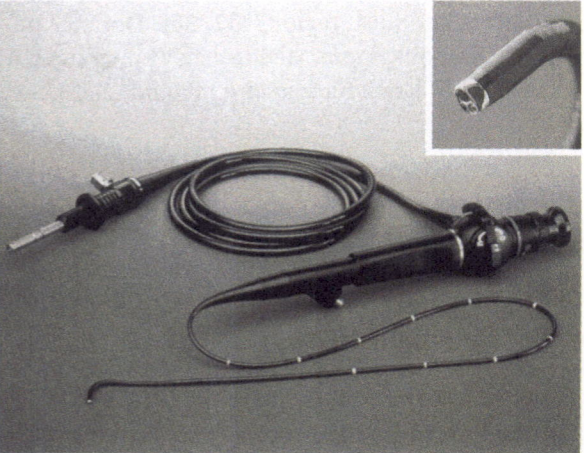

b

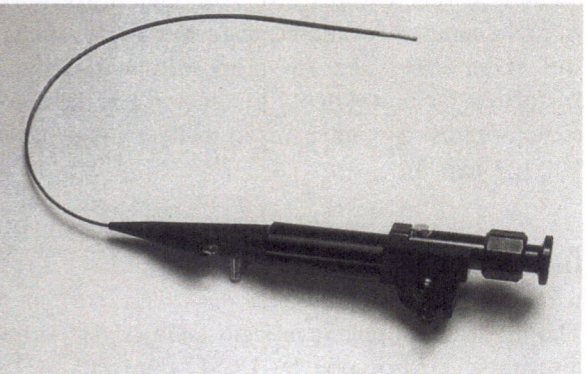

c

Stereoscopes

In addition to the stereo telescope of transanal endoscopic microsurgery (Wolf) stereo laparoscopes manufactured by Aesculap (Tuttlingen, Germany) Olympus Winter&Ibe (Hamburg, Germany) and Opticon (Karlsruhe, Germany) and others are available. However, they are only useful in combination with two cameras for three-dimensional video techniques. Stereoscopes are comprised of two high-quality optical systems integrated into one tube. As high-precision optic adjustment and additional parts such as lenses and prisms are required, the manufacturing is difficult and more expensive than monocular endoscopes [40]. The two optics should be distortion-free, because this is important for a maximum correspondence of the two images.

Fig. 1.8. a Flexible endoscopes are being used increasingly in endoscopic surgery, e.g. for common bile duct exploration and intraoperative lithotripsy (Endomedix). **b** Photographic representation of a flexible choledochoscope (URF-P 2, Olympus Optical). Comparable scopes are available from Storz, Wolf, Pentax and others. **c** Semi-disposable scopes (Endomedix) can be resterilized using ethylenoxide or formaldehyde a limited number of times, depending on care and handling

Flexible Endoscopes

Flexible endoscopes are being used increasingly in endoscopic surgery, e.g. for common bile duct exploration (Fig. 1.8a). Flexible scopes (Storz, Wolf, Olympus Optical, and Pentax, Tokyo, Japan) can only be reliably sterilized by EO or formaldehyde processing which is time consuming and involves an additional risk of damage to these expensive devices. Semi-disposable scopes, (Endomedix; Fig. 1.8c) can be resterilized a limited number of times using EO or formaldehyde. The problem is

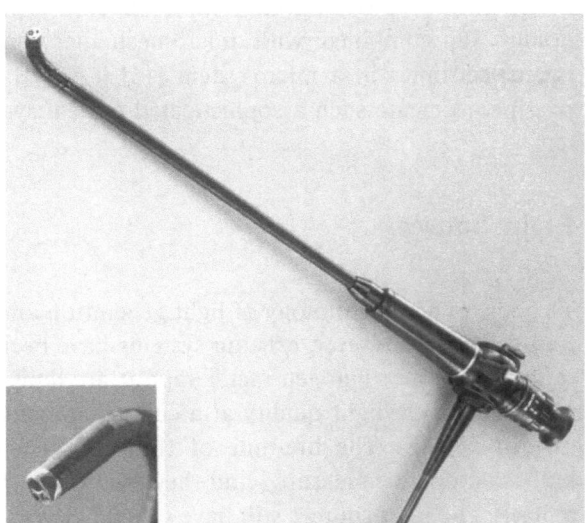

a

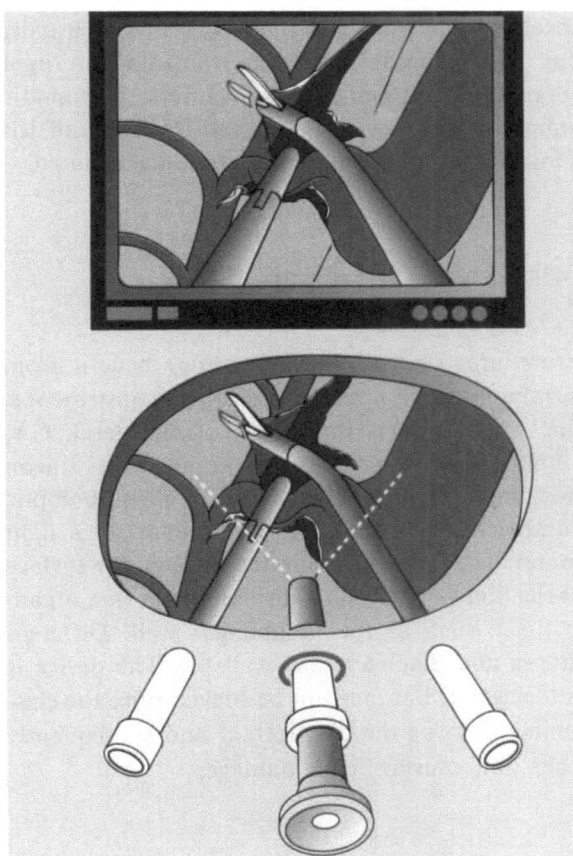

b

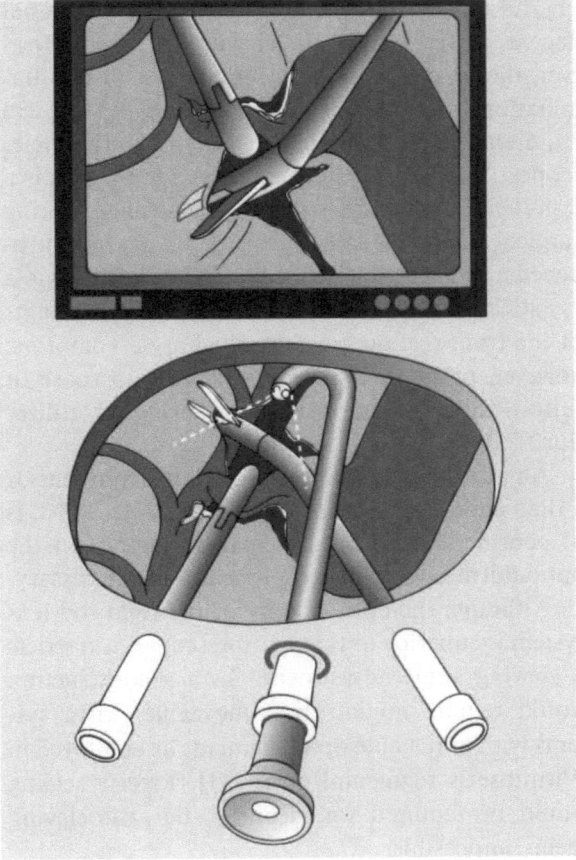

c

Fig. 1.9. a The new thoracofibrescopes have a rigid shaft but are flexible on the distal end (LTF, Olympus, Optical). Although the optical quality is inferior compared to rod lens endoscopes, the deflecting is of considerable benefit for diagnostic thoracoscopy. Schematic comparison of surgical manoeuvres using rigid (**b**) versus semiflexible (**c**) telescopes. Surgical manoevers are more difficult to conduct when the endoscope is deflected because the eye coordination axis is reversed

that these thin and delicate endoscopes are easily damaged, which, considering their price, is a major disadvantage for general use in endoscopic exploration of the bile duct. However, direct optic imaging of the biliary tract is desired and of considerable benefit for lithotripsy of common bile duct stones.

The use of a semi-flexible introduction sleeve through which the scope should be inserted through the cannula into the abdominal cavity is one way of preventing breakage.

Semi-flexible Endoscopes

To construct a semi-flexible endoscope the conventional flexible endoscope was shortened and modified by a rigid intersection (e.g. Olympus Optical; Fig. 1.9a). Such a construction permits additional degrees of freedom of the viewing direction. However, the image quality of fibreoptics and the illumination do not fulfil all the endoscopic surgical requirements because they are inferior to rigid telescopes. The use of these flexibles scopes requires experience and care to prevent mishaps during surgical manoeuvres (Fig. 1.9b, c). Baxter has introduced a semi-flexible scope which is operated via a joy stick placed at the hand-piece. The movements of the front section are controlled by servomotors; however, orientation problems similar to those of fully flexible endoscopes occur during its utilization.

An adjustable viewing angle of the front lens of a rigid endoscope, for example, from 0°to 90°C, is of considerable advantage, making change of the optic during complicated procedures unnecessary.

Although the optic quality of the rigid rod lens system is superior to that of fibrescopes, it restricts a viewing angle adjustment. Such a construction would require miniaturized moveable prism systems with adjustable optic segments as employed in Wittmoser's segmental optic [41]. Precise sealing would be required for cleaning, but autoclaving seems impossible.

An optical system which allows three-dimensional viewing with auto iris, auto focus, zoom and auto convergence combined with optimal resolution and colour reproduction is almost like the human eye. Such a system is required to provide the image quality that permits the highest possible safety during an operation. With CCD chip technology [6] combined with micromechanics and microelectronics in a microsystem [15] it may be possible to create such a sophisticated optical system.

Light Sources

There is no new technology of light generation and transmissions; however, existing systems have been refined. The new halogen metal vapour arc lamps emit light of daylight quality at a colour temperature of 5700 K. The life-time of these advanced bulbs can now be measured and they are simple to replace. The light sources still have some disadvantages: light cables can only be interchanged with special connectors, and the iris control is usually not interchangeable between cameras and light sources of different manufacturers. Automatic lamp changing and standardized interfaces of iris control and light cable connection are required.

Intraluminal Illumination

Procedures such as cardiomyotomy benefit from intraluminal illumination with the gastroscope. The EndoLumina (BioEnterics, Carpinteria, CA, USA) includes a soft and transparent silicon elastomere bougie connected with a glass fibreoptic bundle that is designed to be attached to a light source. The light is transmitted through the surface of the bougie and thus transilluminates thin organic tissue such as the oesophagus wall. Different shapes and diameters are available. The device is autoclavable, but may not be soaked since the elastomere absorbs the disinfectant and subsequently leaks out, causing tissue damage.

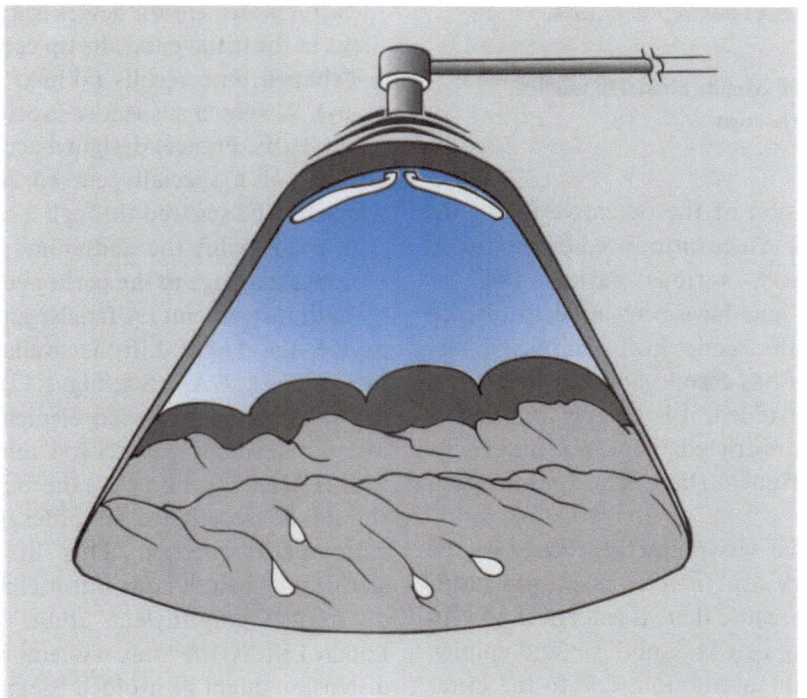

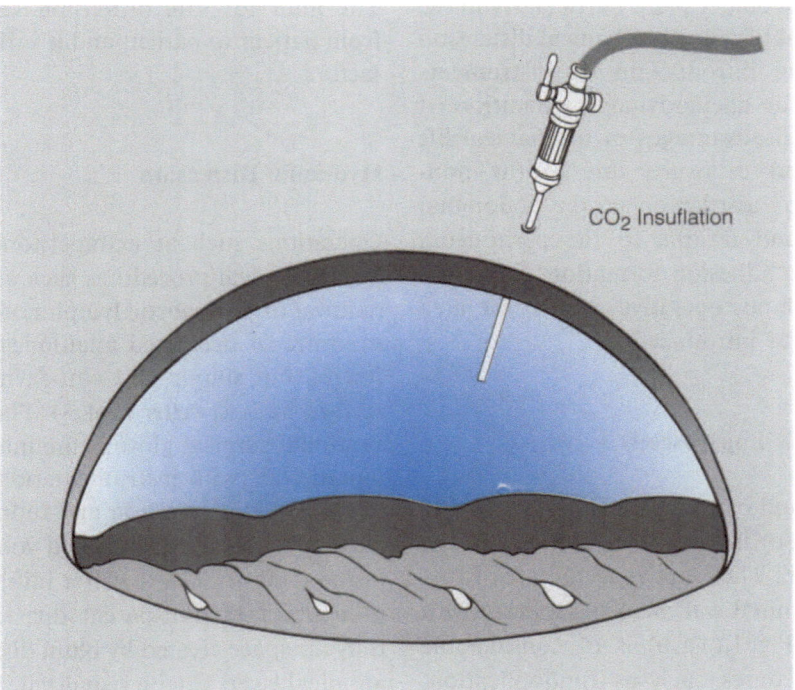

Fig. 1.10 a, b. Mechanical (**a**) versus gas pressure (**b**) distension of the abdominal wall. With mechanical lift there is insufficient exposure due to the non-uniform "tent-like" distraction of the abdominal wall, whereas gas insufflation provides an adequately exposed operative field. However, gasless laparoscopy entails advantages for high-risk patients and in cases of trauma

Exposure of the Operative Field

New Technology of Mechanical Distension and Gasless Laparoscopy

Mechanical distension of the operative field is as old as surgery itself. Since introduced by Mouret in laparoscopic surgery, various devices such as hooks, barbs and fans have been used to distend the abdominal wall. Aside from simplicity, mechanical distension has certain advantages: gas insufflation can be avoided, it is reliable and instrument design is less restricted. Thus, a round cross-section of the instrument shaft is no longer essential.

From the clinical viewpoint the elderly or the trauma patient may benefit if extensive gas insufflation is avoided because there is less effect on ventilation and the risk of CO_2 embolism and emphysema are decreased. In addition, due to the intra-abdominal pressure the phrenic nerve may be irritated and cause shoulder pain. Particularly in the event of substantial bleeding mechanical distension permits immediate introduction of instruments without altering the haemodynamic condition of the patient. The disadvantages of mechanical lift include insufficient exposure, due to the non-uniform "tent-like" distraction of the abdominal wall (Fig. 1.10), and trauma to the peritoneum which may lead to adhesion formation. Some patients complain of postoperative pain in the area where the hook was introduced.

Devices for Gasless Laparoscopy

The simplest method of mechanical lift is to apply sutures to the skin or insert a thick thread through the abdominal wall. The Dundee technique of suspending the abdominal wall by using a drain with an inserted rod (Fig. 1.11 a, b) is of considerable help during procedures such as fundoplication, vagotomy, etc. The soft plastic tube reduces traumatization of the peritoneum and postoperative pain in the suspended area. However, since this technique does not contain built-in safety features such as automatic release or spring gauge it has to be used with care.

Semm's suspension device is a simple rod with a hinge at the distal end. The tip can be deflected and a T-shaped barb results (WISAP, Sauerlach, Germany). A French suspender (Societe 3X, Caluire & Cuire, Paris, France) designed according to Mouret consists of a specially curved stainless steel rod which can be screwed through a small incision and than used to lift the abdominal wall (Fig. 1.11 c). However, damage to the peritoneum may be caused by both instruments. A fancier and more expensive device, the LaparoLift, is available from Origin (Menlo Park, CA, USA, Fig. 1.12). The principle is the same; a hook-shaped element (LaparoFan) is inserted through an incision and the abdominal wall is lifted. In our view the blades of the hook should be redesigned in order to improve their "atraumatic" design. This lift system is not sterilizable as it is large but it can be covered with a sterile polyethylene tube. Although, the LaparoLift is the only system with which over-distension might be avoided because of an integrated spring gauge, this is not achieved automatically. The limit for safe distension varies considerably from patient to patient and is influenced by several factors.

Hydraulic Distension

Operations such as extraperitoneal hernia repair and urological procedures such as nephrectomy or removal of para-aortic lymph nodes require precise exposure of dedicated anatomical regions. An effective, but simple and cost-saving method is described by Rassweiler (Vol. 3). The finger of a conventional surgical glove is mounted at the tip of a laparoscope with instrumentation channel. Subsequent to blunt insertion and tunnelling, the finger is filled with a predetermined volume of saline solution (500–1000 ml). After initial filling, the balloon becomes transparent due to distension and thus the space created by blunt dissection of the anatomical layers can be visualized. Subsequent to aspiration of the balloon via standard suction and removal the scope can be positioned and the extraperitoneal operative field insufflated at 5–8 mmHg. Similarly functioning disposable balloons are available from Origin, General Surgical Innovations (Portola Valley, CA, USA) and others.

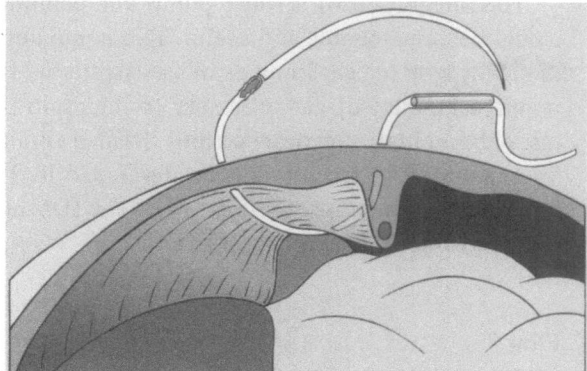

1.11a

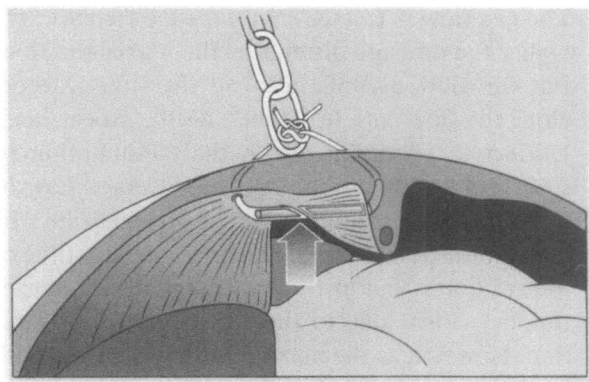

b

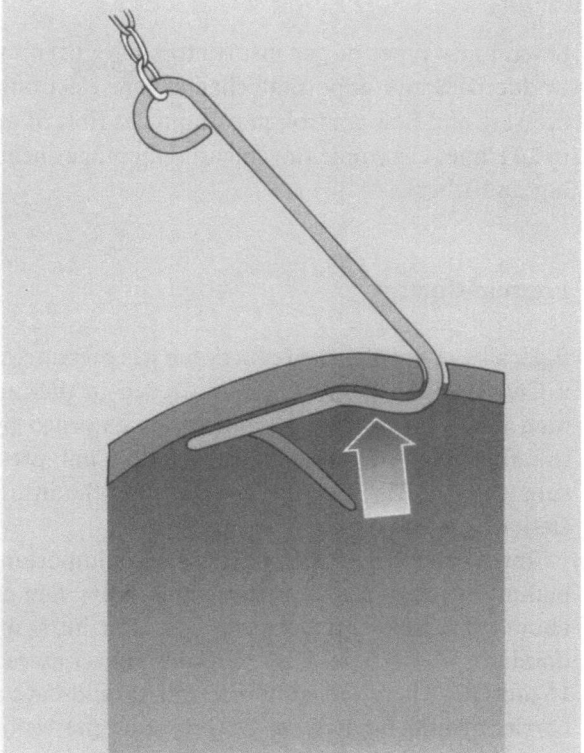

c

▲
Fig. 1.11a–c. Suspending the abdominal wall using a drain with an inserted rod (Dundee technique). **a** The first step includes the insertion of a drain trocar mounted with a silicon tube. **b** The stainless steel rod is then placed between the insertions and the tube is fixed to a gallow. **c** The suspender according to Mouret (Societe 3X; Caluire&Cuire, Paris, France) consists of a specially curved stainless steel rod which can be screwed into the abdominal cavity through a small incision

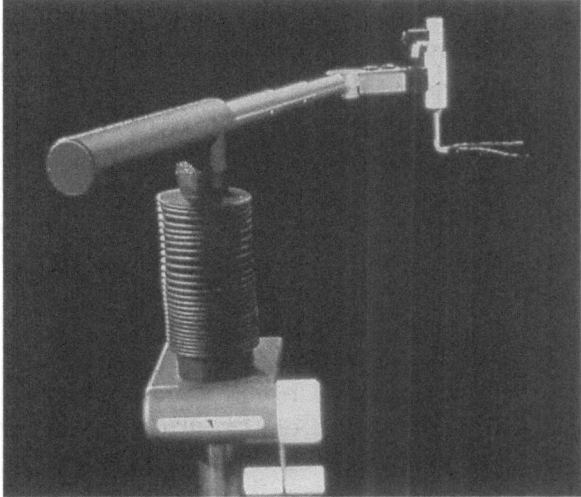

◄
Fig. 1.12. The Laparo Lift device by Origin is electrically driven

Gas Insufflation[1]

Several new types of gas insufflators have been introduced. Some important changes are electronic pressure and flow control, maximum gas flow of up to 20 l/min, electronic flow measurement, gas heating and filters.

Pressure Control

Basically, an insufflator reduces the gas pressure of a CO_2 cylinder to low pressure needed in the human body. This pressure reduction is governed by the following parameters: intra-abdominal pressure, the insufflation (driving) pressure, the insufflation flow, and the gas temperature.

Intra-abdominal pressure is the most important parameter to control. Due to the blood pressure of about 10 mmHG in the vena cava, the intra-abdominal CO_2 pressure should not exceed 15 mmHG. Therefore, an insufflator should have a barrier against inadvertent CO_2 pressure preset for over 15 mmHG and a pressure relief system (Fig. 1.13).

Exact pressure control is of importance during suction and especially during argon beam spray coagulation. The use of argon beam coagulators, in particular, can cause major elevation of the intra-abdominal pressure. Furthermore, conventional irrigation and aspiration devices with piston pumps and imprecise adjustment also cause significant fluctuation of the intra-abdominal pressure.

Roller pumps, by contrast, are precisely adjustable to determined volumes (Fig. 1.14). For instance, if an argon beam spray coagulation device is used it insufflates approximately 4 l/min. The roller pump suction can then be adjusted to equilibrate pressure, provided a sucker is introduced. By contrast to the conventional suction device which aspirates ca. 2.4 l liquid per minute and sucks ca. 20 l air, a roller pump aspirates approximately the same amount of liquid and air (2.9 l/3.1 l).

---

[1] In co-operation with S. Sawatzki, WOM, Berlin.

The integration of a roller pump and aspirator would be more reliable and useful. This could automatically stop the gas input as well as aspirating the required amount of gas necessary to maintain the intra-abdominal pressure within defined limits. Such a system has recently been developed in Tübingen, the Operating System OREST I (Dornier Medizintechnik, Germering, Germany).

Flow

The gas flow is created by pressure difference: the higher the pressure difference, the higher the flow. But the flow depends also on the flow resistors along the flow path (e.g. tubes, needle, trocar, etc.). During an operation of 1 h the consumption of CO_2 is about 60 l, resulting in an average flow of 1 l/min. The maximum flow of 20 l indicated by the manufacturers not only reduces the life-time of the gas bottle, but also represents potential danger for the patient due to the risk of overpressurization. However, as the maximum flow depends both on the driving pressure and the diameter and length of the supplying tubes, the maximum flow of the device is never achieved at the output site of the cannulae. Our examinations indicate a real flow of up to 6−9 l/min. A flow higher than 9 l/min seems unnecessary and carries considerable risks.

To prevent insufflation in the event of incorrect insertion of the Verres needle, e.g. intra-arterially, the driving pressure should not exceed more than 50 mmHg, which consequently reduces the maximum flow. In order to achieve both safe and stable pneumoperitoneum, an adequate pressure and flow control is necessary (which can be described as soft approach pressure control, SAPC). In addition, the output site (cannula) requires optimization and standardization. Most of the current insufflators work intermittently to obtain intra-abdominal pressure by means of pressure equalization. With a powerful controlling algorithm the average flow of such a device reaches 90% of a comparatively continuously working device. The advantage of the intermittently working device is the elegant pressure measurement without additional tubes. From the point of view of safety, the high-flow gas insufflation itself may cause severe complications, due to the lack of a safety valve, which would automati-

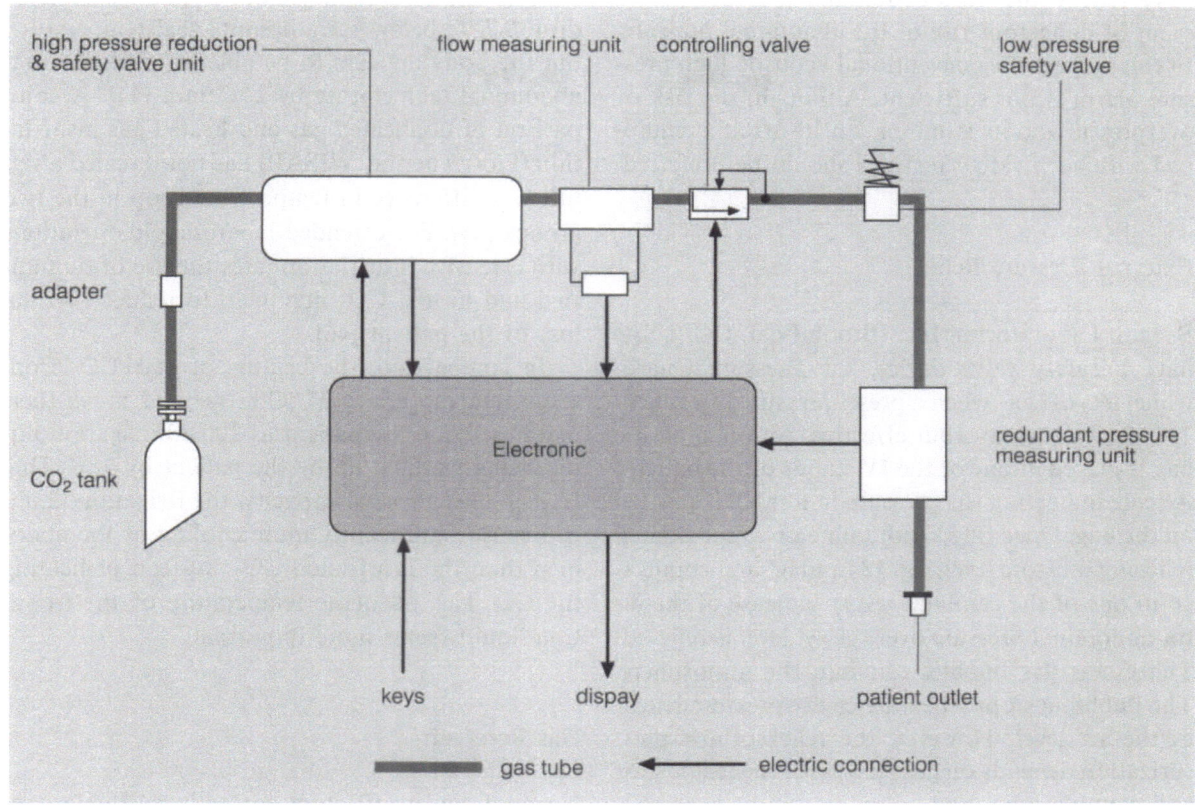

▲
Fig. 1.13. A modern insufflator with safety valves and electronic control of all functions

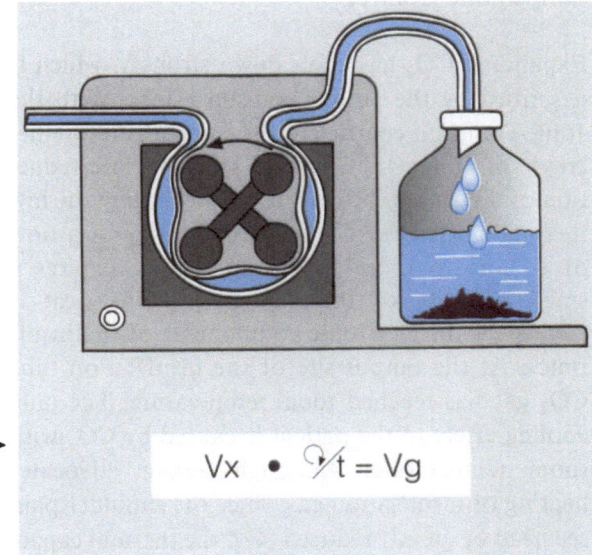

$$Vx \cdot \frac{\%}{t} = Vg$$

Fig. 1.14. The roller pump suction allows adjustment to determined volumes of either gas and liquid. Depending on the rotation speed of the roller, certain volumes are squeezed through the tube. Thus, excessive aspiration of gas is abolished ►

cally reduce the intra-abdominal pressure in the event of dangerous rise of the abdominal pressure. In this respect the conventional acoustic high pressure alarm is not sufficient. Although, the risk of overpressurization is minor, an insufflator equipped with such safety features should be preferred.

External Pressure Relief

Beacon Laboratories, Inc. (Broomfield, CO, USA) have a safety valve device, the Pressure Guard, which lets off gas when a preset pressure is reached. The device is simple but effective. An open plastic bag is placed at one of the IV stands of the patient. A scale indicating the pressure in mmHg is printed on the bag. Once filled with saline up to the desired relieving pressure level, e.g. 13 mmHg, and connected to one of the cannulae, every increase of the intra-abdominal pressure over the set level is relieved. The excess gas bubbles out into the atmosphere. The bubbling stops when the cavity pressure reaches the set level. However, the relief of overpressurization depends on gas flow from the insufflator and cannula type used.

Temperature Control

Expanding CO_2 gas cools down strongly, which is described by the Joule-Thomson effect. With the Joule-Thomson coefficient the gas temperature decrease of about 45 °C caused by a pressure reduction of 60 bar can be calculated. Regarding the low thermal capacity of CO_2 gas, the heating of a flow of 9 l/min to room temperature only requires a small quantity of thermal energy. The heat is created by the electronic components of the insufflator. At the output site of the insufflation tube CO_2 gas has reached room temperature. The only cooling effect to the patient is caused by CO_2 with room temperature. Although Semm advocates heating of insufflation gas, since the shoulder pain seems to be greatly reduced [42], the thermal capacity of CO_2 is not sufficient to decrease the body temperature significantly. A core temperature drop of 0.3 °C is caused by 40–50 l insufflated gas at room temperature [43]. Only in case of high flow

(ca. 9 l/min) does the intra-abdominal temperature drop 0.7 °C below intra-oesophageal temperature, but the body appears to be able to increase intra-abdominal temperature by 2 °C/min [44]. A comparison of nonheated gas and heated gas insufflation (Flow Therme, WISAP) has not revealed a significant difference in temperature drop in the two groups [45]. For extended laparoscopic operations with extensive insufflation rates the use of humidified and heated CO_2 may help to reduce thermal loss of the patient [46].

In comparison, the heating of 100 l CO_2 from room temperature to 37 °C extracts as much thermal heat from the patient as 200 ml irrigation liquid being warmed up by the patient by 3 °C. Due to its higher thermal capacity, the irrigation liquid can cause significantly more cooling of the abdomen than the insufflated CO_2. Instead of heating the CO_2 gas, adequate temperature of the irrigation liquid seems more important.

Gas Reservoir

None of the insufflators currently available contains an additional gas reservoir. It is often noticed that it is necessary to change the gas bottle when the abdomen collapses. Aside from the hazardous risk, changing the gas cylinder causes a delay. The solution is quite simple: a main reservoir and a reserve cylinder. An acoustic or optic signal would indicate that the pressure in the main cylinder is decreasing and the reserve cylinder would then automatically be switched on. A manometer placed at the back of the insufflator should constantly show the actual reserve pressure. This additional reservoir would eliminate the inconvenience and danger of sudden decompression of the pneumoperitoneum during the operation.

The right choice of purchasing an insufflation device should be based on a through understanding of the clinical significance of several tests and evaluations [47] as well as the individual requirements of endoscopic operations. Besides technical specifications the insufflator should be easy to use, operate fully automatically, display intra-abdominal pressure and flow values clearly, and have a pressure relief system.

Exposure Maintenance

During the operation the front lens is often stained by condensation and blood. Several useful antifog solutions are available for maintaining a clear view. To clean a stained optic and external instruments the laparoscopic scope warmer (Applied Laparoscopy; Laguna Hills, CA, USA) is useful. This sterilizable thermos bottle contains 500 ml of irrigation fluid which is kept hot for 3–4 h (Fig. 1.15). A more expensive telescope warmer, an electrically heated device is manufactured by Wolf; however, it cannot be sterilized and care has to be taken to cover it sufficiently with sterile polyethylene film.

Optic Irrigation

Only few telescopes have integrated irrigation channels for maintaining the operative view. These are the TEM stereoscope and the Mediastinoscope (both by Wolf). The hydrolaparoscope (Circon ACMI, Stamford, CT, USA) has recently been introduced which permits both rinsing of the lens and irrigation of the operative field (Fig. 1.16a). Optic irrigation is imperative in delicate dissections, because accidental bleeding from a large vessel can quickly obscure the view. Bleeding was the most common cause for conversion from endoscopic procedure to open surgery in a multicentre study in major European centres [48].

Combination of Insufflation, Irrigation and Suction

Since irrigation fluid drops at the front lens can impair the view until they dry, the Tübingen system combines suction, insufflation and irrigation to maintain a clear lens (Fig. 1.16b). The gas is introduced via a channel of an outer sleeve which fits to conventional 10-mm telescopes. The gas stream of the CO_2 is led over the objective lens and, hence, condensation is avoided (Fig. 1.16b_4). In addition the front lens can be irrigated by means of an separate rinsing channel (Fig. 1.16b_2). The front lens is immediately dried due to the constant gas output. This exposure maintenance system has been tested experimentally and clinically and is manufactured by Wiest (Munich, Germany).

Energy Systems

High-Frequency Devices and Instruments[1]

The quality of cutting and coagulation and the prevention of undesired side effects are of central importance during high-frequency (HF) surgery. Major prerequisites are the instruments and suitable generators as well as application techniques and their adequate execution. Once the surgeon is acquainted with the specific characteristics of HF surgery it becomes a versatile and safe technique for operative endoscopy.

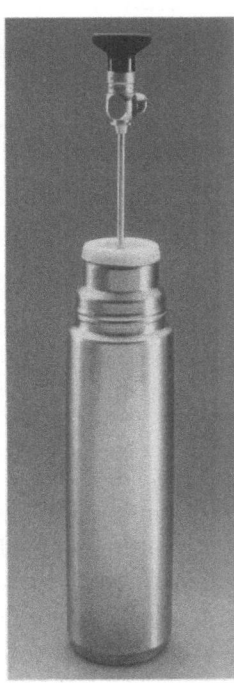

Fig. 1.15. The scope warmer (Applied Laparoscopy) is a sterilizable thermos bottle which keeps 500 ml irrigation fluid hot for 3–4 h

---

[1] In co-operation with G. Farin, Erbe Elektromedizin, Tübingen, Germany.

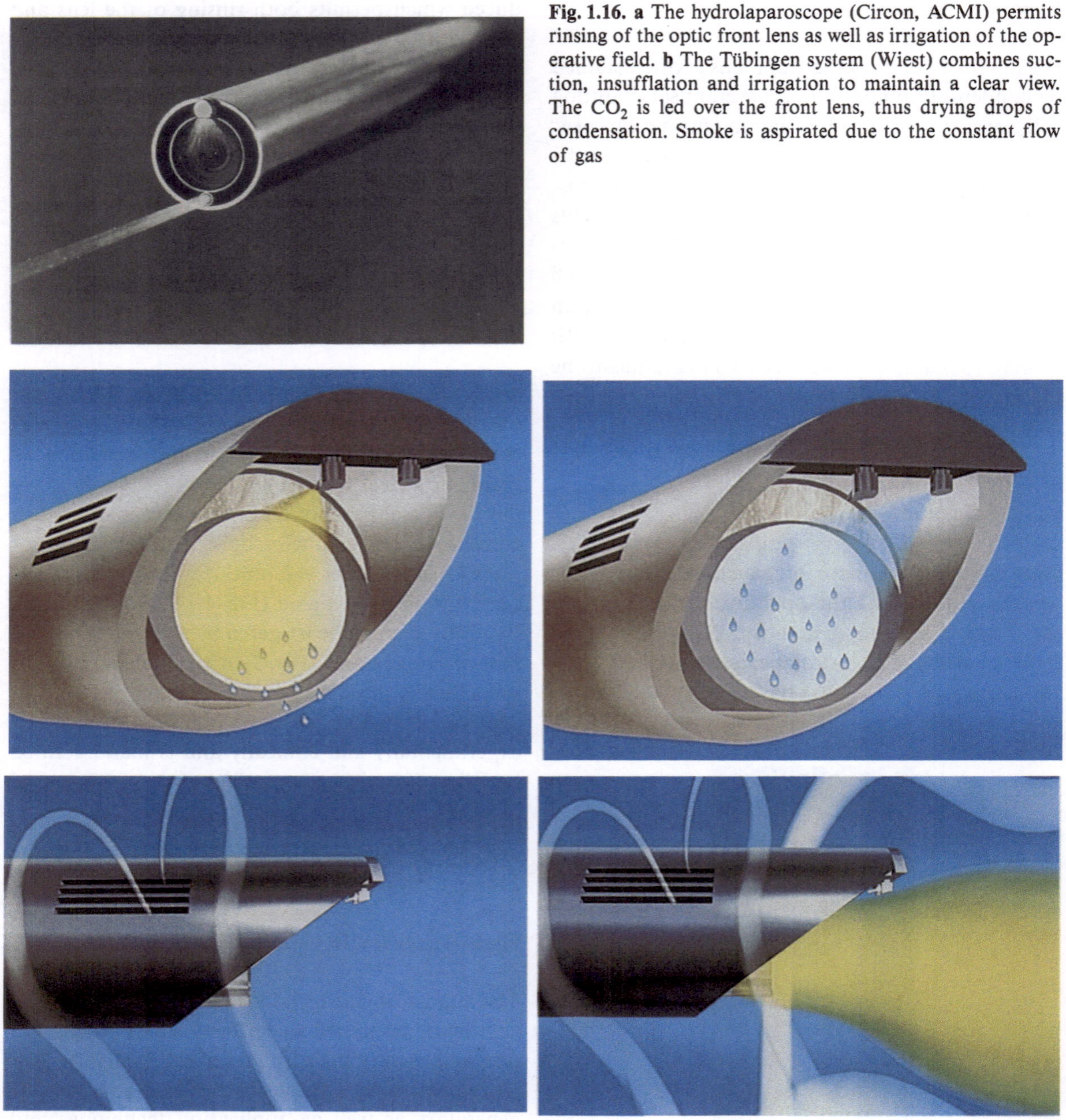

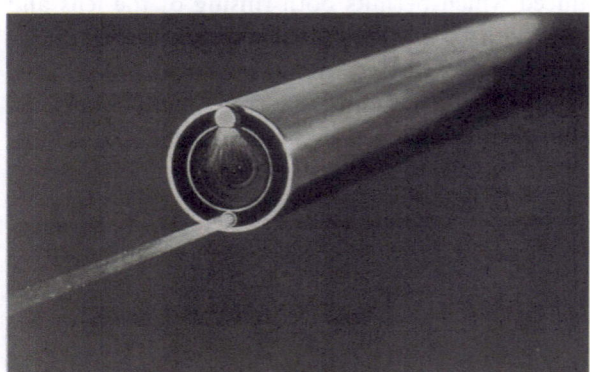

a

Fig. 1.16. a The hydrolaparoscope (Circon, ACMI) permits rinsing of the optic front lens as well as irrigation of the operative field. **b** The Tübingen system (Wiest) combines suction, insufflation and irrigation to maintain a clear view. The CO_2 is led over the front lens, thus drying drops of condensation. Smoke is aspirated due to the constant flow of gas

b_1 b_2

b_3 b_4

Quality of the Cutting

The quality of the cutting is determined by the type and extent of the thermal damage to the cutting margins. The tissue along the cutting margins should suffer as little thermal damage as possible so as to promote postoperative wound healing. Particularly, the delicate dissection of vascularized structures requires adequate differentiation of tissue layers. For histopathological examination of the specimen, precise cutting is mandatory. However, the cutting margins should be coagulated sufficiently to ensure efficient haemostasis while cutting. Carbonization of the cutting margins should be avoided under all circumstances, and tissue vaporization should be kept to a minimum because the vapour and smoke obscure the endoscopic view.

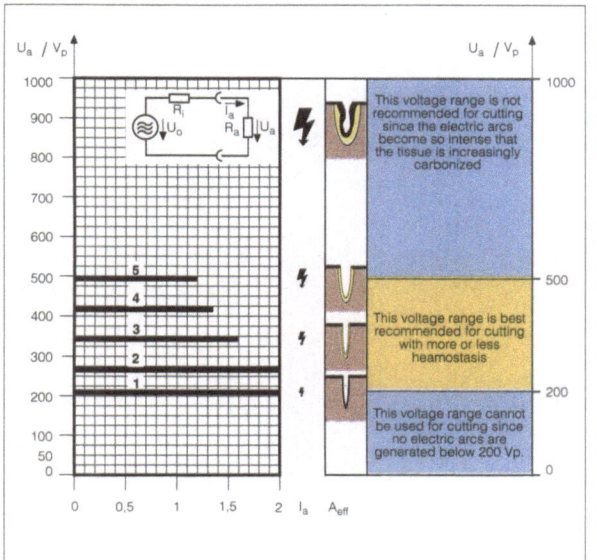

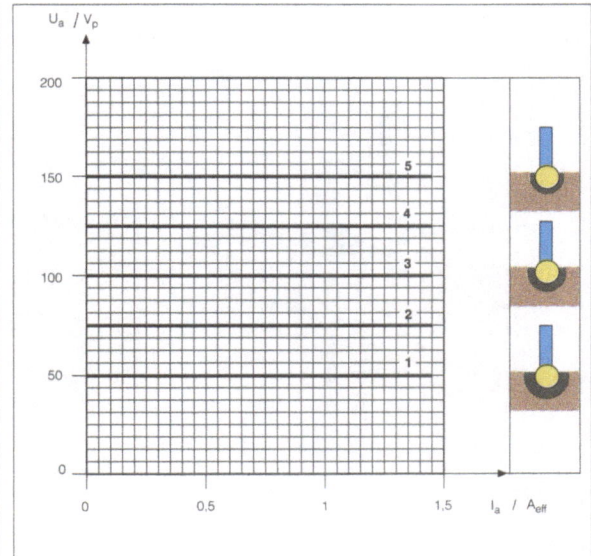

a

b

Reproducible Cutting

The quality of the cutting depends on the intensity of the electric arc between the cutting electrode and the tissue, and the electric arc on the level of the electric voltage, the shape of the cutting electrode and the cutting procedure. The amplitude of the HF voltage between the cutting electrode and the tissue must reach at least 200 V, since the electric arc cannot be ignited at lower voltages. The higher the HF voltage, the greater the intensity of the microelectric arc and thus of the thermal damage to the cutting margins (Fig. 1.17a). "Low-coagulation" cutting can be achieved with low, unmodulated HF voltages, thin-cutting electrodes and swift incision. "High-coagulation" cutting is achieved with high HF voltages, thick-cutting electrodes and slow movement during cutting. However, the amplitude of the HF voltage should not exceed 500 V, since the electric arc between the cutting electrode and the tissue becomes so intensive that carbonization and vaporization develop.

Since the amplitude of the HF voltage and the intensity of the electric arc between the cutting electrode and the tissue determine the quality of the cutting effect, HF surgery devices with automatic voltage or arc control should be used in order to ensure a reproducible and constant quality of cutting. This also precludes the undesired side effects such as carbonization and vaporization.

Fig. 1.17. a The relationship between high-frequency (HF) voltage, intensity of the microelectric arc and thermal damage to the cutting margins. HF devices with automatically regulated HF output provide reproducible quality of the cutting effect. **b** The relationship between HF voltage and intensity of the coagulation effect. HF devices with automatically regulated HF output voltage in the "soft coagulation" mode ensure absence of electric arcs and maintain a soft and moist coagulum

Quality of the Coagulation

An important criterion for the quality of the coagulation is, again, the type and extent of the thermal damage to the tissue. As regards the extent of the coagulation zone, the reproducibility of the intended effects and the prevention of the unintended effects play an important role. It should always be ensured that only as much tissue as is needed for therapeutic purposes is coagulated. Desiccation (dehydration) of the coagulated tissue leads to shrinkage, which thereby supports haemostasis. However, desiccation can also lead to adhesion of the coagulated tissue to the electrode, thus incurring the risk of tearing it off from the surrounding tissue and inducing bleeding [49]. Carbonization represents a considerable risk for postoperative adhesion and should therefore be avoided [50].

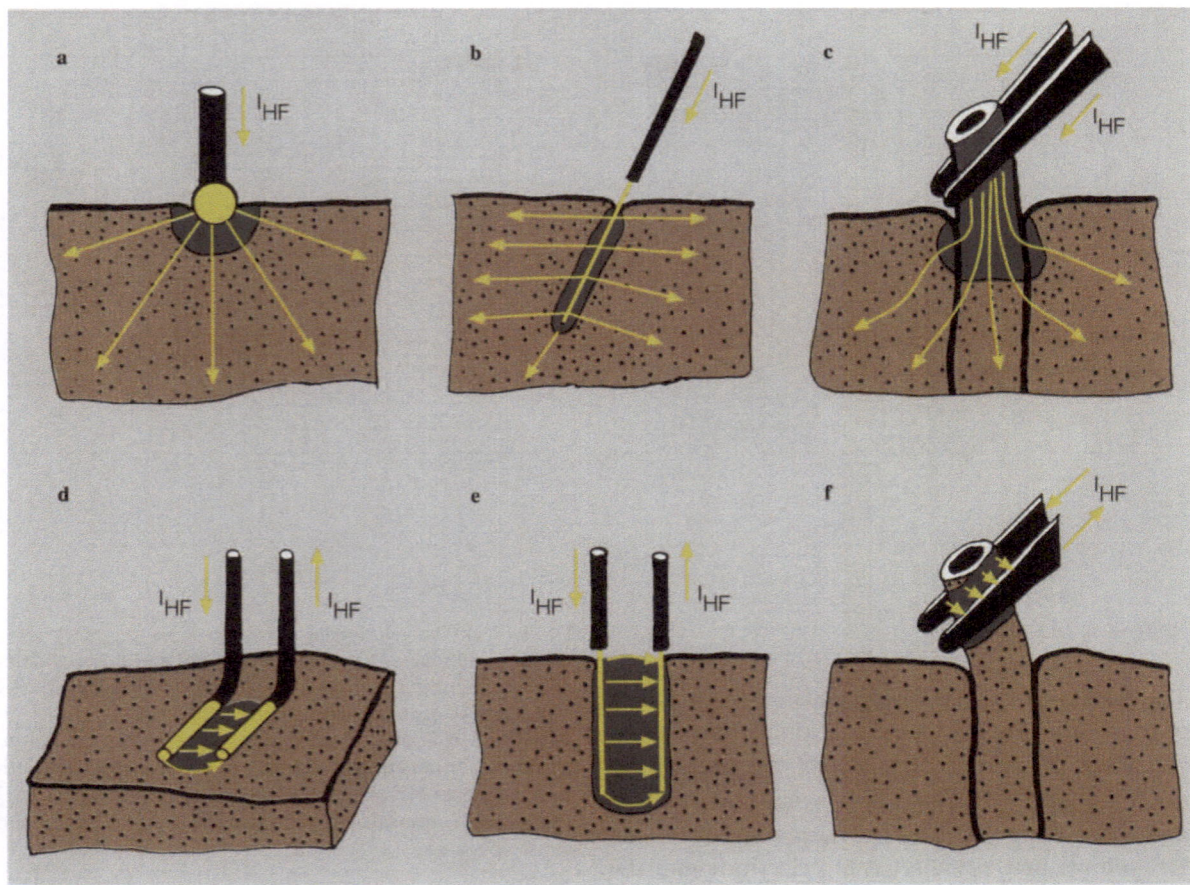

Reproducible Coagulation

Coagulation depends particularly on the level of the electric voltage between the coagulation electrode and the tissue. Pure coagulation with adequate desiccation, minimal vapour formation and without carbonization can be achieved with HF voltages of amplitude ranging between 20 V and a maximum of 190 V. If the amplitude of the HF voltage exceeds 200 V, then electric arcs are formed which produce carbonization and smoke. As the coagulum remains soft and moist in the absence of electric arcs, this coagulation mode is termed "soft coagulation" (Fig. 1.17b).

In monopolar coagulation, the spatial development of the coagulation zone is proportional to the effective surface of the contact and inversely proportional to the square of the electric voltage between the coagulation electrode and the tissue (Fig. 1.18). In bipolar coagulation, the spatial de-

Fig. 1.18a–f. Comparison of the spatial development of the coagulation zone of monopolar (**a–c**) and bipolar (**d–f**) high-frequency (*HF*) current. **a, d** contact coagulation; **b, e** puncture coagulation; **c, f** spread coagulation

velopment of the coagulation zone is largely limited to the tissue between the poles of the bipolar coagulation instrument. Because of the strong influence of the voltage on the spatial development of the monopolar coagulation zone, HF surgery device with automatic voltage control should be used.

Excessive desiccation and adhesion between tissue and electrode can largely be avoided by means of the automatic switch-off of the coagulation process when the vapour phase has been reached in the coagulum. This is related to the change of the tissue's electrical features and lowered water content.

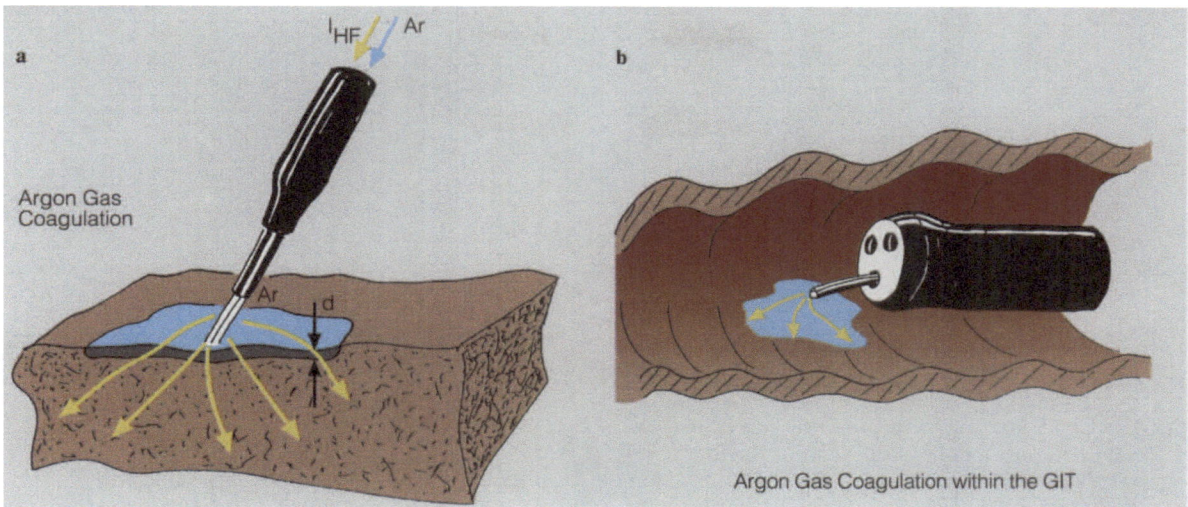

Since sometimes a relatively large area must be coagulated with a small monopolar electrode, the electric voltage between the electrode and the tissue must exceed 200 V. Electric arcs have to be generated which sufficiently penetrate electrically insulating layers of dried out tissue. This coagulation mode is termed "forced coagulation". When applying "forced coagulation" in the presence of air, desiccation, carbonization, vaporization and the adhesion effect must be expected. However, when applying forced coagulation or other HF modes in combination with irrigation fluids such as water, these unintended side effects become minor or entirely nonexistent [51].

Voltages with amplitudes above 2000 V generate electric arcs of such length that contact of the active electrode with tissue becomes unnecessary. Although a surface coagulation can simply be gained by moving the electrode over the tissue at a distance, a reproducible coagulation effect is not possible. In the presence of oxygen this "spray coagulation" leads to considerable carbonization, vaporization and adhesion, which limits its application during endoscopic operations.

Inert Gas Coagulation

Argon gas coagulation is the preferred method for contact-free coagulation of tissue surfaces. Here the HF current is applied to the tissue by means of

Fig. 1.19 a, b. The different application techniques of inert gas coagulation. **a** The argon gas is ionized due to the high-frequency (*HF*) electrical field and thus forming the electric arc which leads to a relatively constant coagulation depth of the tissue without significant carbonization. **b** Flexible application of argon gas coagulation within the gastrointestinal tract

an electrically ionized argon gas jet [52]. Argon is suitable for this because it is naturally relatively ionized and it has a high electric conductivity. The chemically inert argon prevents the carbonization and vaporization of the coagulum. Correct application technique leads to a relatively constant coagulation depth and well-controlled desiccation of the tissue surface, which permits adequate haemostatis (Fig. 1.19 a, b). Once a HF generator with a sufficiently controlled constant HF voltage is used, the depth of the coagulation zone is reproducible.

Argon gas coagulation is now a proven method for haemostasis in the gastrointestinal tract [53] as well as being useful for pulmonary [54] and splenic surgery [55]. In addition to a HF surgery device, argon gas coagulation requires a controlled argon source and an argon gas coagulation probe suitable to the specific application.

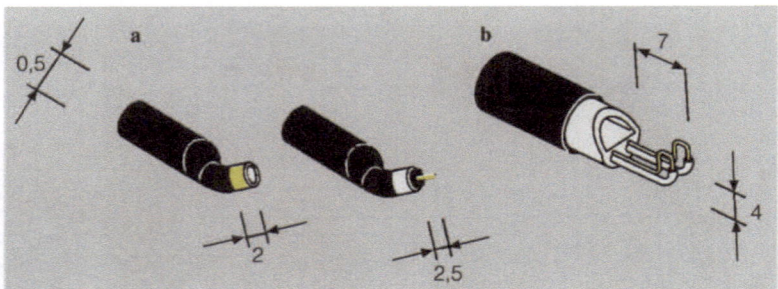

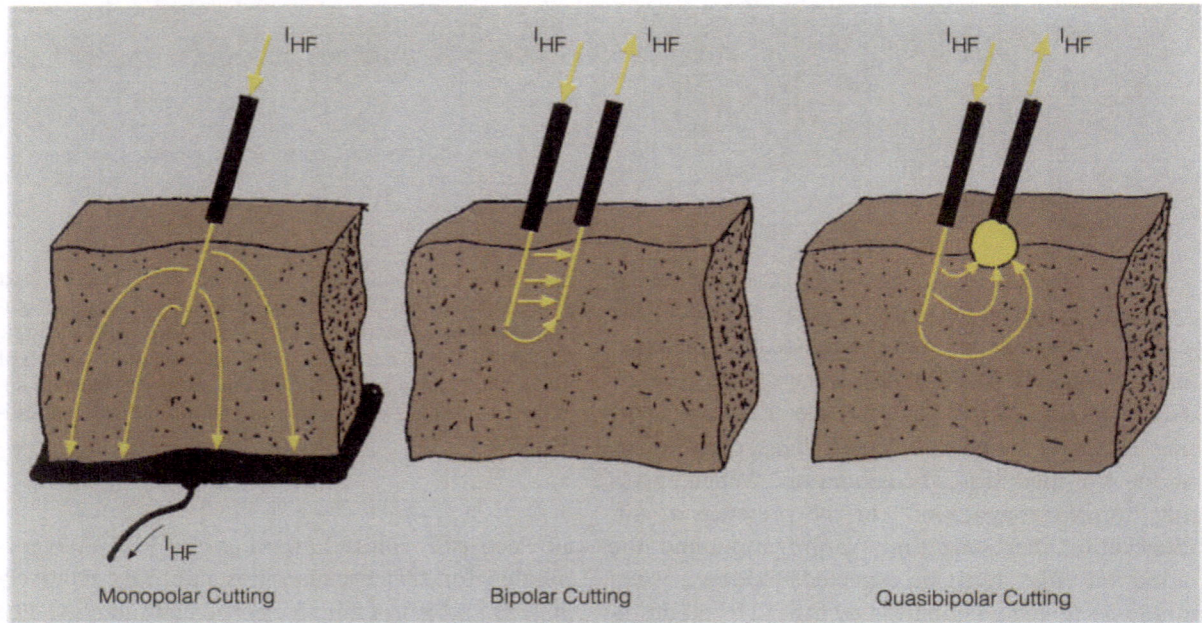

Fig. 1.20 a–c. Examples of bifunctional cutting/coagulation instruments. **a** The needle is used for cutting, the distal ring for coagulation. **b** The two thin wires are used for bipolar cutting, the two thicker wires for bipolar coagulation. This instrument is additionally equipped with an irrigation channel. **c** The three different cutting techniques; monopolar (*left*); bipolar (*middle*); quasibipolar (*right*). *HF*, high frequency

Instrumentation for HF Surgery

Today, a broad spectrum of monofunctional, bifunctional and multifunctional HF surgery instruments is available for cutting and coagulation, and also in combination with other functions (Fig. 1.20).

Cutting Instruments

The simplest cutting instrument regarding design and application is the monopolar cutting electrode in needle form. In endoscopy surgery the thin-needle electrode can function as a scalpel for precise dissection and cutting. The advantage of thin-needle electrodes is that the HF current required for cutting is so low that there is only minimal thermal

damage to lateral tissue structures. A HF surgery device with automatic maximum voltage or arc control carries advantages for the use of HF needles. If the minimum voltage of 200 V necessary for cutting is not achieved, thin-needle electrodes may easily bend or even break and stick in the tissue. At voltages with amplitudes higher than 500 V a thin needle can quickly glow away. In order to abolish this risk, bipolar and quasi-bipolar cutting elec-

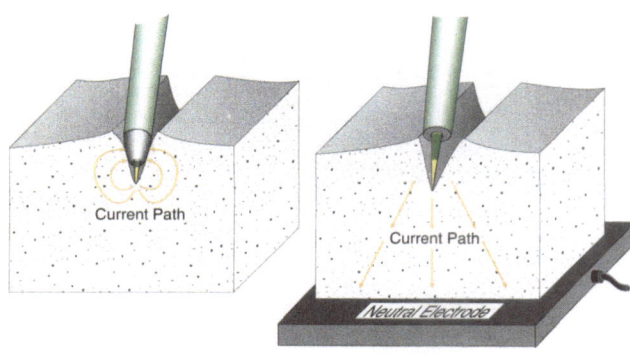

A. Quasi-Bipolar Cutting   B. Monopolar Cutting

Fig. 1.21. Monopolar (*right*) and quasibipolar (*left*) needle electrodes with adjustable needle length are available for preparation cuts with critical incision depth. (From: Endoscopic Surgery Allied Technologies 1 (1993) 103, Thieme Verlag, Stuttgart)

trodes have been developed. The "quasi-bipolar" needle electrodes combine both the above-mentioned advantages in application of a thin-needle electrode and the safety advantages of a bipolar electrode. Figure 1.20c gives a schematic representation of the three different cutting techniques. Monopolar and quasi-bipolar needle electrodes with adjustable needle length are available for preparation cuts with critical incision depth (Fig. 1.21).

Coagulation Instruments

As opposed to conventional surgery and flexible endoscopy, instruments designed specifically for coagulation are rarely used in endoscopic surgery. In order to save the time needed for changing instruments, suction tubes or forceps are often used as monopolar or bipolar coagulation instruments. Hooks primarily designed for blunt manipulation of preparation are also used as cutting and coagulation instruments in arthroscopy and laparoscopy. The utilization of these instruments represents a compromise between optimal function and time saving. Figure 1.18 shows various coagulation techniques which can be carried out with both monofunctional, bifunctional and multifunctional instruments.

Bifunctional Cutting/Coagulation Instruments

Bifunctional cutting/coagulation instruments incorporate principally two surgical techniques. An instrument primarily designed for cutting is used for coagulation, such as practised in transurethral resection (TUR) with the resection snare, or the instrument is equipped with separate cutting and coagulation electrodes. Coagulation with an instrument designed primarily for cutting entails the risk of unintended cutting. This can be ensured if the "soft coagulation" mode described above is applied. If "soft coagulation" does not provide sufficient haemostasis due to too small an effective contact area, "forced coagulation" can be applied. However, due care must be taken, as "forced coagulation" carries the risk of a cutting effect due to the electric arc. In order to reduce this risk, the diameter of the cutting instruments is increased as is necessary for a low-coagulation cutting quality. Bifunctional cutting/coagulation instruments are equipped with a cutting and a coagulation electrode (Fig. 1.20, 1.21). Figure 1.22 represents a sectional drawing of a multifunctional cutting-coagulation instrument. The needle electrode is advanced automatically by means of a pneumatic actuator which is activated prior to the HF current.

Multifunctional Instruments for HF surgery

Cutting and coagulation have been combined with other functions, such as suction, irrigation, grasping, mechanical dissection, ultrasound dissection etc. to produce multifunctional instruments. As multifunctional instruments are not only connected with a HF surgery device, but also with suction and irrigation equipment, complex systems are formed that must be co-ordinated with regard to ergonomy and safety (Fig. 1.22).

HF Surgery Device

Today, HF surgery devices are available for operative endoscopy that meet the requirements for reproducibility of cutting and coagulation effects and in the prevention of undesired side effects. By means of automatic monitoring, regulation and

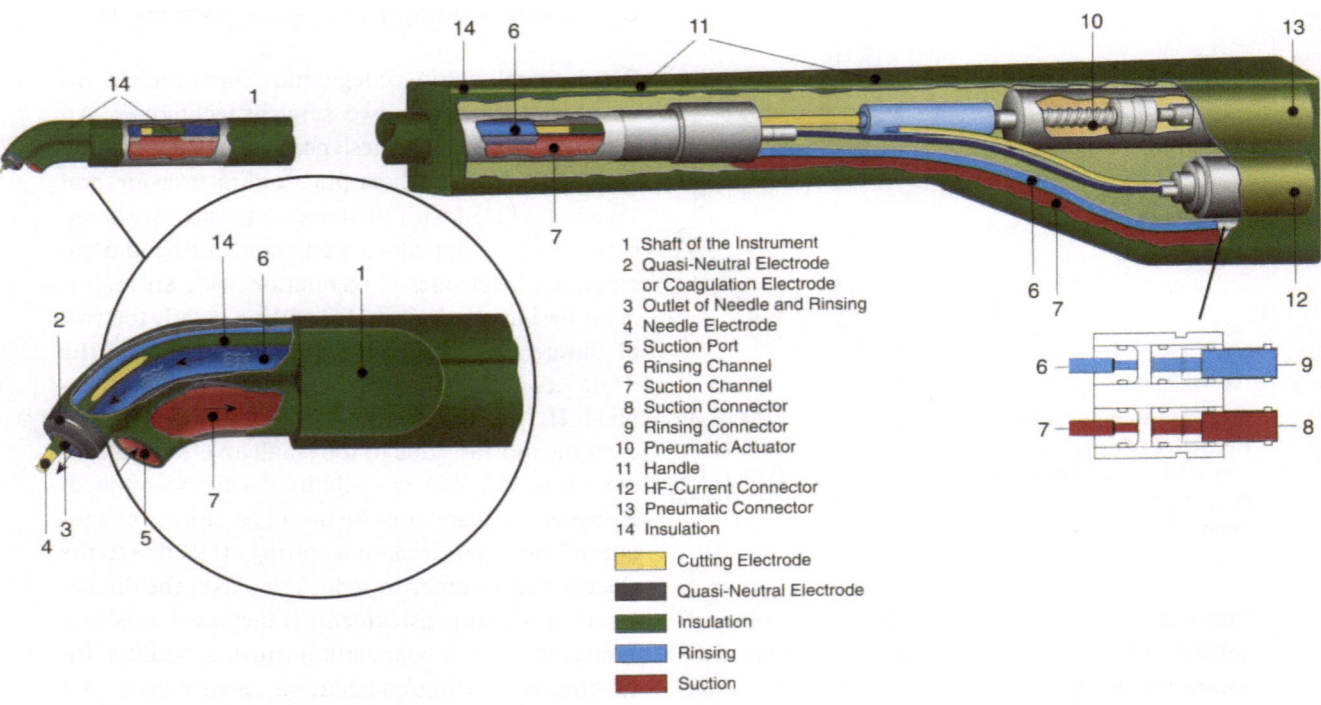

1 Shaft of the Instrument
2 Quasi-Neutral Electrode
  or Coagulation Electrode
3 Outlet of Needle and Rinsing
4 Needle Electrode
5 Suction Port
6 Rinsing Channel
7 Suction Channel
8 Suction Connector
9 Rinsing Connector
10 Pneumatic Actuator
11 Handle
12 HF-Current Connector
13 Pneumatic Connector
14 Insulation

Cutting Electrode

Quasi-Neutral Electrode

Insulation

Rinsing

Suction

Fig. 1.22. Sectional drawing of a multifunctional instrument with pneumatic actuator. (Multifunctional instrument from Erbe, Tübingen, Germany, designed for endorectal surgery). When the cutting mode is activated, the bipolar cutting needle is pneumatically advanced. (From: Endoscopic Surgery Allied Technologies 1 (1993) 98, Thieme Verlag, Stuttgart)

control of the electrical parameters the quality of the cutting and/or coagulation effects are ensured. As multifunctional instruments require complex control and monitoring functions to operate, these instruments and devices should be equipped with interfaces through which they communicate with each other. In order to assure sustained availability of the systems, the relevant devices should be equipped with automatic error detection and report functions. In operative endoscopy, a HF surgery device or a corresponding surgical instrument can no longer be viewed independently of each other, but must be treated jointly as components of a system [56].

Therapeutic Ultrasound

The use of vibrations in ultrasound frequency is not limited to diagnostic imaging purposes. Several reports of liver surgery with ultrasonic dissection have been positive [57, 58]. A recent introduction has been the use of vibrations in the harmonic range, leading to a cutting and coagulating instrument for endoscopic surgery, the "harmonic scalpel" (Ultracision, Smithfield, RI, USA).

Ultrasonic Dissection

With ultrasonic dissection damage to vessels ducts and nerves can be avoided whilst soft tissue such as fat or glandular parenchyma are separated or cleaved. This is achieved through a cavitational effect which occurs at the tip of the vibrating rod of the device (25000/s). The ultrasonic high energy converts water to steam. Thus, the efficacy depends on the water content of the tissue and the cells which are in contact with the dissection tip. Fat and parenchymatous cells contain more water than connective tissue, thus the cavitational effect causes

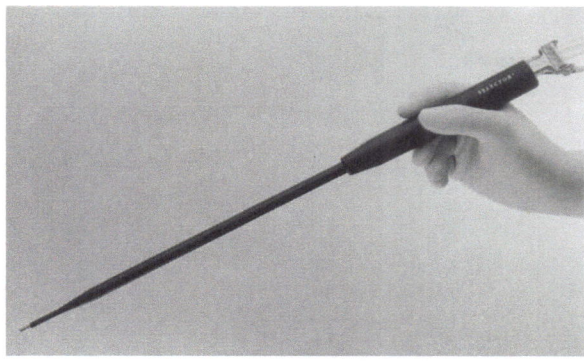

Fig. 1.23. The ultrasonic dissector by Surgical Technology Group (Andover, Hampshire, UK) carries significant advantages for dissection of parenchymatous organs. Similar devices are available from ValleyLab/Pfizer and Söring

fragmentation of parenchymatous cells and fat but structures containing significant amounts of collagen such as vessels and nerves are left intact. Figure 1.23 shows the ultrasonic dissector by Surgical Technology Group (Andover, UK). Similar devices are available from ValleyLab/Pfizer (Boulder, CO, USA) and Söring (Quickborn, Germany). Additional electrocoagulation functions are optionally available. The ultrasonic and HF current can be activated simultaneously. Their effects are additive and as the HF is conducted in electrolytic solutions, vessels, ducts and nerves are coagulated. The

HF should, therefore, be applied carefully and certainly reduces the safety margin of the ultrasonic probe. A combination of a HF hook with an ultrasonic dissection probe is available from Erbe.

Ultrasound Cutting

If the frequency of the vibrating tip respective to the central rod is increased up to 55 000 Hz (harmonic range), the energy applied to the tissue which is in contact with the probe generates sufficient heat for coagulation. The thermal effect is dominant. If the tip is shaped like a scalpel, cutting and slightly coagulating effects are produced. The increased frequency, however, causes technical difficulties, including interference and resonance, especially when the vibrations are transmitted over a long distance (40 cm). The "harmonic scalpel" (Ultracision) is remarkable, because the knife is not really sharp and only cuts when the tip is vibrating in the harmonic range. The coagulating effect is, however, not deep and seems to be insufficient to prevent bleeding. Variant instruments are available with coagulation tips; spatulae and even a scissors have recently been introduced. All instruments have been clinically tested [59] and are available in 5-mm sizes (except the scissors). Figure 1.24 illustrates the thermal effect of ultrasound, HF and laser.

Fig. 1.24. Comparison of the thermal effect of ultrasonic (*left*), high-frequency (*middle*) and laser (*right*)

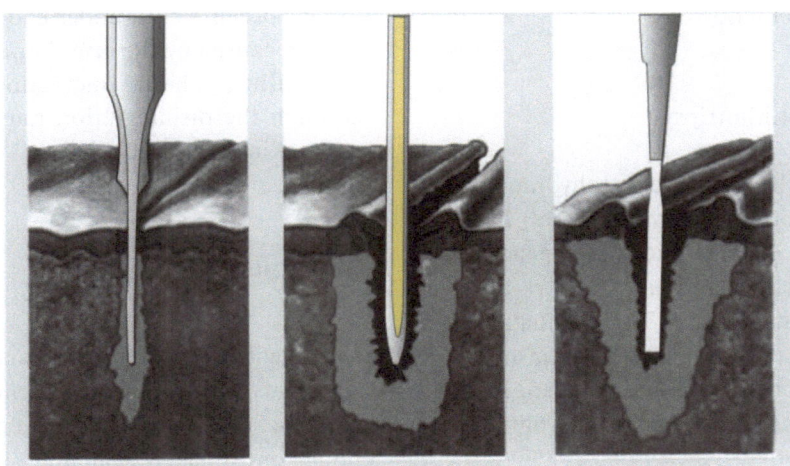

Gallstone Lithotripsy

Gallstone fragmentation techniques vary from simple mechanical disintegration to ultrasound, piezoelectric and laser fragmentation [60, 61]. For endoscopic purposes all these techniques have both advantages and disadvantages.

In mechanical lithotripsy soft stones are grasped and crushed with a forceps or using the Dormia basket. More sophisticated lithotripsy can be performed using unique and very effective motor driven systems such as LaproLith and RothoLith (Endomedix). The RothoLith is flexible and was developed for percutaneous gallstone fragmentation, the LaproLith mainly for disintegration of gallstones prior to removal of the gallbladder. When switched on, the stones are completely fragmented within seconds and the residual liquid mixture can be aspirated easily. However, very large stones cannot be fragmented because they do not rise in the vortex caused by the rotating blade.

Ultrasonic Lithotriptors

The ultrasonic desintegration of stones is based on the cavitational effect which was explained above. The shock impulses create shock waves which disintegrate the stone. The difficulties in transmitting the vibrations to the tip limit the length and the flexibility of ultrasound lithotripsy probes. The efficacy is low and depends on the composition of the stones, so that only the stones with high bilirubin and calcium content are fragmented efficiently by this technique.

Electrohydraulic Lithotripsy

Shock waves can be created electrohydraulically by means of two exposed electrodes (wires) at the tip of the probe. An electrostatic charge generated by a piezoelectric element produces a spark at the tip which creates a shock wave. The disintegration effect is greater than that caused by ultrasound and 60% – 80% of stones can be fragmented. However, direct tissue contact of the probe may damage soft tissue.

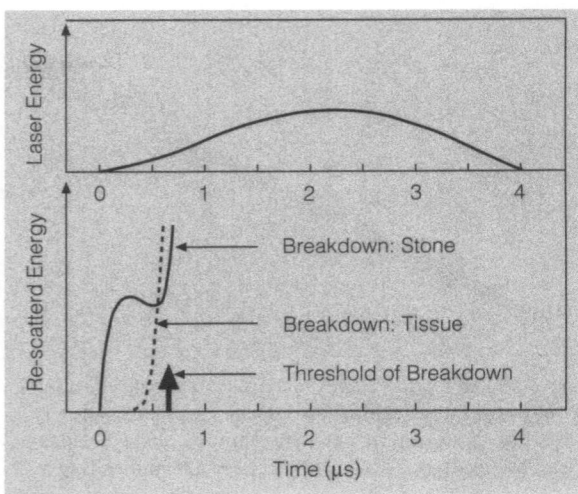

Fig. 1.25. The "Lithognost" laser (Telemit; Munich, Germany) produces a low, intensive laser light impulse prior to the main shot. The reflected light is analysed and the characteristic absorption of calculi is a preconduction for activating the main pulse

Laser Lithotripsy

Laser lithotriptors are very expensive but stones can be detected by means of light absorption. The Telemit laser "Lithognost" (Telemit, Munich, Germany) creates, when activated, a low, intensive laser light impulse which is absorbed, depending on the material illuminated (Fig. 1.25). The reflected amount of laser light is immediately, within nanoseconds, measured and if no specific light absorption characteristic of calculis is indicated, the main laser impulse is not activated. This principle is important because even under endoscopic view tissue damage caused by the laser impulses cannot totally be abolished. The fragmentation rate is adequate, although the disintegration rate of large stones is slow, taking up to 20 min.

Instrument Holders

Instrument holders are not mandatory for routine operations. However, in emergency gallbladder surgery, for example during the night and if not enough assistance is available, an instrument holder can be very useful.

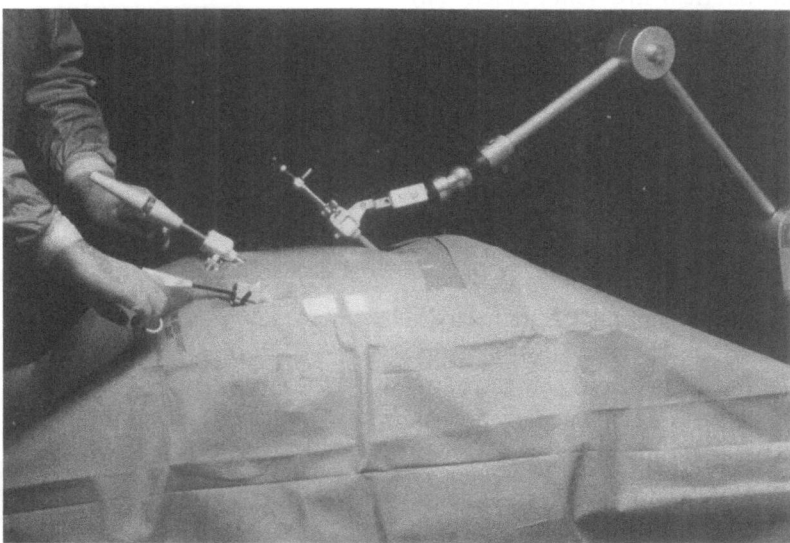

Complicated surgery, e.g. colonic resection, requires five or even more access channels. The surgeon who has to cope with several instruments making extensive movements is often hindered by the close proximity of his assistants. Hence, we have evaluated the feasibility of mechanically assisted operations. The one-man operation is, in fact, possible and with some experience easy to perform. However, its feasibility depends on the quality and features of the instrument holder. The Robotrac (Aesculap; Tuttlingen, Germany) has an inherent disadvantage: it collapses when both joints are unlocked. In addition the Robotrac is not autoclavable, but its holding force and position maintenance are excellent.

The autoclavable "first assistant" from Leonhard Medical (Huntington Valley, PA, USA) operates by vacuum locks which use conventional operating theatre suction and passive retraction so that it cannot collapse. Due to the vacuum principle, there is less holding force than with the Robotrac but the force is adequate for most applications [62–64]. The "little brother" has the same features (Fig. 1.26). The mechanical interfaces to the Leonhard arm enable adaptation of different instruments in addition to the telescope.

Having to control and adjust mechanical holders during a complex surgical procedure disrupts the continuity because frequent change of the position of the optic is required. Hence, the ideal holder

Fig. 1.26. The autoclavable "first assistant" from Leonhard Medical is operated by vacuum locks using conventional operating theatre suction

should have a voice-controlled locking function and manoeuvrability. However, such an intelligent holder is comparable to a manipulator and requires delicate technology. Computer Motion Inc. (Goletta, CA, USA) has developed the first robotic positioning system for endoscopes – the automated endoscopic system for optimal positioning, AESOP. The system comprises an arm with three segments interconnected with joints that are driven by servomotors. The arm needs protection with a sterile polyethylene tube. The movements can be programmed both by remote control and with a foot pedal. One of six programmable buttons simply has to be pressed at an important position and subsequent AESOP remembers operative sites by pressing the buttons correspondingly. However, as both patient position and anatomy vary, the programming has to be repeated, which is time consuming. The system can be activated via a foot pedal while the other instruments are operated simultaneously. However, as HF is controlled by a foot pedal, the foot control of the AESOP may lead to confusion.

From an educational point of view the assistant should not be replaced by holders or robot arms. However, as voice recognition and eye-tracking are

under development robotic instrument holders may
enhance the efficacy of endoscopic surgical manipulations.

Access Instruments

Trocars and Cannulae

Several types of trocars and cannulae have been developed. The new features include valve systems,
safety mechanisms, flexible trocars, new introduction principles and adapters which allow instruments of varying cross-sectional diameter to be employed without the need for reducer flops or tubes.
The importance of safer penetration of the abdominal wall has led to several developments such as:
the insertion of a needle scope into a Verres needle
[65], complex access cannulae [66] and the principle of using an "optic scalpel" [67]. It seems likely
that access and port problems will be resolved within the next few years. However, standardization of
the trocars and cannulae remains an important
consideration.

Passive Dilatation

Passive dilatation of the access channel is achieved
via a blunt trocar with cone-shaped tips. This system is used mostly in reusable cannulae (see Vol. 1,
Chap. 2).

Active Cutting

Penetration by means of sharp pyramidal trocars
reduces the force required to traverse the abdominal
wall. However, the sharp tip of the trocar may
cause severe injuries [68] if the shield does not deploy quickly enough (Fig. 1.27a, b). The principles
of the safety shield, described in Vol. 1, Chap. 2,
have been extended by new designs. A trocar from
Dexide (Fort Worth, TX, USA) is a sharpened tube
with a blind rod inside which moves forward when
the abdominal wall is negotiated (Fig. 1.28a). The
trocar (developed by Origin) retracts within approximately 1 ms subsequent to the penetration of the
abdominal wall (Fig. 1.28b). This adds consider-

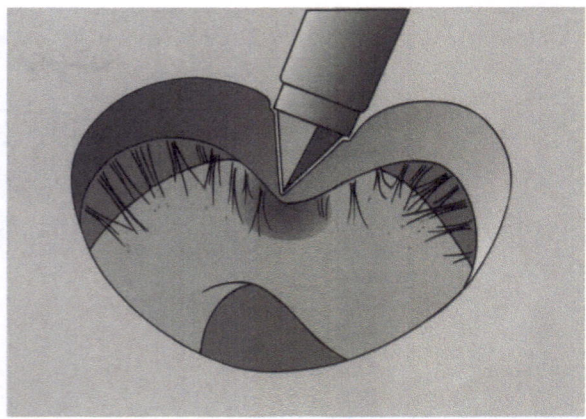

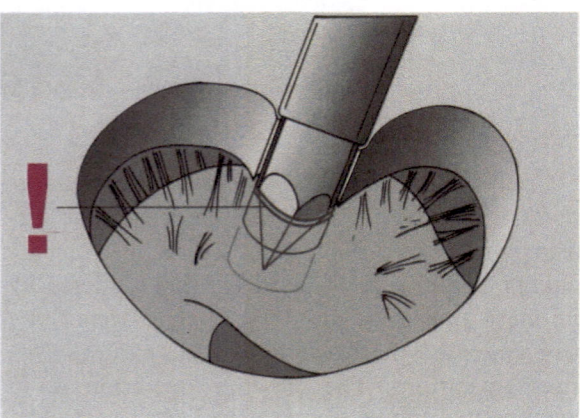

Fig. 1.27a, b. Safety trocars may help to avoid severe damage
of intra-abdominal organs. However, the sharp tip of the
trocar may cause severe injuries if adhesions are present

able safety because the retraction can be hampered
by adherent structures. Bühler (Tuttlingen, Germany) markets a reusable safety shield trocar.

Although all these trocars are considered "safe",
the bowel may be injured in the presence of adhesions. Hence, the use of sharp trocars demands experience and great care, even although recent studies [69, 70] indicate fewer bowel injuries.

The electrosurgical trocar Accucise is marketed
by Applied Laparoscopy. The trocar consists of a
plastic rod with a diathermy loop mounted on the
tip (Fig. 1.29). The introduction force is approximately the same as with sharp trocars. Because the
current is not automatically switched off when the
abdominal cavity is reached, the internal organs
may be injured, particularly in the presence of adhesions. These electrosurgical trocars are best intro-

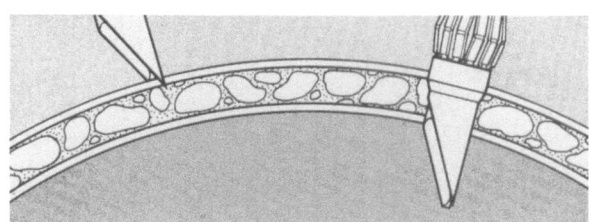

1.28 a

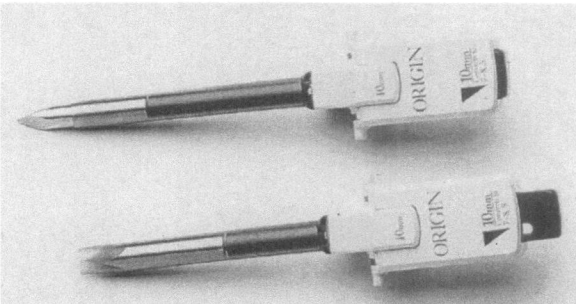

b

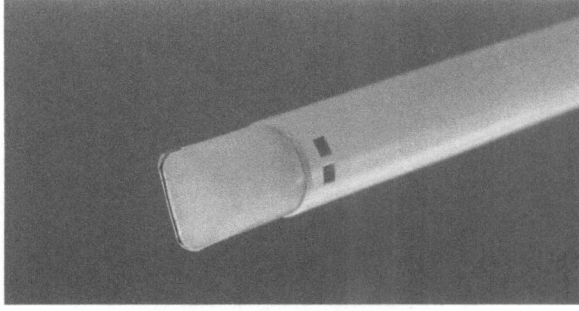

1.29

Fig. 1.28. a Dexide (Fort Worth, TX, USA) markets a trocar which employs a sharpened tube with a blind rod inside which moves forward when the abdominal wall is negotiated. **b** Disposable cannula with retracting trocar (Origin)

Fig. 1.29. The Accucise trocar (Applied Laparoscopy) incorporates a plastic rod with a diathermy loop mounted on the tip

duced under vision. Their advantage is reduced bleeding from the stab wound caused by the trocar.

Controlled Active Cutting

The new "optic scalpel" (Olympus Winter&Ibe) consists of a special endoscope which allows simultaneous contact view with transillumination of tissue and a focus on objects at a distance [67]. The focus is adjusted via a separate ring at the ocular site. The 5-mm, 30° telescope is introduced into a stainless steel tube scalpel which has a sharpened distal end and fits in a trocar. This trocar allows a

dilatation up to 10 mm (Fig. 1.30a–e). The puncture is performed using the tube scalpel which can be moved via a hinge at the handgrip of the system.

Investigations on the abdominal wall of pigs in phantom and animal experiments have revealed a certain "colour code" that permits identification of the anatomical intersections (Table 1.1).

The puncture channel can be visualized by moving the endoscope to and fro and the layers distinguished by their "colour-coded" anatomical structure. However, both colour intensity contrast are low, thus the orientation requires considerable experience. The contact view is afforded by a special optic adapter for tissue transillumination, so that large vessels can be detected and spared. In addition to the colour code, the resistance of the anatomical structure is useful in identifying the layer reached while performing the insertion: fat and muscle allow easy passage, whereas the fascial intersections require active dissection. The reflection intensity of the peritoneum (white in an adhesive bowel loop or vascularized tissue; translucent in free intra-abdominal space) indicates the possibility to provide a "safe window" for entry into the cavity. The optic scalpel also seems useful for preperitoneal approaches because the surgeon can access the area of interest under visual control.

Valves

Active Valves

Among the active valves are the manually controlled trumpet or flap valves. Flap valves are mainly used in disposable devices. In reusable trocars, cleaning and maintenance of flap valves is difficult

Table 1.1. "Colour code" of the anatomical structures of the abdominal wall

Anatomical structure	Colour
Fat	White reflection
Muscles	Light red
Fascia	Bright white reflection
Peritoneum	
Adherent internal structure	Opaque/bright reflection
Free abdominal cavity	Translucent/vascularized

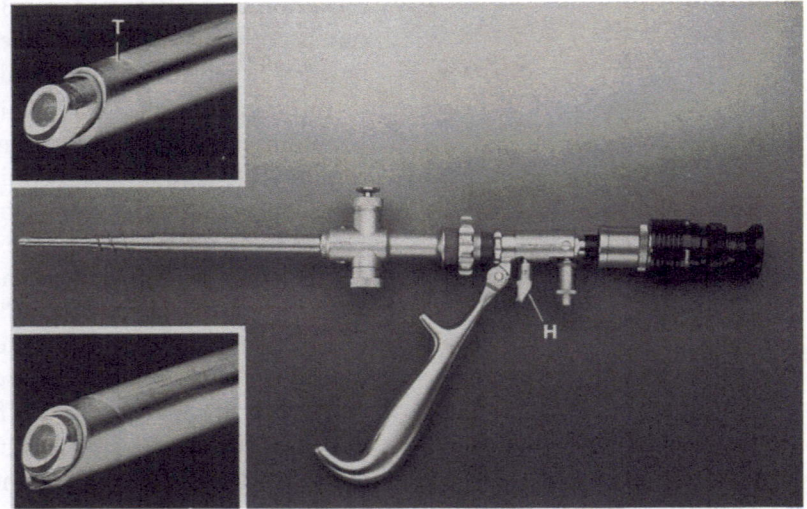

a

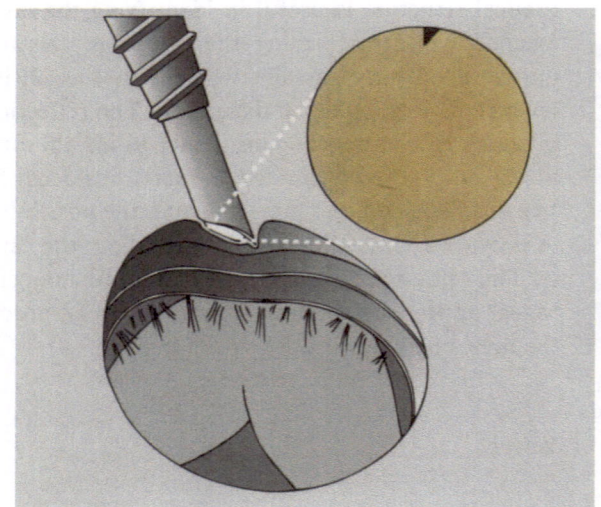

b

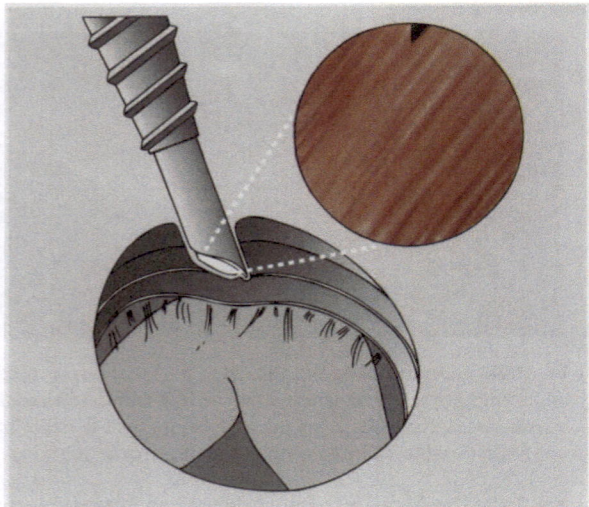

c

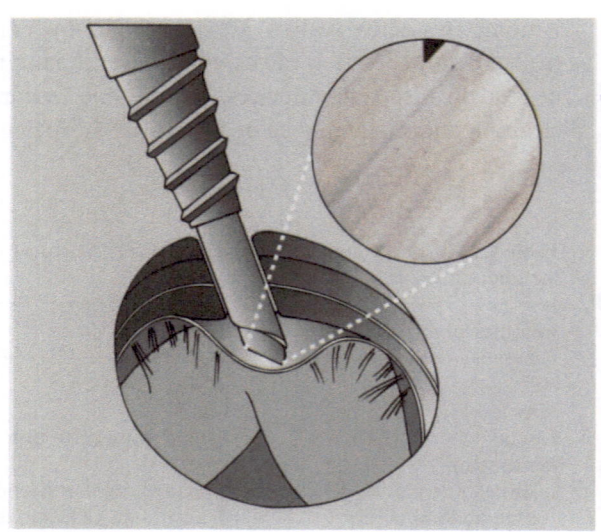

d

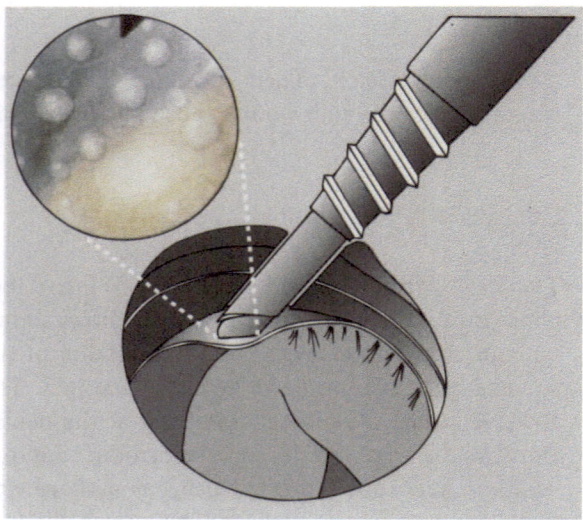

e

and time consuming. The small springs are the major weak point. They do not seal sufficiently when tissue fragments lodge between the flap and its seat.

The sealing quality of trumpet valves is excellent even under dirty conditions. However, the sharp-edged piston of the valve has to be kept fully open during insertion and withdrawal of instruments, otherwise the cannulae may be removed or the insulation of the instruments scratched (Fig. 1.31a), and this may lead to a complete blocking of the cannula. A solution to this problem has been offered by Aesculap by means of the locking piston (Fig. 1.31b). The piston can be withdrawn, secured and subsequently released by pressing the small button.

In general, trumpet valves can damage instruments and thus some experience and concentration is required when using them. The passive silicon valves are best; they do not require any controlling mechanism and seal adequately under most circumstances.

Passive Valves

The silicon rubber seal made by Apple (London, UK) is simple and reliable (Fig. 1.32a). The trocar sleeve is made of plastic which is temperature resistant. However, the company does not allow it to be reused because the autoclaving does not meet standards. The hot steam and EO may affect the internal structure of the material, which can weaken it considerably and leave toxic residues. The rubber sealing provides easy insertion of any instrument and sufficient friction to keep it in place. The cannulae is screw shaped, which protects it from being accidentally removed while withdrawing an instru-

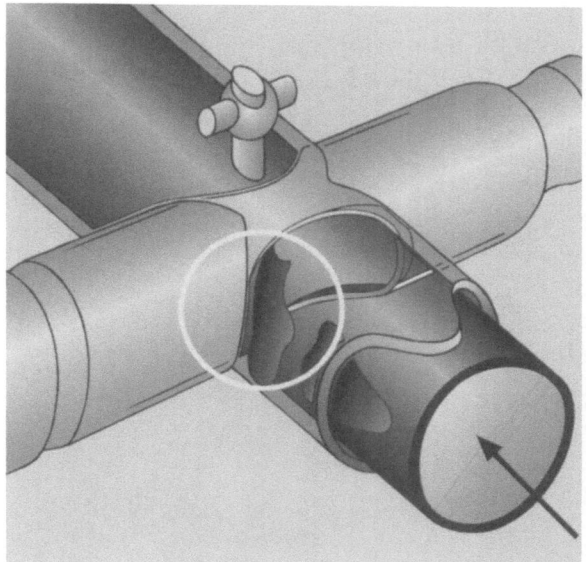

a

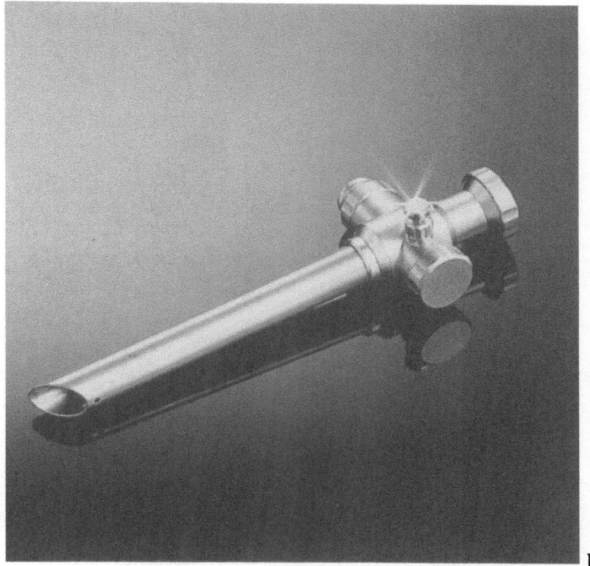

b

Fig. 1.31. a The piston of the trumpet valve has to be kept fully open during insertion and withdrawal of an instrument, otherwise the cannulae may be removed or the insulation of the instrument scratched and damaged. b Aesculap, uses a locking piston that permits free movements of the instruments. Simply pressing the button releases the piston

Fig. 1.30a–e. The "optical scalpel" (Olympus Winter&Ibe) permits an active, controlled, sharp penetration of the abdominal wall. The optic is inserted into a tubular scalpel (T) which can be operated from outside by a small hinge (H). Due to the colours of the different anatomical layers of the abdominal wall: fat, yellow (b); muscle, red (c); fascia, white; peritoneum, vascularized translucent or bright reflecting opaque, orientation is provided while penetrating the abdominal wall. The colour of the peritoneum indicates whether there is a free intra-abdominal cavity (e upper left) or whether there is an adhesion (e lower right)

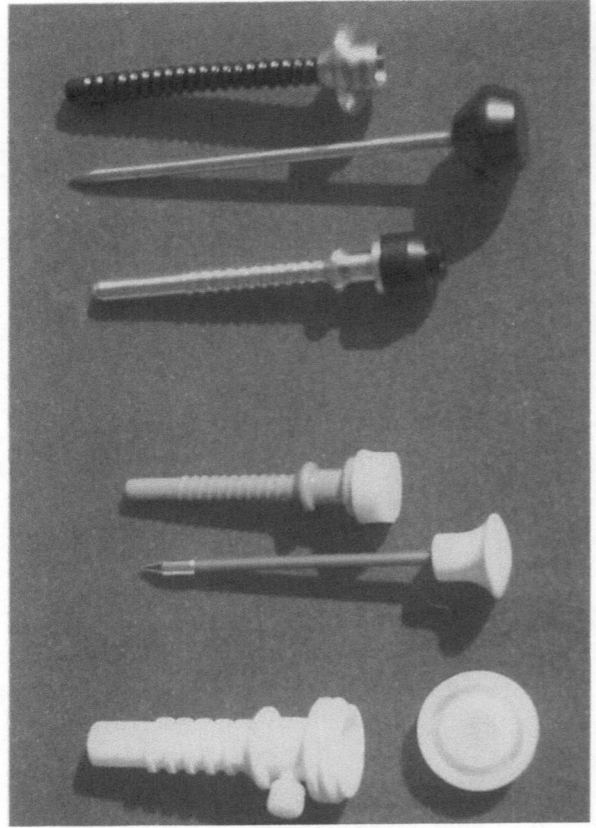

a

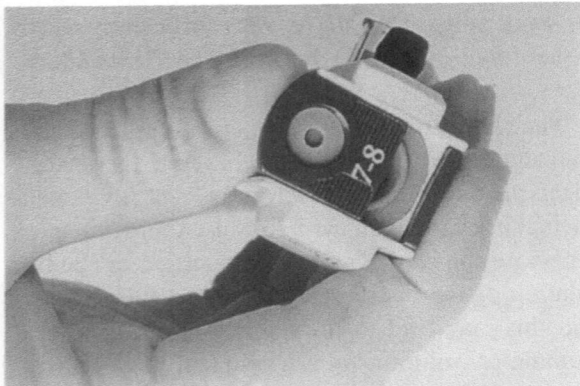

a

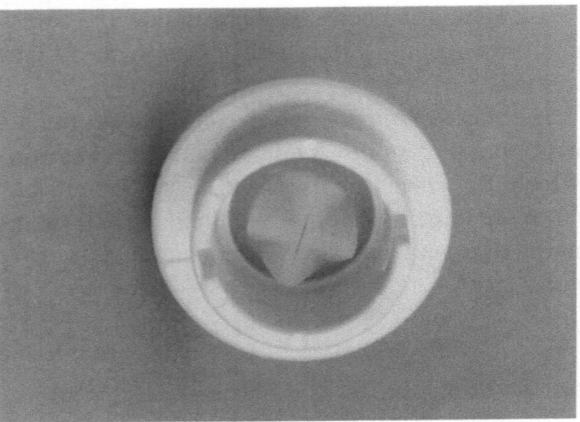

b

Fig. 1.33. a Origin markets cannulae with built-in converters that allow simple one-hand transposition. **b** A variable diameter seal (Applied Laparoscopy) permits the insertion of instruments from 4.5 – 10.5 mm in diameter without changing reducer caps

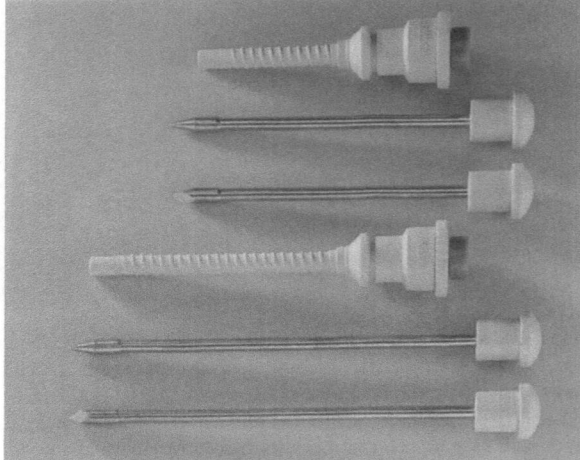

b

Fig. 1.32 a, b. Disposable trocars (Apple, London, UK; PCI, Liptingen; **a**) and Wolf (**b**) are equipped with simple silicon valves. The friction at the instrument is sufficient and only minimal gas leakage occurs during insertion or withdrawal of the instrument

ment. Similar reusable cannulae are marketed by Wolf (Fig. 1.32 b).

Diameter Seal

All cannulae incorporate a seal at the entrance of the valve. Apple use this entrance seal as a part of the valve itself. However, the 10-mm cannula can only take around 10-mm instruments with adequate seal leakage. If a 5-mm instrument is introduced and moved from side to side, there is loss of gas. Hence, the 5-mm instrument must be used with an adapter, either with a reducing tube or with additional seals. The latter is included in the Origin trocars as a set of seals and can be changed easily with one hand (Fig. 1.33 a).

The excellent variable diameter seal is made by Applied Laparoscopy (Fig. 1.33 b). It seals adequately within a range from 4.5 to 11.5 mm and the instrument can be moved from side-to-side without leakage. However, the cannulae are disposable.

Anchorable and Self-retaining Cannulae

The Hasson cannulae are anchored with sutures to keep them from sliding out of the abdominal wall [70]. This principle is quite useful and most of the available trocars allow the fixation of thread at the valve housing (Fig. 1.34 a).

Screw

The screw shape of the trocar sleeve may allow easy and reliable fixation of the cannula in the abdominal or thoracic wall, provided that the screw flanks are adequately designed. The majority of cannulae screws have simple elevations similar to conventional screws [71]. The soft human tissue, however, requires relatively deep threadings with smoothed edges. In particular for dilatation from 5 to 10 mm such a design alleviates the screwing considerably.

Balloon

The balloon anchoring of cannulae is exemplified by the Marlow (Willoughby, OH, USA) and Origin devices (Fig. 1.34 b). The major restriction is the minimal space for the balloon. However, the smooth surface may reduce trauma to the peritoneum. These cannulae are disposable as the balloon fixative precludes resterilization.

Mechanical Sheath Expansion

Mechanical spread cannulae have some advantages in terms of firm anchoring (Dexide). They are simple and reliable and their space requirement is low. In Fig. 1.34 c various products are shown. Regrettably, this useful type of fixation is only available as a disposable cannula. Cleaning problems impede reuse.

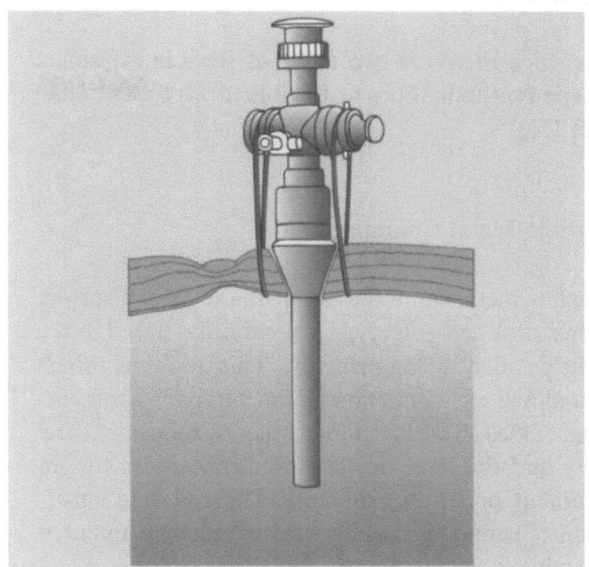

a

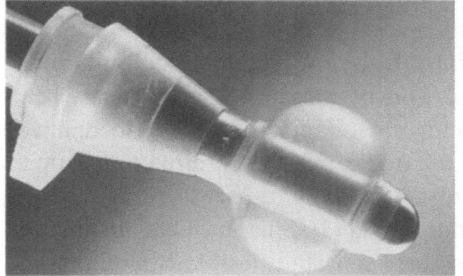

b

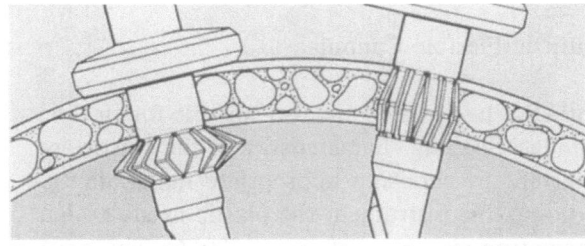

c

Fig. 1.34. a The Hasson cannulae are anchored with sutures to the abdominal wall, preventing gas leakage and accidental withdrawal of the cannula. **b** Marlow and Origin deploy balloons retaining the cannulae in place. **c** Mechanical sheath expansion keeps the Dexide cannulae from sliding out

Flexible Trocar Cannulae

Basically, there are two types of flexible cannulae: elastic synthetic tubes or flexible metal tubes (Table 1.2) [72].

Flexible Metal Cannulae

Flexible metal cannulae can be made from a spring. Storz produce this type of cannula based on a tightly coiled spring principle. This design is robust and allows easy insertion of the curved instruments (Fig. 1.35 a). The instrument has to be insert carefully and the jaws firmly closed, otherwise the instrument penetrates the coil. The coils are subsequently separated, while the curved instrument is introduced or negotiated. The immediate recoil ensures that there is only a momentary leakage of gas, which is not a particular problem once the cannula is fully introduced. Acceptable fixation is achieved after insertion of the curved instrument, because the opening slits clamp the tissue. To remove the cannula the trocar must be inserted to ensure exact alignment of the coils, otherwise they retract and may be damaged [73]. Silicon valves are going to be added to these reusable flexible cannulae.

Synthetic Flexible Cannulae

Synthetic elastic tubes are also suitable for flexible cannulae. Shaping characteristics of the plastic are important in choosing appropriate material, e.g. for a reusable instrument the plastic needs a high temperature resistance of about 200 °C. The most suitable material is polytetrafluoro-ethylene (PTFE; Teflon, Fig. 1.35 b). However, its elasticity

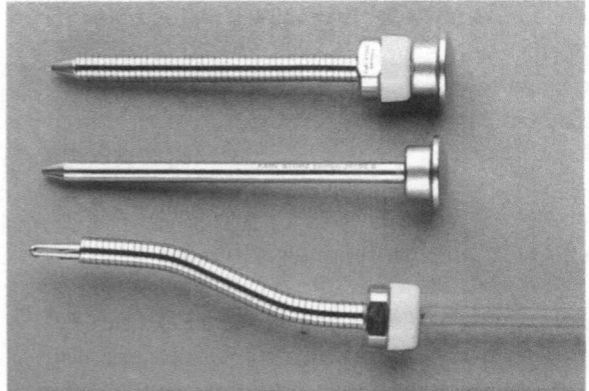

a

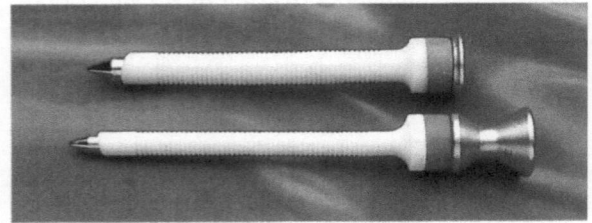

b

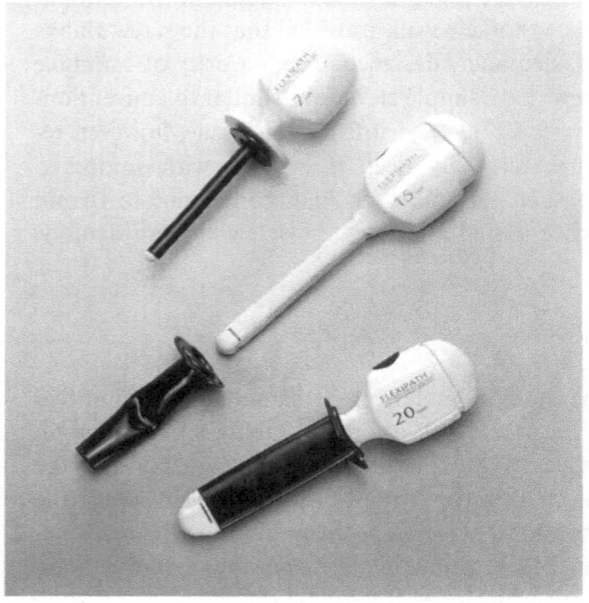

c

Fig. 1.35. a Storz produces flexible cannulae based on the tightly coiled spring principle. For removal of the cannula the trocar has to be fully inserted to ensure alignment of the coils. **b** Flexible cannulae made from Teflon tubes (Wolf). **c** Soft plastic cannulae with special introducer (Ethicon, Cincinnati, OH, USA)

Table 1.2. Basic requirements for flexible cannulae

Cleanability
Biocompatibility
No kinking while the instruments are being introduced
Minimal deformation
Minimal altering of length or diameter
Minimal friction between material and instrument
Adequate friction between cannula and tissue
Reasonable price

is not optimal. Hence, those flexible trocars do not exhibit optimal features.

Teflon is also used by Olympus Winter&Ibe. The flexible tube of the cannula is made of Goretex. This material is a thin foil, with pores 20000 times smaller than a drop of water and 700 times the size of a H_2O molecule. Goretex film is used to line the tubes, which are very flexible. The disadvantage is that the tube is disposable because the pores cannot be cleaned sufficiently after use.

Quite soft, flexible, disposable cannulae (Ethicon; Cincinnati, OH, USA) are made from polyethylene. Their introduction is facilitated by using a trocar that can be distended within the cannula, tightly fixing it.

Percutaneous Instruments

The "Quicksert" disposable instruments by Kinsey Nash (Nashville, TN, USA) are 3.7 mm in diameter. A piercing pin permits quasi self-seating, whereby the cannula is eliminated. These instruments include graspers, scissors and dissectors and can be reinserted without requiring additional incisions for cannulae. Thin, directly insertable instruments may provide considerable improvement in endoscopic surgical procedures and if they are reusable save costs as well. The smaller puncture sites may cause less pain and scar formation as an advantage for the patient.

Instruments for Laparoscopic Cholangiography

Laparoscopic cholangiography usually starts with the cannulation of the cystic duct with a catheter, e.g. a 4–5 Fr ureteric catheter. After the catheter has been inserted through the small incision into the cystic duct, Heister's valve is passed into the common bile duct [30, 74].

The surgeon can choose from a variety of forceps. These forceps, originally designed for urological procedures, combine a small instrument channel and grasping jaws at the distal end (Fig. 1.36). When approximated these jaws keep the cystic duct watertight as the catheter is impacted. However, all these forceps are delicate and break easily if not maintained adequately and it is hardly possible to clean them sufficiently.

Insertion of the catheter into the incision can be facilitated by using a preshaped, bent catheter guiding sleeve (Rüsch; Kernen, Germany). The deflection can be adjusted by moving the sleeve back and forth within the outer tube (Fig. 1.37a). A guide wire can be used; however, this is usually unnecessary. Marks at the catheter's tip permit a precise introduction depth of 2–3 cm. The catheter can be temporarily anchored to the cystic duct by a slightly approximated titanium Ligaclip.

Fig. 1.36. Forceps for intraoperative cholangiography consist of a small instrument channel and grasping jaws at the distal opening of the channel

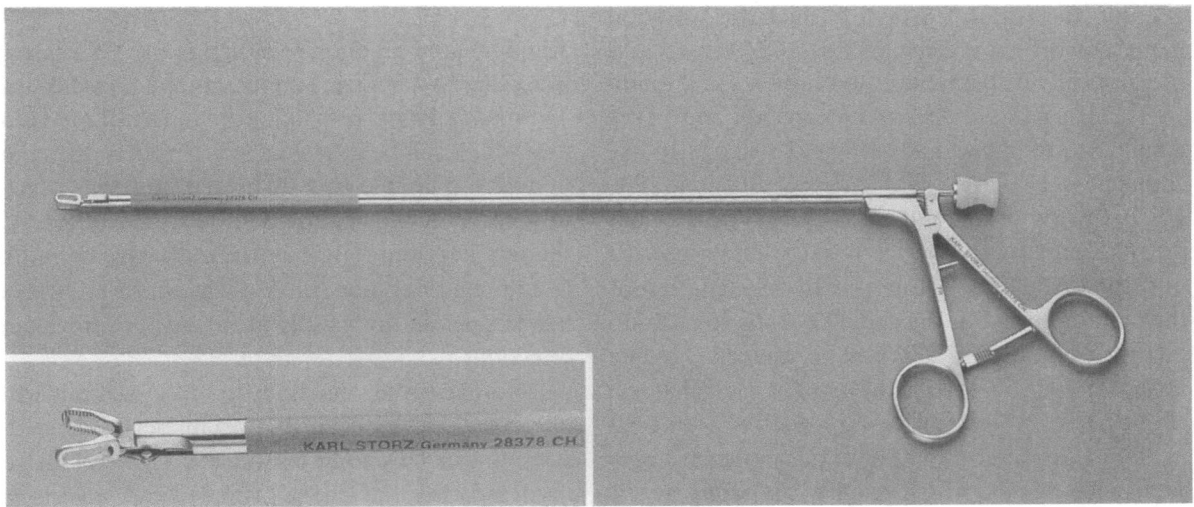

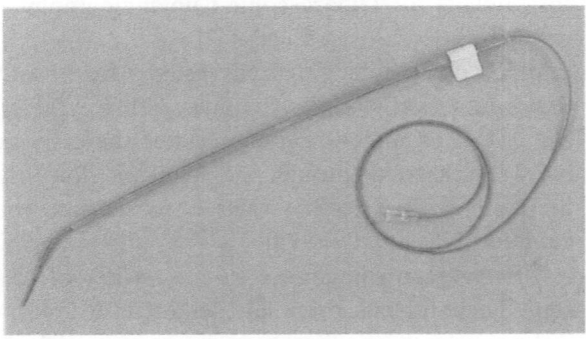

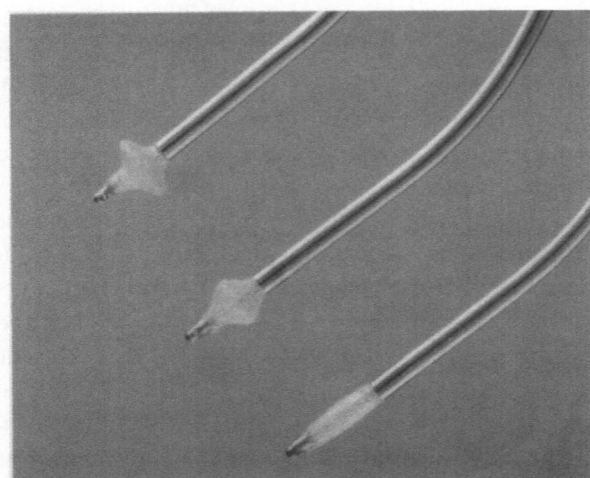

Fig. 1.37. a The preformed guiding sleeve (Tübingen and Rüsch, Kernen, Germany) facilitates the guidance of the conventional radiology catheter into the cystic duct. b Catheters manufactured by Applied Medical Resources or Origin employ a mechanical retention tip which can be adjusted via a ratchet handle

There are special catheters available in three sizes (Taut; Geneva, Il. USA) with which extravasation is prevented by a cone-shaped tip. However, these mechanically distendable cones have a small diameter, which limits their sealing capacity and hence a balloon would be an advantage. This Fogarty-like catheter is available from Arrow (Reading, PA, USA). Since a ballon catheter is employed, care has to be taken that the device is sufficiently inserted into the cystic duct. Otherwise the insufflation of the balloon pulls out the catheter. Catheters manufactured by Applied Medical Resources (Laguna Hills, CA, USA) or Origin, employ a mechanical retention tip which can be adjusted via a ratched handle (Fig. 1.37b). These rigid catheters have preformed angles, which require a separate access

or a flexible trocar. However, they reduce the need to suture or clip the catheter in place.

Another design is available from Lapromed (Irvine, CA, USA), the "PortSaver", with which the abdominal wall can be electrosurgically penetrated. This should only be undertaken under endoscopic control from inside the abdominal cavity. The disposable "cholangiographic device" has a rectangular open tip in which a hollow needle is inserted. If the cystic duct is placed in the opening, a vacuum keeps it in place and then the needle is pushed, puncturing the duct, and contrast can be injected. This procedure will only work if the cystic duct is of a normal size and perfectly skeletonized.

Hand Instruments

Grip and Handle Design

Basically, the handle function can be described by coaxial and transaxial actions (Fig. 1.38a-c). Transaxial action handles are most common. The grips have finger rings and are positioned at 90° to the longitudinal axis. Hence, the action of fingers relative to the hand are transmitted in longitudinal movements. As a result the whole instrument moves. This unintended movement must be compensated for. However, it can be minimized when the grips are positioned in longitudinal direction. The opening actions then are 90° to the axis, hence, the force vector in longitudinal direction is zero.

Ergonomic Grip Design

A unique and ergonomic design is the Polaris grip by ValleyLap/Pfizer, manufactured by DaVinci. The main advantage is that grip and shaft are modules which can be interchanged. However, the ergonomics are limited to a dedicated position, which, in fact, can only be used in a few procedures. Although, left- and right-handed users have been taken into consideration, most of the time the surgeon has to operate the handle in various positions and directions.

In order for all functions to be carried out with one hand, drives such as pneumatic cylinders or servomotors have to be considered. However, drives need switches, an energy supply, and additional

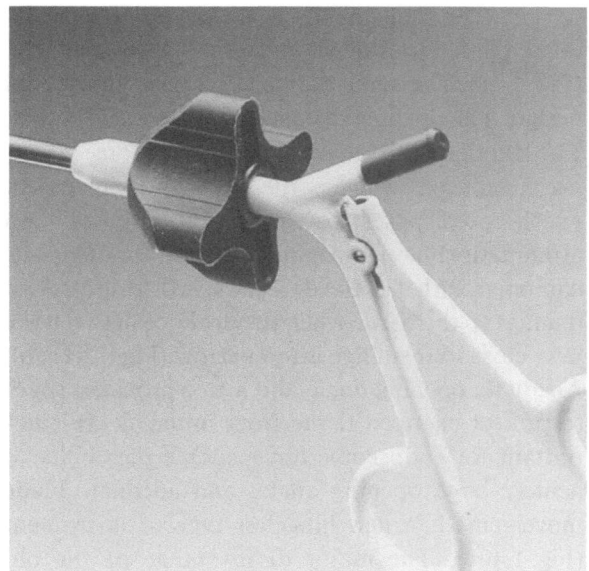

a

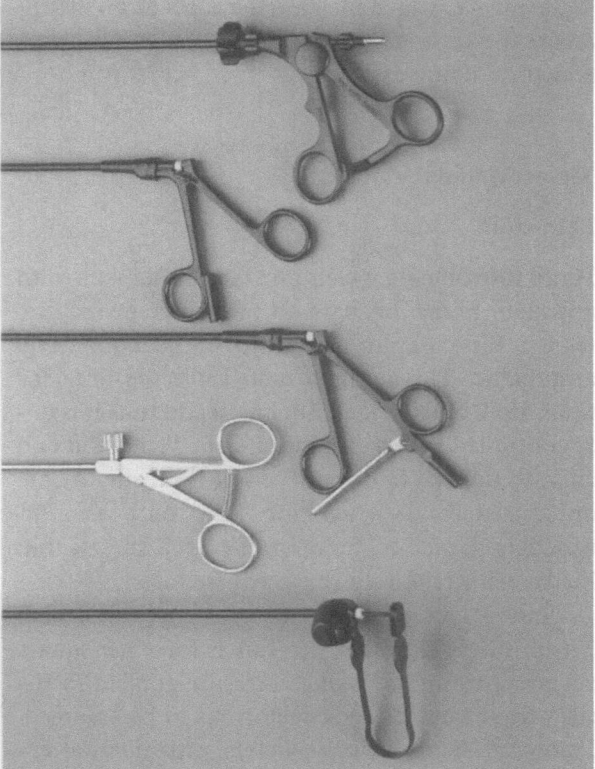

c

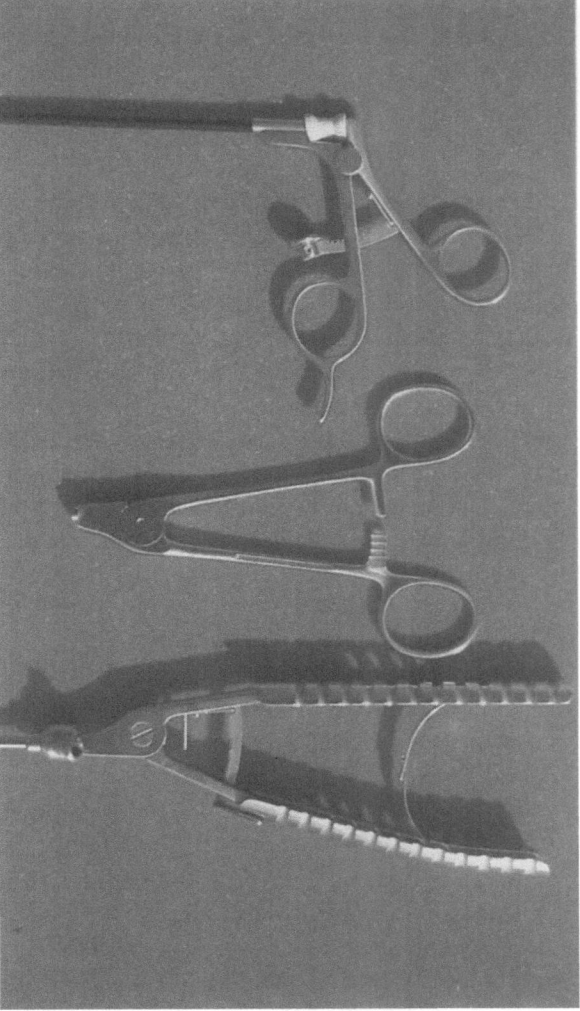

b

Fig. 1.38 a – c. Different types of handles. The principal functions can be classified into "coaxial" and "radial" action

maintenance, which increase the costs of an instrument; the priority, however, is to accomplish fast and precise operations.

Tissue Manipulation

Retractors

Hand instruments which provide the surgeon with adequate retraction have to meet certain requirements. First of all they have to be completely atraumatic. This is important, since the retractor tip is often outside the visual field and thus it is only controlled by sensorial feedback. The broad and smooth flanked hooks utilized in open surgery are appropriately designed for that purpose. Endoscopic retractors, however, have flanks and thin blades with relatively sharp edges (Fig. 1.39).

Only a few retractors are adequately designed. The principle is simple; pressure is force per square surface area and to reduce pressure applied to tissue, the square of the retractor has to be enlarged. Retractors made from segments with internal cables (Surgical Innovations; London, UK) are excellent as they are relatively stiff once the inner cable is strained by means of the handle. However, the cleaning of the segments is delicate and cumbersome.

An interesting concept of organ retraction is the "joy stick" by Origin. It was designed for cholecystectomy. The organ is punctured, the device inserted and then a balloon inflated. The gallbladder can be handled easily; however, the dissection is more difficult because the bladder slips around the balloon.

Considerable facilitation of organ dissection and retraction are the Dundee "variable curvature instruments" (reusable, Storz; disposable USSC; Fig. 1.40). A circular, preshaped retractor blade introduced in a straight shaft recovers once pushed out of the shaft. The instrument allows precise adjustment of the curvature. Thus retraction and mobilization are facilitated considerably [75].

Forceps

The design of the forceps currently available is similar to that of the forceps employed in conventional surgery. The shape of the jaws, for example, reproduces the features of De Bakey, Allis, Russian, etc. (Fig. 1.41). The small diameter restricts an optimal design. The opening distance of the jaws is limited. The length and the maximum possible force is very much reduced, whereas the stiffness is increased, which predisposes to accidental injuries. An atraumatic bowel grasping forceps, for instance, equipped with De Bakey's jaws, will cause severe damage to the tissue when the distance between the jaws close to the hinge is too narrow (Fig. 1.42a, b). Adequate opening angle and a free proximal space to protect clamped tissue from injury is most important for endoscopic forceps. One possibility to achieve large opening angles and adequate blade movements is a new hingeless type of instrument (Fig. 1.42c). The major disadvantage of the old type of hingeless graspers and bipolar forceps is the relatively longitudinal movement of the blades (Fig. 1.43a). The new hingeless instrument has an intermediate tube which approximates the blades when advanced (Fig. 1.43b). The jaws are connected with the grip, thus maintaining the jaws' position while in operation.

The superelasticity of nickel titanium alloy offers the required elasticity for hingeless instruments such as atraumatic forceps, scissors and needle holders. Superelasticity describes the property of recovering an initial shape subsequent to loading and substantial deformation. Superelastic Nitinol has an approximately ten-fold higher elastic deformability than common spring stainless steel [76, 77]. Those instruments combine adequate performance with a simple design, which facilitates the cleaning process as well as repair and maintenance.

Using superelastic materials in the production of endoscopic instruments offers important safety features:

- The graspers have a built-in pressure limit between the jaws, which reduces the risk of tissue damage.
- The needle driver has two locking positions: first lock adjusted exactly to hold the thread without damaging and second lock firm but also adjusted grip of the needle.
- The scissor blades slide with optimal elasticity along each other to facilitate excellent cutting and various curvatures.

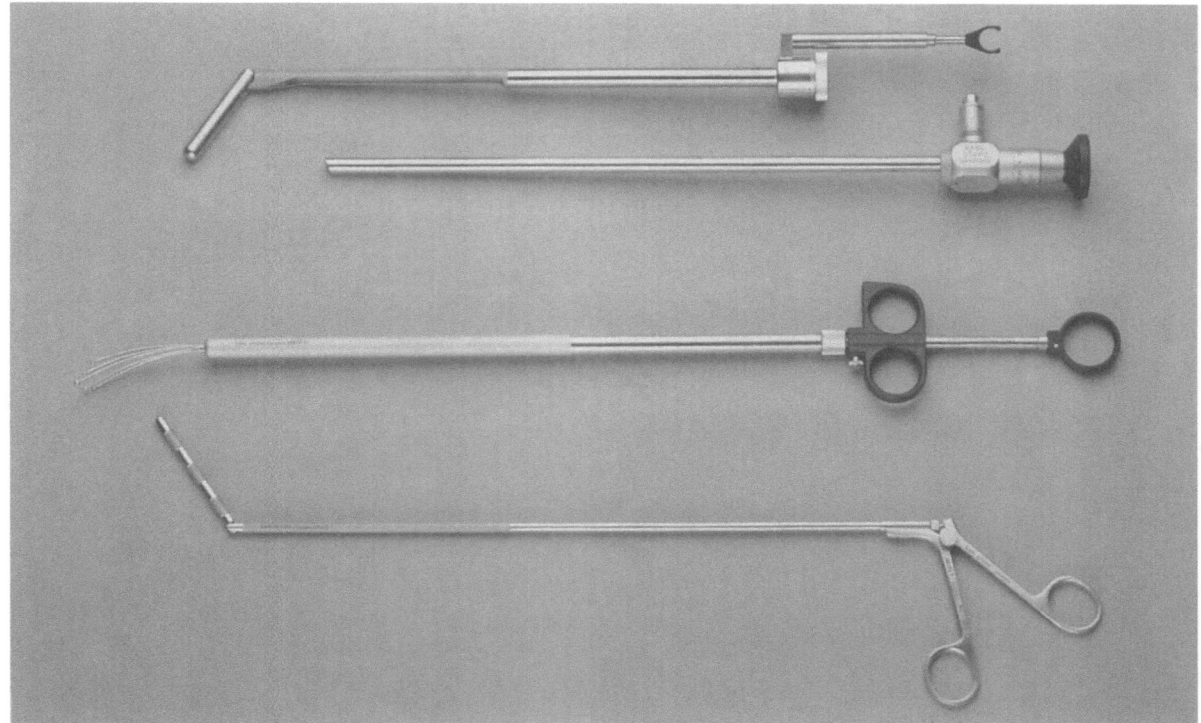

a

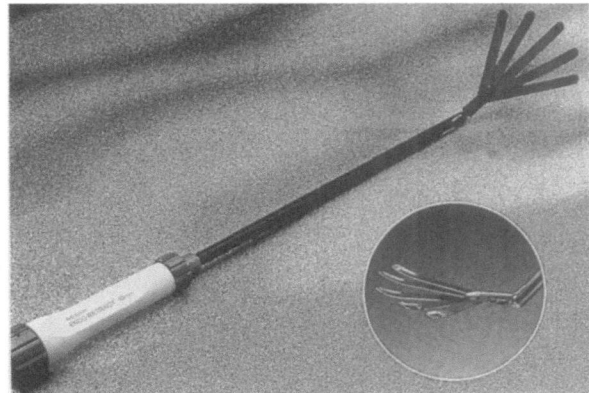

b

◀ **Fig. 1.39 a, b.** Variety of retractors. **a** Storz; **b** USSC

Fig. 1.40 a, b. Dundee "variable curvature instruments", reusable by Storz **a** and disposable by USSC **b** employ a circular, preshaped, superelastic blade that recovers once pushed out of the shaft
▼

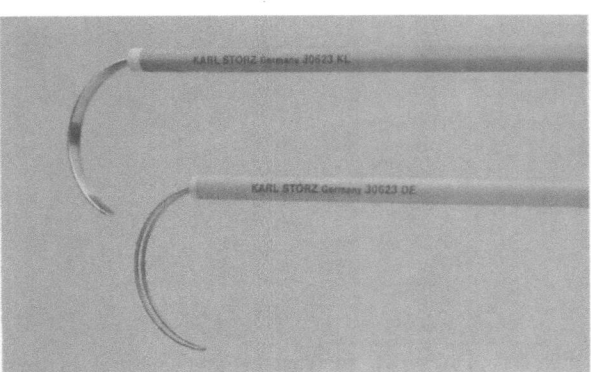

a

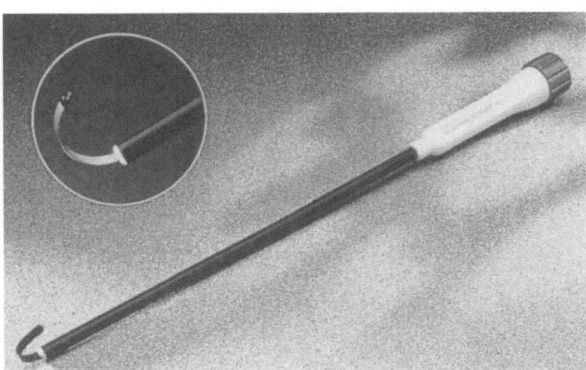

b

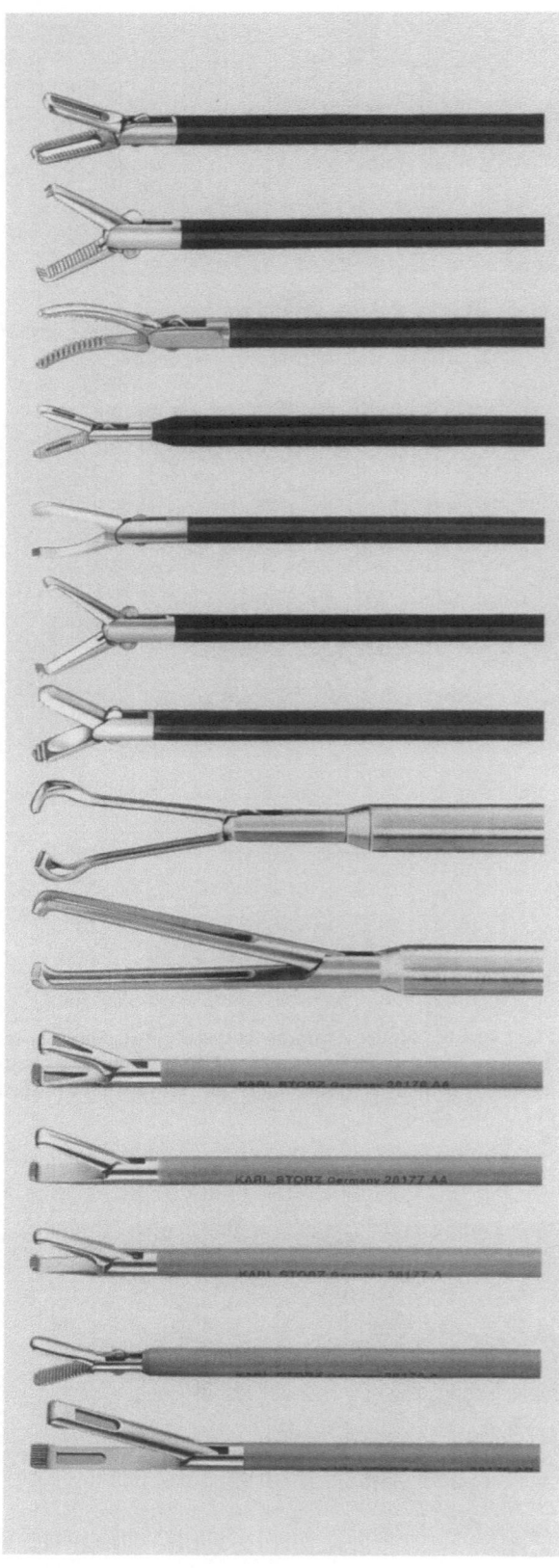
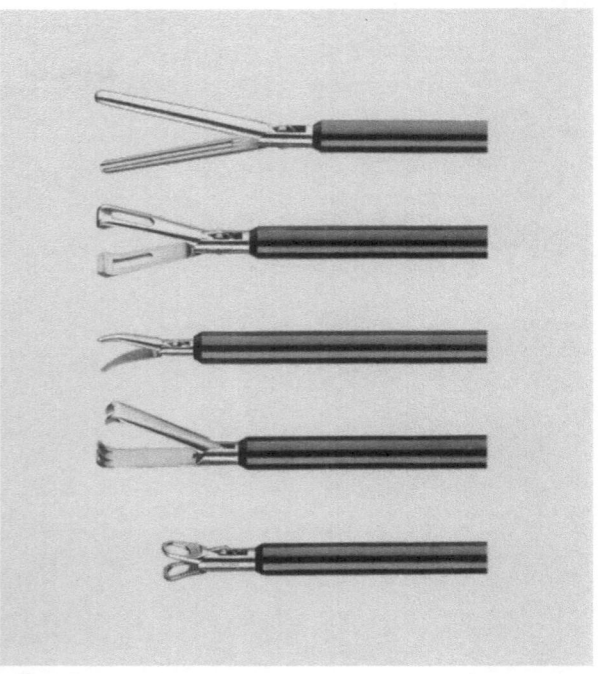

Fig. 1.41. The variety of types of jaws employed in endoscopic surgery

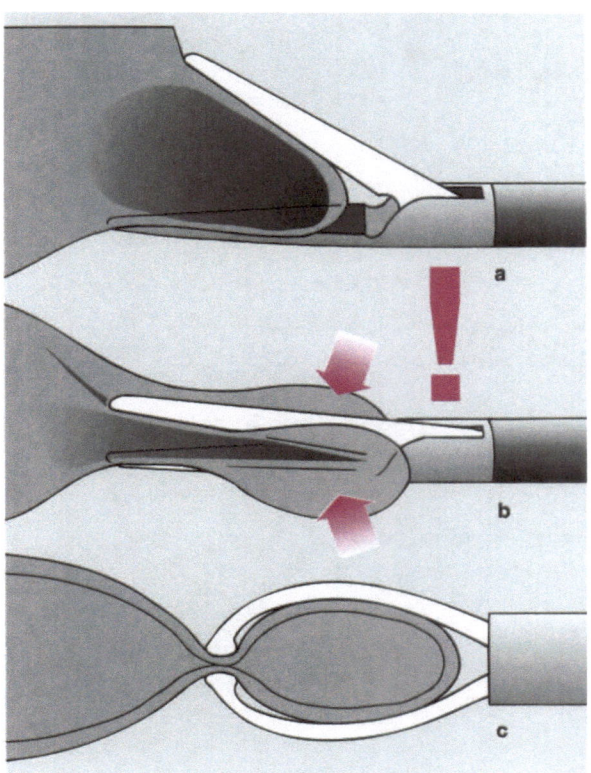

◀ **Fig. 1.42. a, b** A conventional forceps may cause severe damage to the tissue when the distance between the jaws proximal to the hinge is too narrow. **c** Adequate opening angle and a free proximal space to protect clamped tissue from injury is most important for atraumatic grasping forceps

Fig. 1.43. a Conventional hingeless graspers and bipolar forceps entail relatively longitudinal movement of the blades while in operation, which requires compensating movement. **b** The new hingeless instruments (PCI and NDC) maintain the jaw position. An intermediate tube (*F*) is advanced to approximate the blades which are connected to the grip
▼

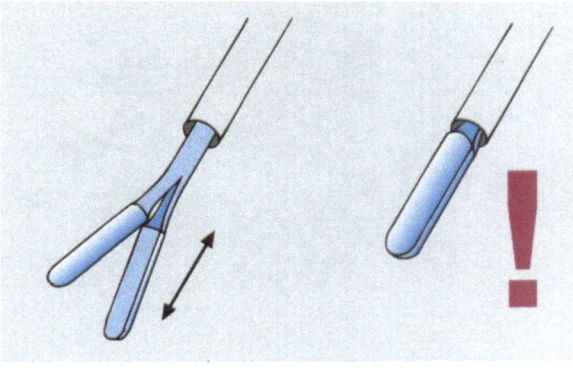

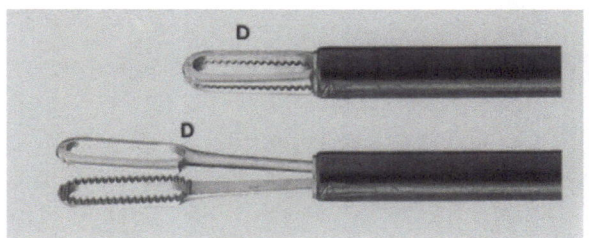

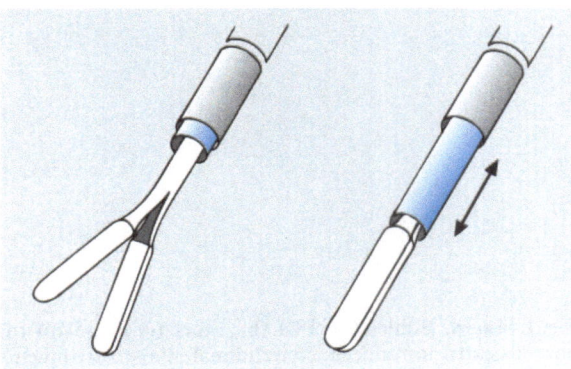

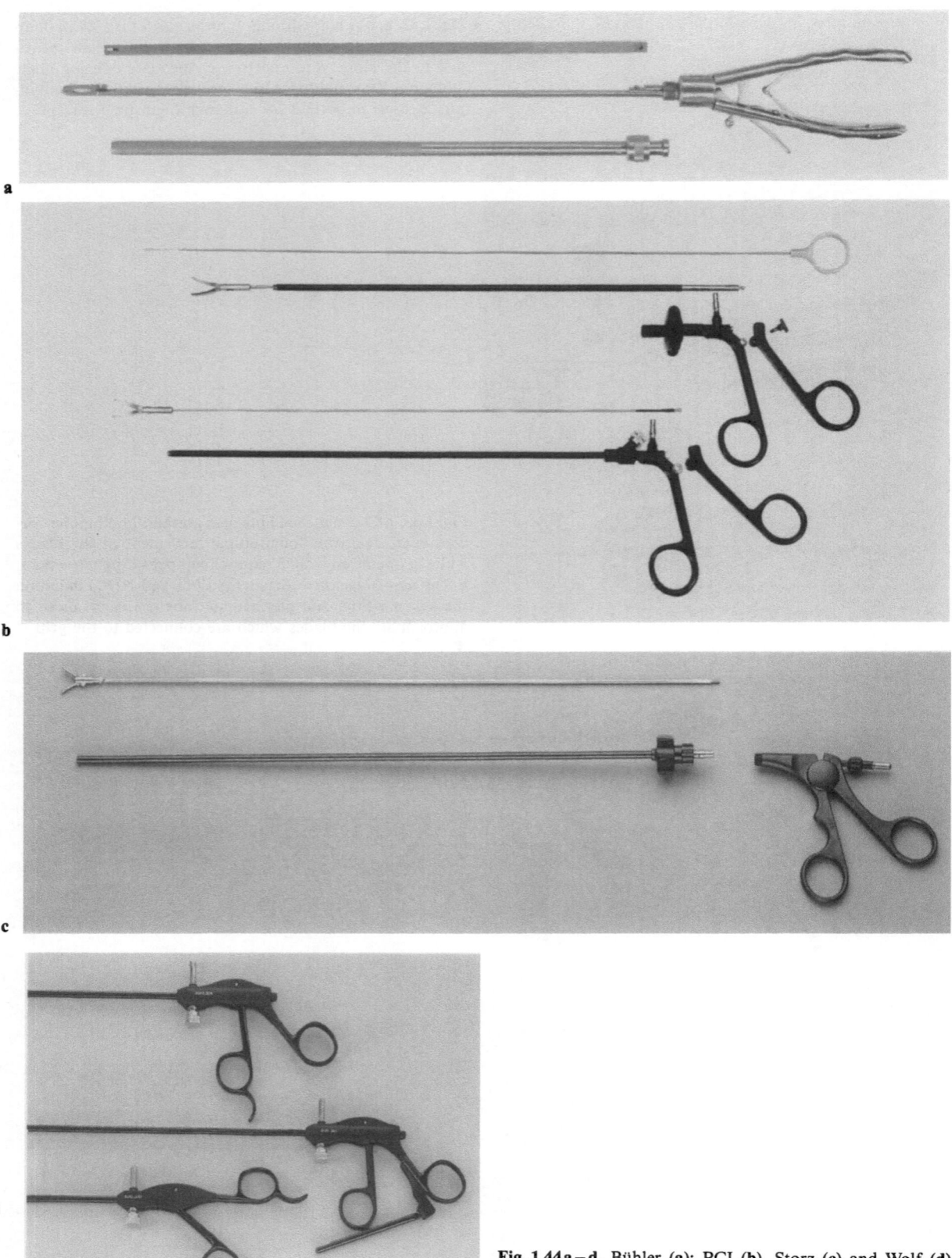

Fig. 1.44a–d. Bühler (**a**); PCI (**b**), Storz (**c**) and Wolf (**d**) have recently introduced conventional hinge instruments which can be disassembled and improve cleaning

For a list of the important features of instruments for endoscopic surgery see Table 1.3.

Bühler, Storz, Wolf, Circon, and PCI have recently introduced instruments which can be disassembled by unscrewing and disconnecting the push rod with the jaws from the outer sleeve (Fig. 1.44 a – d). Most manufacturers offer similarly designed instruments.

Principally, the disassembling permits efficient and usable cleaning prior to sterilization. Furthermore, the functional tip can be replaced when it has worn out. Although cleaning feasibility is improved, this design has weakened the instrument.

Curved Instruments

Curved and bayonet instruments were developed for endoluminal rectal surgery (see Vol. 1, Chap. 25). The narrow operative field requires distally curved forceps, suction probes and needle holders.

For delicate handling of internal organs in advanced laparoscopic surgery, e.g. colonic resections [78] or fundoplication (see Vol. 1, Chap. 23), additional movements and degrees of freedom of the instrument tip are needed. The limited space and movements of the instruments within the thoracic cavity further underlines the need for such equipment. This can be accomplished by simple distal curvature of the instrument (Fig. 1.45 a) [79]. The distal curvature should have a radius of about 25 mm and 45° up to 60° for thoracoscopic interventions and antireflux surgery. Colonic surgery requires a curvature of up to 90°. Figure 1.45 b presents a variety of curved instruments. The handling of bent instruments requires some experience because the instrument tip is moving along a circle as the long axis if the instrument is rotated (Fig. 1.45 c, d).

To introduce curved instruments flexible cannulae are needed. Although curved instruments increase the working area, the degrees of possible distal movement are still restricted to translation, rotation and some movements within the access port.

Table 1.3. Features required for instruments for endoscopic surgery

The instrument position should be stable when the jaws are activated.

The jaws should be adequately elastic so as to permit atraumatic grasping and other jaws functions.

The instrument should be easy to disassemble and reassemble.

The modules should be designed with similar interfaces so that an exchange is possible.

The outer sleeve (insulation) should be replaced easily.

The standardized interface should be connected to cleaning and rinsing devices.

A functional check of all parts should be easy and automatically takes place on each application.

The manufacturer should use a minimal number of parts, which reduces cost and should provide the surgeon with upgrades of the jaw design at a reasonable price.

The simple design for jaw action makes it possible to update the jaw design according to new applications.

The manufacturer should provide the surgeon with all parts so that in case of weakness or breakage only the defective component has to be replaced.

A simple design reduces wear and tear because the number of hinges and bolts are reduced.

Variable Curvature Instruments

A more sophisticated solution is to use steerable, distally deflecting instruments. There are some instruments currently available which allow the transposition of the jaws' action mechanism (Micro France, Paris, France). However, when the jaws are deflected to 90° there is no residual opening angle.

The superelastic property of nickel-titanium is used for the variable curvature spatula and sling passer (Storz) (Fig. 1.40) and in the disposable, variable curvature forceps (USSC). The latter consists of a preshaped Nitinol tube covered by PTFE. The curvature is adjusted by shifting the outer sleeve. The price for the variable curvature is reduced stiffness of the curved part of the forceps. However, it is a useful design which enhances the scope of endoscopic manipulations. USSC is marketing the first deflectable instruments. The disposable roticulator generation incorporates superelastic Nitinol tubes. Although these instruments permit continuous adjustment of the distal end from 0° to 90°, their mechanical stability should be increased.

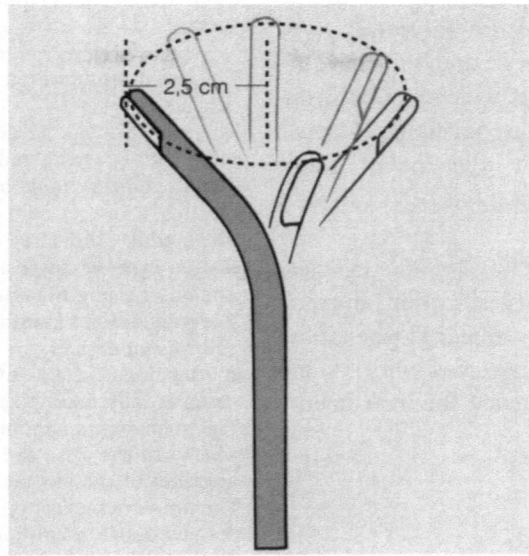

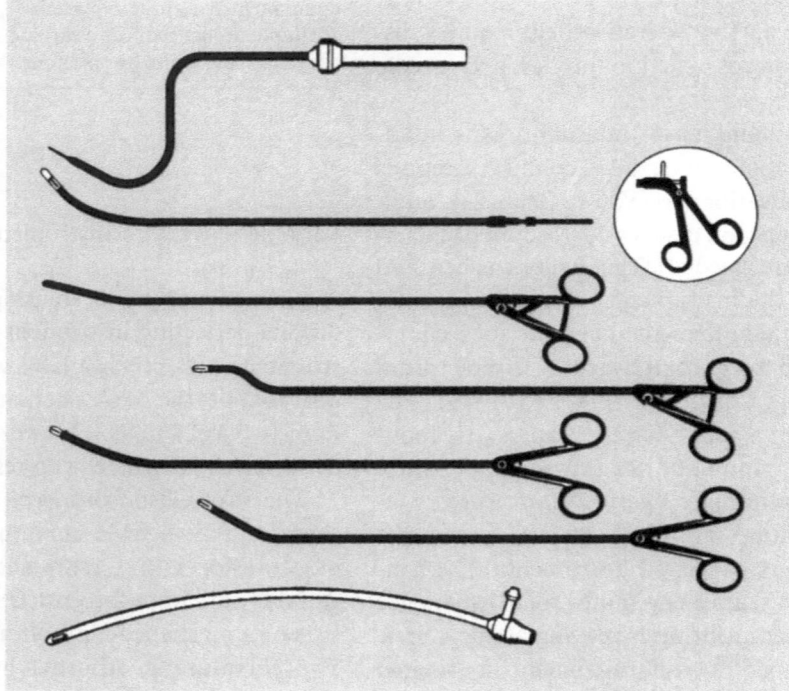

Fig. 1.45. a The ideal circle (radius of 25 mm) that is described by rotation of the functional tip of curved instruments. **b** A variety of available curved instruments (Olympus Winter&Ibe). **c** The geometry which is described by the possible movements of the functional tip of straight instruments within the endoscopic operative field. **d** The handling of curved instruments requires additional training due to the complex geometry which is described by the movements of the functional tip

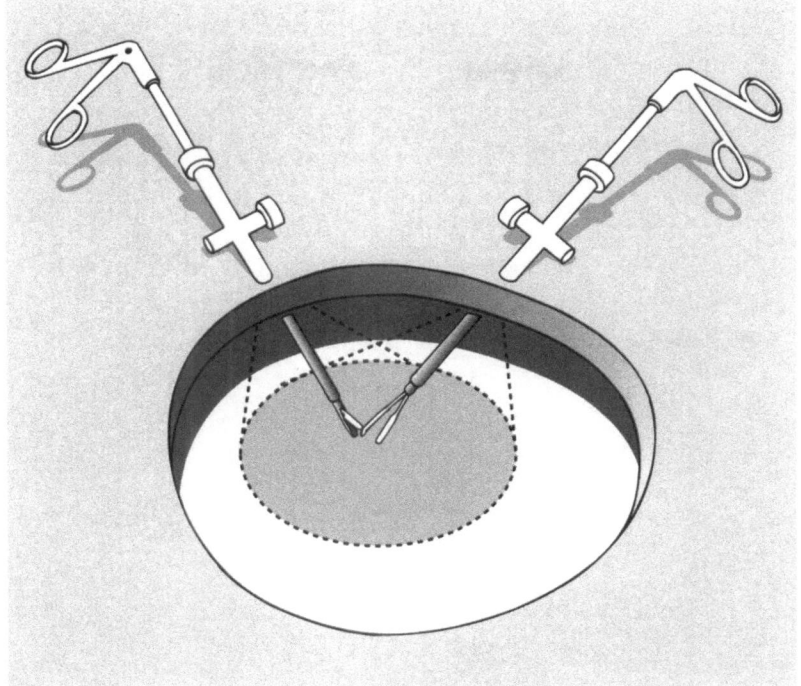

c

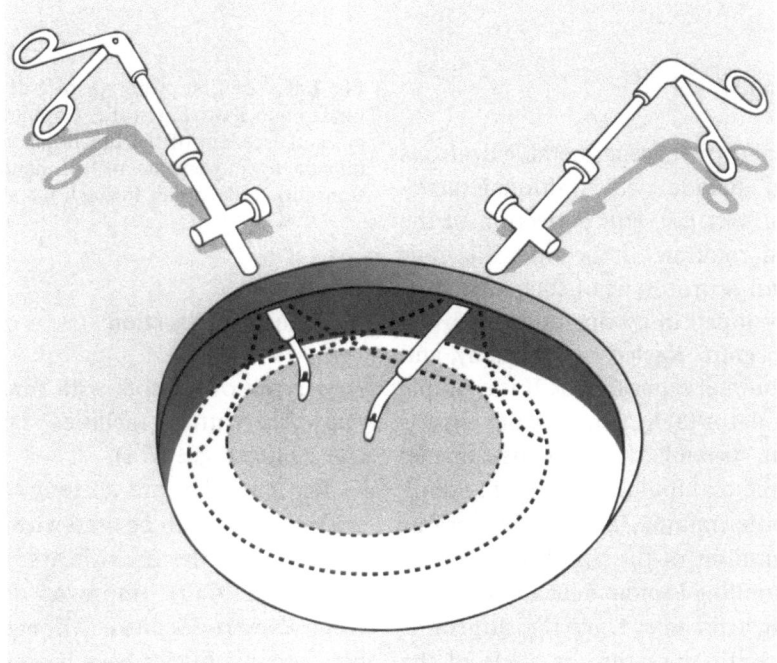

d

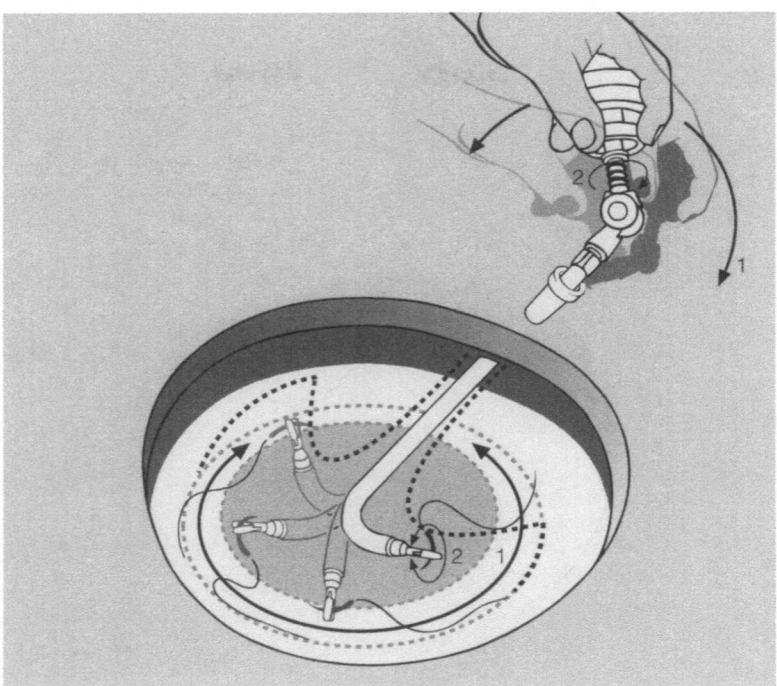

Dextrous Instruments

In our experimental experience a steerable dextrous instrument should include two additional movements of the distal part [79, 80]: deflection of the tip by ±120° and rotation of the tip while it is deflected (Fig. 1.46). A prototype of such an instrument has been developed in co-operation with the Nuclear Research Centre, Karlsruhe, Germany, and has been tested in animal experiments. It is a simple mechanical manipulator [81]. Although our experience indicates that steerable dextrous instruments facilitate endoscopic manipulation, their handling requires considerable training. Due to the various geometric configurations of the tip of dextrous instruments, their handling is more delicate than that of simple curved instruments. Once the surgeon is familiar with a specific curvature or angle of the shaft, he can correctly perform converted movements. Variable distal curvatures during endoscopic operations increase orientation problems. The integration of energetic drive such as pneumatic elements or servomotors will enhance the applicability of dextrous instruments [79, 80].

Fig. 1.46. The first prototype of a dextrous instrument (Tübingen and KfK, Karlsruhe, Germany). Two additional degrees of freedom of the functional tip (*1, 2*) are controlled outside by movements of the handle which are directly transmitted via cables through the shaft to the tip

Mechanical Dissection

New types of scissors with tungsten inlets and remarkable cutting facilities have been developed (Aesculap; Fig. 1.47a).

Because there are no long-term sharp, reusable scissors which can be used with HF disposable scissors, such as the Endoshears by USSC are widely used (Fig. 1.47b). Improved designs are available from Everest Medical (Minneapolis, MN, USA); here ceramic blades have been incorporated in disposable bipolar scissors. Ceramic provides superior cutting, but it is expensive and should therefore be considered as a material for reusable scissors.

Principally, bipolar HF coagulation is preferable to monopolar diathermy due to the reduced risk of unintended side effects.

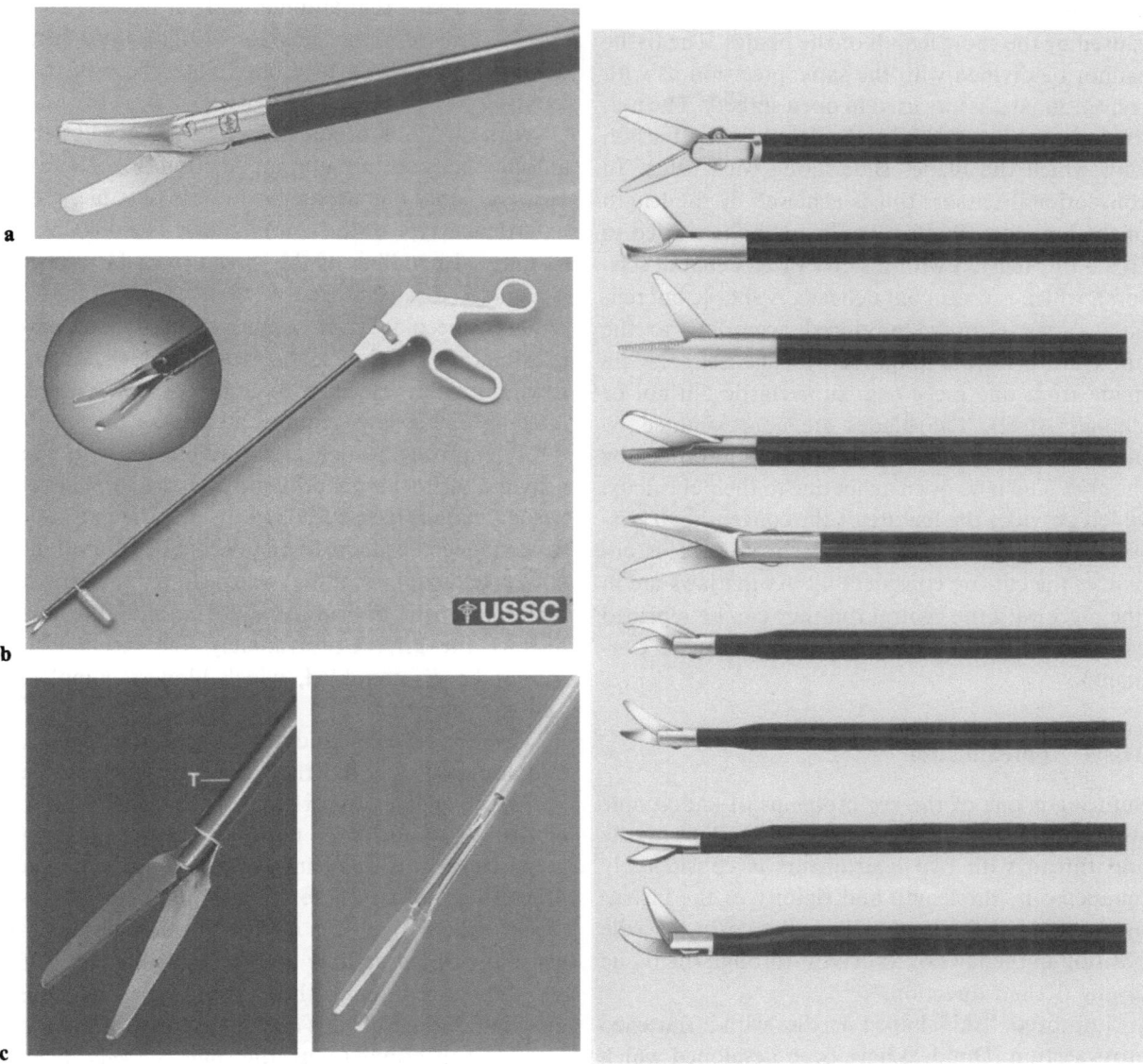

Fig. 1.47. a Aesculap (Tuttlingen, Germany) markets scissors with tungsten inlets in the blades which provide remarkable cutting capability. **b** Disposable scissors such as the Endoshears (USSC) should not be reused due to inadequate cleaning and functional mishaps subsequent to sterilization. **c** Re-posable hingeless scissors are made from one piece (superelastic Nitinol or stainless steel). The reposable blades are approximated by means of an intermediate tube (*T*) that is advanced by the grip. Shaft and handle are fully reusable (PCI, NDC). **d** Range of reusable scissors

A principal problem of endoscopic scissors is caused by the short length of the blades. The tissue cannot be divided with the same precision as with conventional scissors used in open surgery. The major prerequisite of the ideal scissors is the tension with which the blades slide along each other. In conventional scissors this is achieved by the length of the branches. Some manufacturers have tried to create this tension with a screw (Metzenbaum scissors), which is useful but delicate. A simple but reliable scissors can be produced according to the hingeless principle (Fig. 1.47c). The scissors are made from one piece (e.g. superelastic Nitinol or stainless steel). The blades are approximated by means of an intermediate tube that is advanced by the grip. The jaws open again due to their elasticity, which provides the feature of the conventional scissors: the blades slides along each other. This enhances the cutting considerably. As the jaws are in one piece with the central rod they can be replaced easily at a reasonable cost (PCI, Liptingen, Germany).

Tissue Approximation

Suturing is one of the key problems of endoscopic surgery. The remote technique of handling needle and thread with two instruments is considerably hampered by the length and rigidity of the instruments. It is difficult to achieve the correct needle position in the jaws or to drive it through the tissue in any desired direction.

Improved, "ski"-shaped needles with a flattened cross-section (Dundee) have been developed which can be easily erected by simply grasping them (Fig. 1.48a). The flat cross-section has another advantage: the lock is improved, which increases the fixation within the jaws. This form lock is very important for the spring-loaded needle holder without a locking mechanism. The better the form lock, the better the needle remains in position. Technically, the best congruence between jaw shape and needle cross-section is a triangular needle and prism grooves in the jaw (Fig. 1.48b). However, with such a design the thread may be damaged. The best compromise would be a diamond-dusted inner surface of jaws with smooth edges.

The needle holder from transanal endoscopic microsurgery (Wolf) has congruently concave-convex-shaped jaws that automatically swivel a curved needle into upright position (Fig. 1.48c). Endoscopic suturing is facilitated with these instruments.

With the Cook needle holder curved needles are automatically set into upright position (Fig. 1.48d). However, only one needle position is possible with a particular type of the Cook holder. The difficulty of internal handling of the thread to make a knot is a major disadvantage.

Some needle drivers entail spring-loaded approximation of the jaws. Although high spring force provides excellent fixation of the needle, opening of the jaws requires additional force.

To improve the delicate handling of both the grip and the locking mechanism classical and novel design features have been introduced. The most advanced mechanism created by Wolf (Fig. 1.48e) involves telescopic locking which functions like a ball-point pen: one pressing locks and the next releases the grip. Unfortunately, the mechanism cannot be disassembled, which hinders complete and easy cleaning.

The new needle holder by MBG (Gembloux, Belgium) probably has the firmest gripping of the holders available. Its principle is quite simple; it consists of a tube and a pushrod and two tungsten metal rings which are simply pressed against each other (Fig. 1.48f). There are two major disadvantages to the design: it is difficult to tie a knot, because the tip is too long and the opening depth of jaws is reduced due to the central rod. Hence, the grasping of the thread is difficult. A monofilament suture when gripped with the rings is likely to be damaged. Handling of needle and thread is more practical with the conventional needle holder than with the one made by MBG. Although the MBG design is novel and fascinating it needs some practical refinements and improvements to facilitate cleaning after usage.

Z. Szabo and G. Berci have designed two instruments, the parrot and the flamingo forceps (Fig. 1.48g) [82], which permit excellent execution of internal suturing and knotting. Although, the handling is not optimal, the congruently shaped jaws of the instruments facilitate grasping and positioning of needle and thread. It must be stressed that the grasping of any suture with all available tungsten-reinforced holders, with the exception the

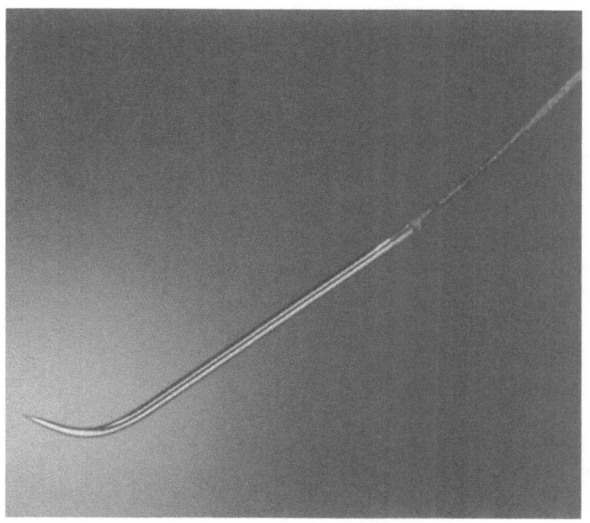

a_1

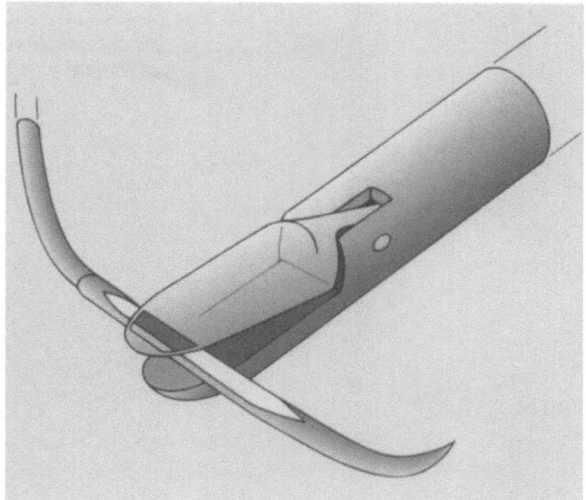

a_2

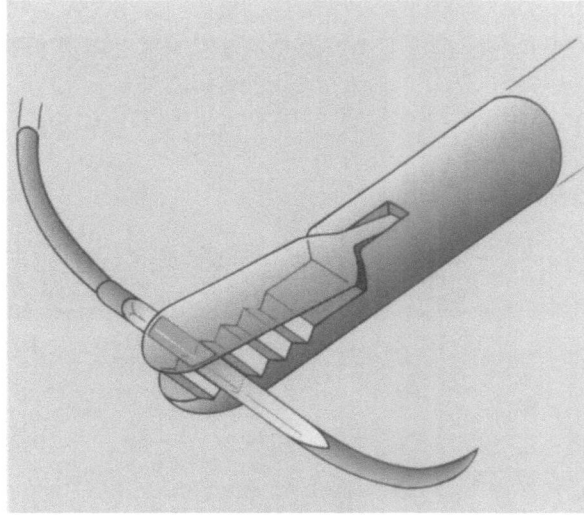

b

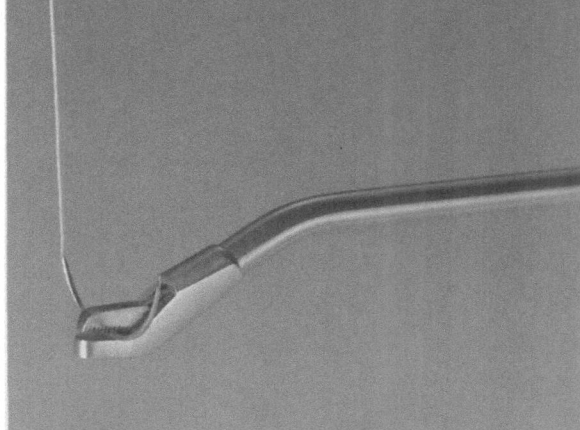

c_1

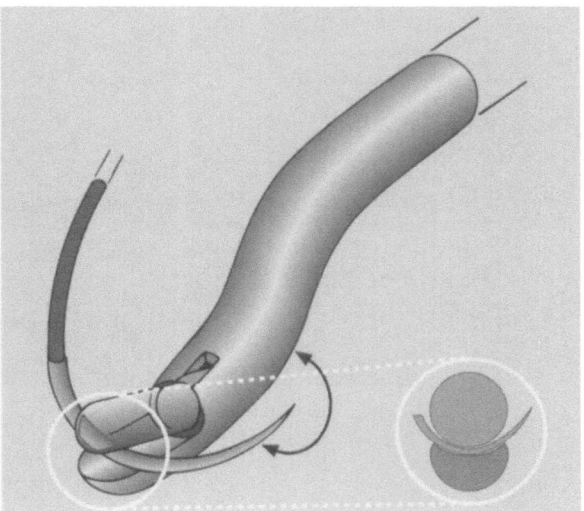

c_2

Fig. 1.48. a "Ski"-shaped needles with flattened cross-section facilitate erection of the needle by simply grasping them. **b** Triangular cross-section of surgical needles and concurrently shaped prism grooves in the jaws provide the best needle fixation; however, self-erection is impossible. **c** Congruently concave-convex-shaped jaws of the needle holder from transanal endoscopic microsurgery (Wolf) automatically swivel a curved needle into upright position

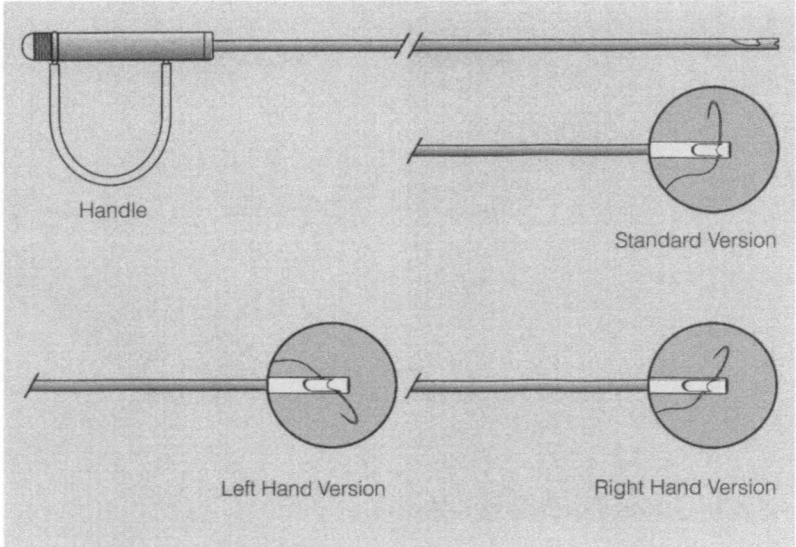

d

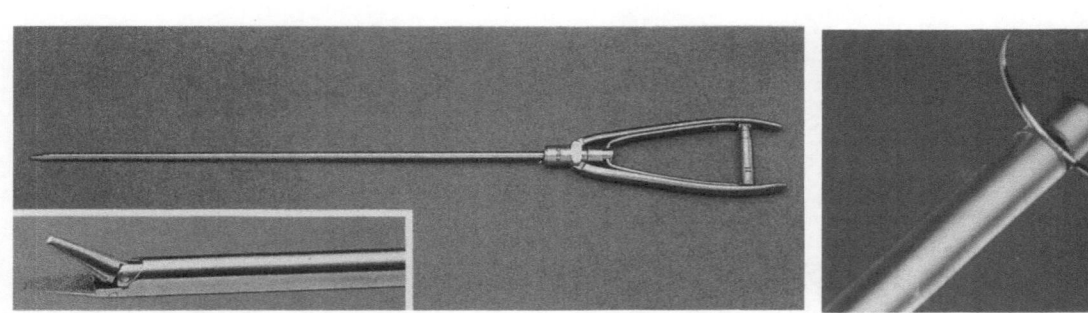

e

f

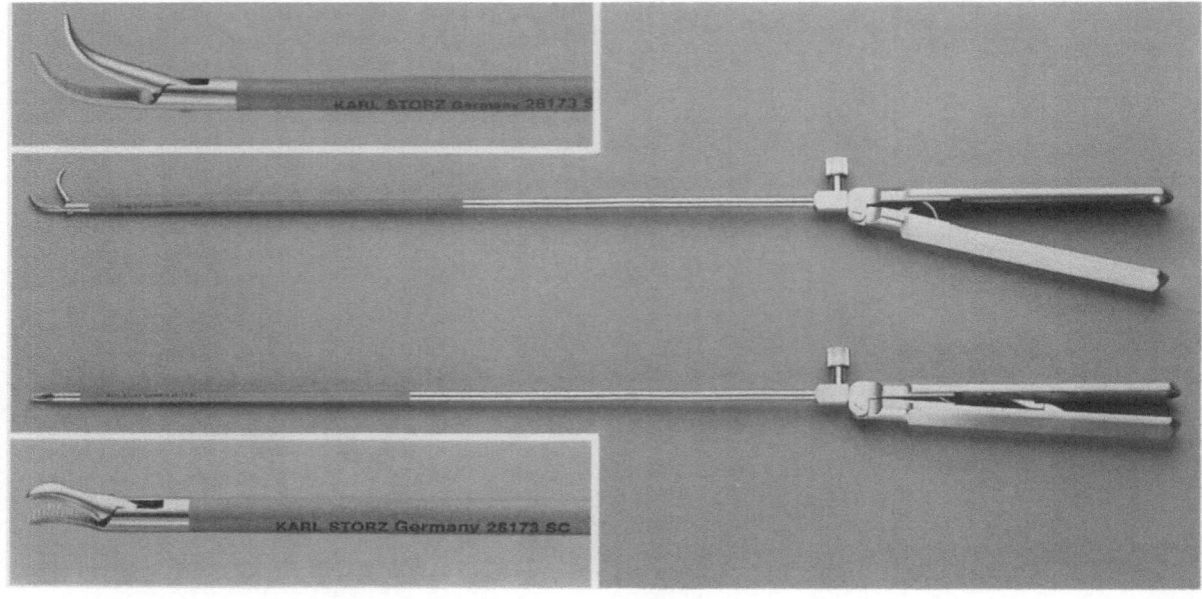

g

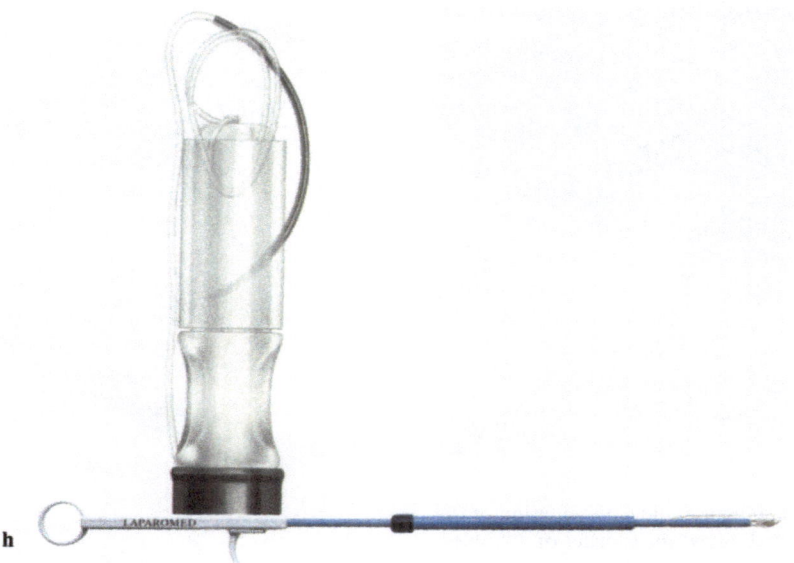

h

Fig. 1.48. d The Cook needle holder automatically sets curved needles into a predetermined position but grasping a thread is difficult. **e** Wolf markets a needle holder with a locking mechanism that functions like a ballpoint pen: one pressing locks and the next releases the grip. **f** The needle holder from a Belgian company (MBG) consists of a tube and a pushrod equipped with tungsten metal rings which are simply pressed against each other. Although needle hold is excellent, grasping a thread is difficult. **g** The "parrot" and the "flamingo" forceps designed by Szabo and Berci (Storz) facilitates internal suturing and knotting. **h** A disposable suture applier (Lapromed) consists of a needle, suture, pretied knot and applicator. Subsequent to suture the needle is simply led through those two loops and the knot then fastened from outside

rubber-shod holder, may lead to severe damage to the structure of the suture with subsequent breakage.

A disposable suture applier (Lapromed) consists of a needle, suture, pretied knot and applicator. The needle with the thread is stored in the tip of the device. After introduction the needle can be grasped. It is attached to a 15-cm-long thread. The knot is pretied and two loops are exposed at the tip of the shaft. To make these slip knots the needle is simply led through those two loops and the knot can then be fastened from outside by means of a retaining band (Fig. 1.48 h). This suture applier is useful for the application of one single knot. If, however, several knots are required, the device increases costs considerably. It has the advantage that

the surgeon does not have to cope with external slip knots.

Complex Suturing Devices

Our experimental work on suturing has led to the development of a new sewing device [83]. A needle holder designed in collaboration with the gynaecologist B. Klemm allows movement from one jaw to the other, which has some advantages in the handling of the needle. The needle can be positioned appropriately by moving the jaw in a longitudinal direction.

Sewing Devices

The shuttle needle and its applicator are almost like a real sewing machine. They were developed by the Tübingen group in collaboration with the Nuclear Research Centre in Karlsruhe, Germany, from 1989 to 1991. With this device a needle can be transferred between two jaws, similar to the sewing shuttle employed in weaving looms. The shuttle needle has a central cross bore for the thread and two trocar point tips (Fig. 1.49 a – d). It can be transferred between the jaws of the instrument and is intermittently docked to miniaturized grip elements

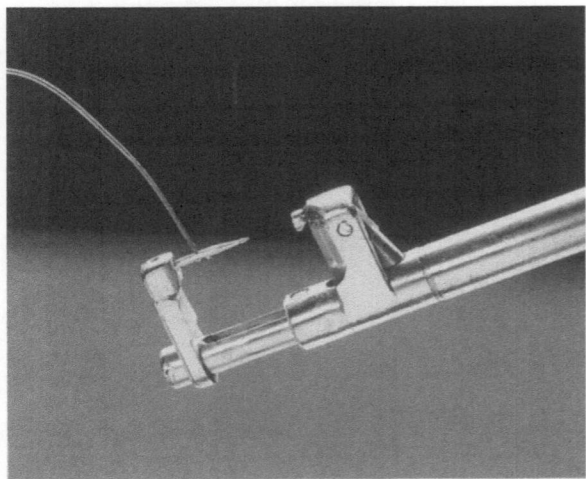

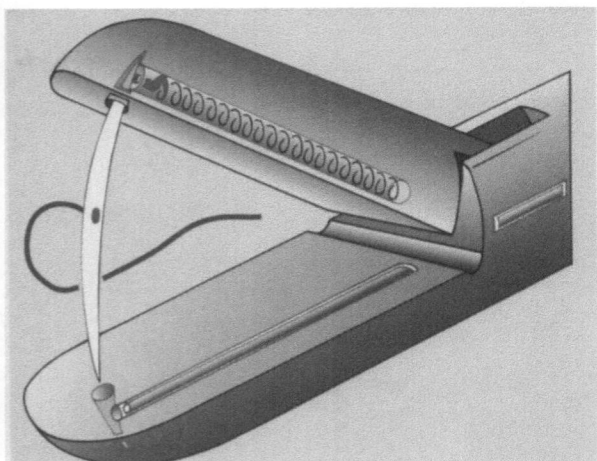

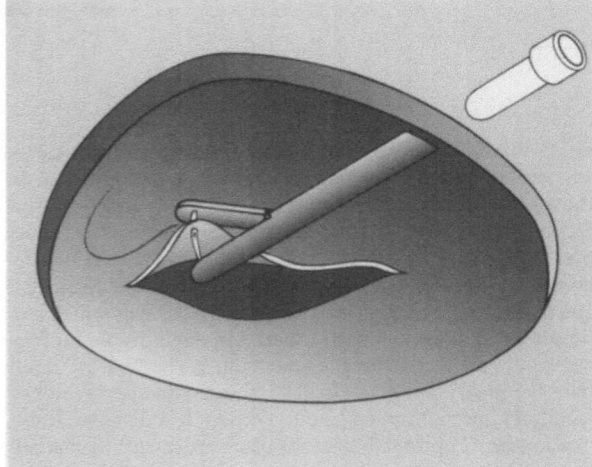

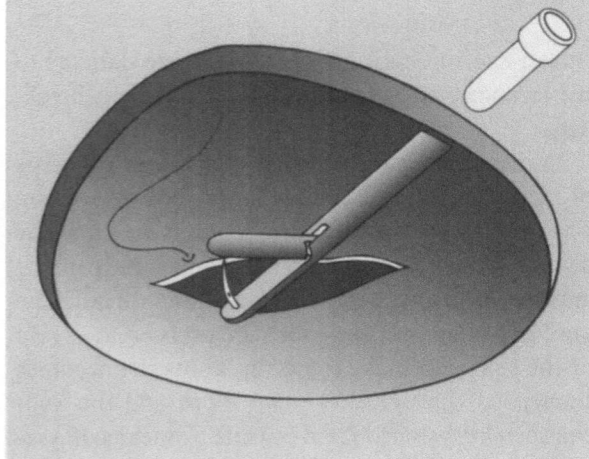

Fig. 1.49. a Photo and **b** diagrammatic representation of the "shuttle needle" device that allows the transfer of a "T-Needle" between the two jaws of the instrument by means of a spring-loaded gripping element within the moveable jaw and gripping element located in the opposite jaw which can be pneumatically operated from outside. **c** The "T-Needle" is stitched through the tissue into the opening funnel of the gripping element. **d** The needle remains in the locked gripper and the thread led through the stitch channel

integrated in the jaws by an active pneumatic gripper controlled by a foot switch. The other gripper is a passive, spring-loaded attachment. If the needle is held with the pneumatic gripper, the force of the spring-loaded grip is overcome and the needle is held in the pneumatic grip. If this grip is released, the needle is fixed in the spring-loaded grip. The elaborate handling of the needle with two holders is no longer required and the transfer can also be used to tie a knot. Different shapes and cross-sections of the needle and two transfer directions "vertical" and "axial" have been designed and tested. The shuttle needle facilitates endoscopic suturing. The device is now marked as "Endostich" by USSC.

Ligating Instruments

The execution of a ligature with thread requires delicate handling with two forceps to pass the tie around the vessel and the creation of an external slip knot. Although the tie can be appropriately passed using curved instruments, the development of instruments especially for ligature is important.

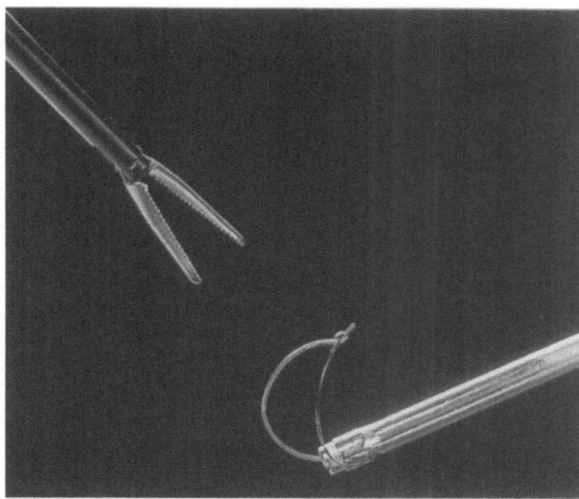

Fig. 1.50. Ligating is facilitated by using a superelastic Nitinol wire which permits the passage of a thread surrounding the pedicle. (EndoLig)

The passage of the thread around a vessel can be facilitated using superelastic material, e.g. Nitinol. In Fig. 1.50 the thread is passed with a superelastic wire surround the pedicle. Nitinol wire, which features stress-induced martensitic phase transformation, can be preshaped using special heat treatment. It can then be introduced in a restraining tube. When extruded it recovers its preformed curved shape [76, 77]. Thread can be inserted through a needle eye at the distal end and then passed around a pedicle. The thread is subsequently grasped by a forceps and the ligature then finished with an external slip knot or a knot clip.

A device similar to the above-mentioned Endolig is the sling passer by Storz (Fig. 1.40a).

Classic Ligature with Tandem Forceps (Endo-overholt)

This instrument works in accordance with the ligature technique of open surgery. Two graspers are inserted in separate channels contained within one port. In between them is a moveable scalpel which can be controlled from outside. Both handles of the graspers are interconnected. Two additional channels carry two pretied polydioxanone (PDS) loops, each with its own plastic pusher. The loops are placed so that each surrounds the forceps tips on

either side (see Vol. 3). After the vascular pedicle is mobilized, it is grasped by the two forceps and then carefully divided by extrusion of the knife. After the knife is retracted the loops are pushed forward such that they surround the vascular pedicle and are then firmly tightened. This procedure is faster than standard endoscopic ligature using external slip knots.

Knot Pushers

Numerous knot pushers have been designed for endoscopy since the push rod was popularized by Semm. Most of the reusable knot pushers have grooves, small terminal slits or forks (Fig. 1.51a), and all of them tend to lose the thread when the knot is pushed down. All disposable pushers consist of a simple plastic tube. Although, it is impossible to lose the thread, reinserting a thread through the long rod is difficult.

A suitable reusable knot pusher should have a terminal concavity at its distal end to accommodate the knot in position. Insertion is then easy and the tie cannot slip off. To save time, for reproducible, safe cutting of the thread and to avoid slipping of the knot, an outer sleeve can be employed to cut the thread immediately after it is tightened (Fig. 1.51 b, c). Such a cutting knot pusher is available from PCI.

Knot Substitutes

It is possible to replace external slip knots by knot clips [84]. However, the silver clip used in transrectal microsurgery (Fig. 1.52a) is not appropriate as an implant in laparoscopic or thoracoscopic surgery. The Lapraty knot clip (Ethicon; Fig. 1.52b) is made of bioabsorbable PDS and can therefore be used in various situations, but involves additional costs. The friction of the Lapraty is only suitable when pressed on size 3−0 polyfilament thread, for example start and end of a running suture. The Lapraty knot clip should be improved so that two threads could be fixed simultaneously, which would add applicability to interrupted sutures and ligatures. However, a properly tied external slip knot is the safest and most reliable way of performing a li-

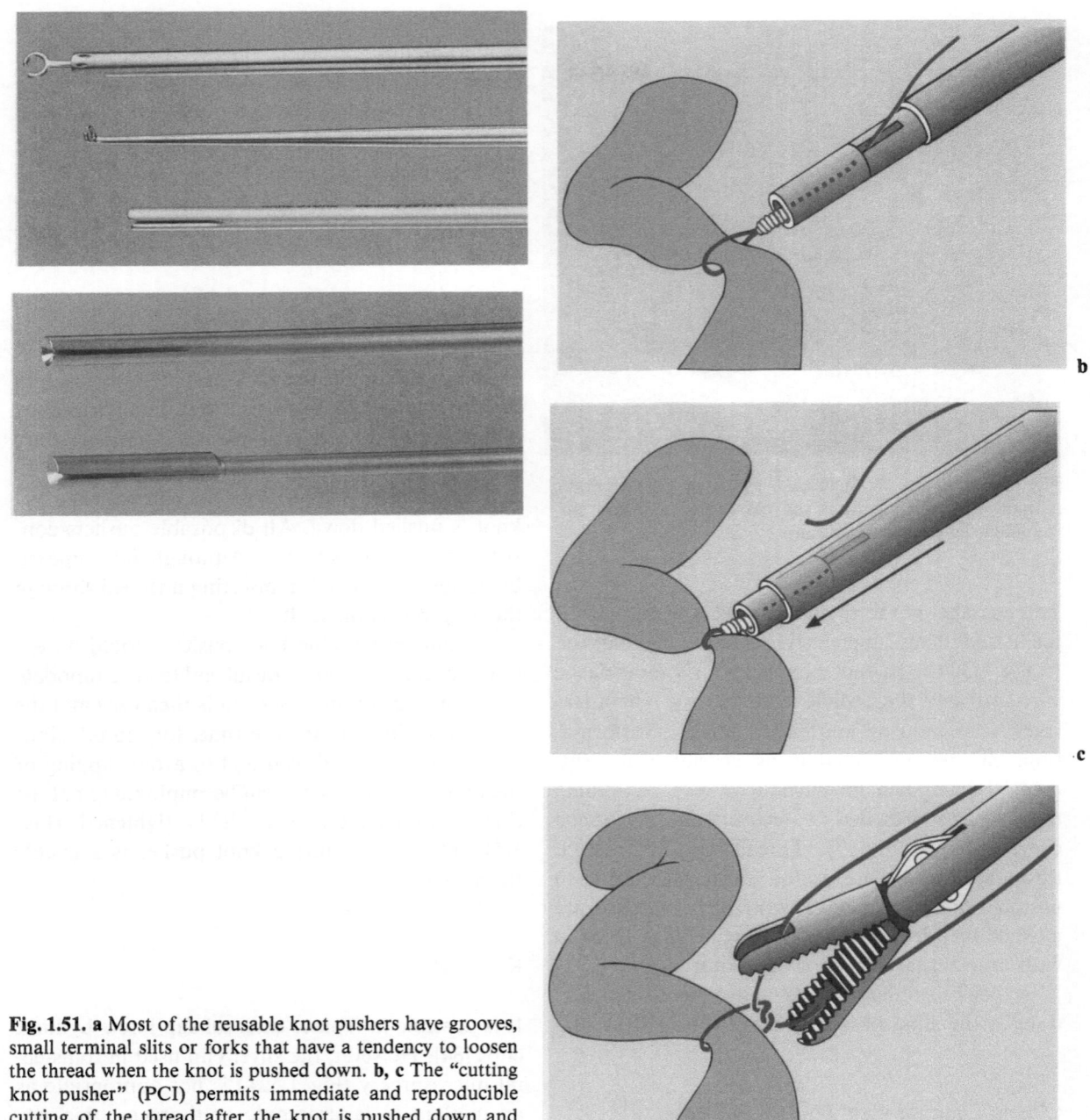

Fig. 1.51. a Most of the reusable knot pushers have grooves, small terminal slits or forks that have a tendency to loosen the thread when the knot is pushed down. **b, c** The "cutting knot pusher" (PCI) permits immediate and reproducible cutting of the thread after the knot is pushed down and firmly locked. (**d**) Knot pushing forceps

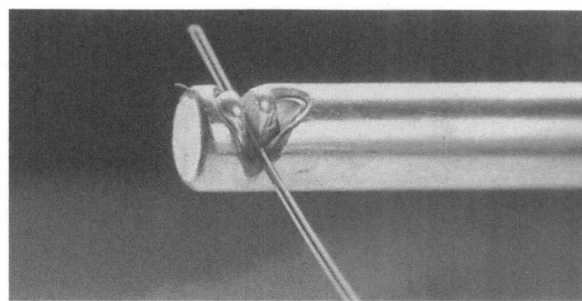

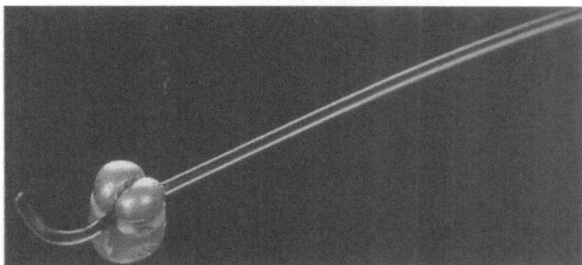

a

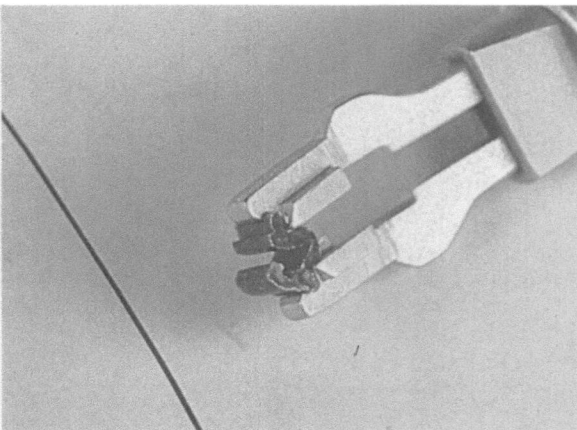

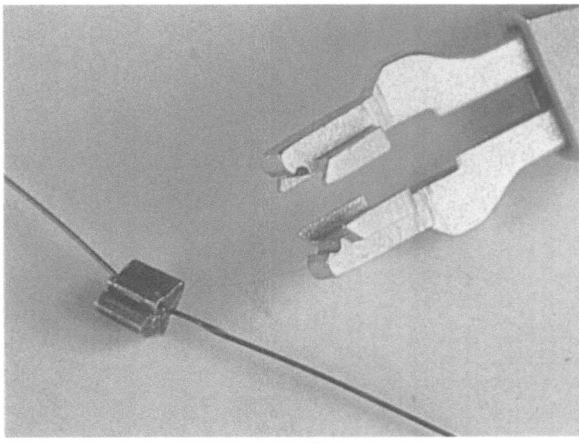

b

Fig. 1.52. a Silver clips are used as knot substitutes in transrectal endoscopic microsurgery (Wolf). **b** Knot clips, Lapraty, made from PDS (polydioxanone) are only suitable for 3:0 PDS to substitute the knots of a running suture (Ethicon; Sommerville, NJ, USA)

gature, although clumsy and time consuming. Electronic tension metering has revealed that only two tying techniques provide sufficient resistance to reverse slipping (up to 40 Newton): the Tayside knot according to Cuschieri for braided non-absorbable, and absorbable material including polydioxanone and lactomen-copolymer (Fig. 1.53 a) and others, and the Melzer knot for PDS II (Fig. 1.53 b).

Clips and Clip Appliers

Ligature Clips

The traditional titanium and the absorbable (Absolock) ligature clips still have some disadvantages. The main problem is their weak grip after application to a pedicle. These clips can slip of easily, especially when they are brushed accidentally during manipulations. However, ligature clips are acceptable for small pedicles, provided they are applied precisely.

The ligature clip produced by Origin works on the principles of the ligature clips of open surgery. The arc-shaped clip captures the pedicle when its tips come in contact prior to full closure (Fig. 1.54 a). The rectangular, hook-like orientation of the clips and applier provides improved control of the actual clipping process.

A new absorbable "lapro clip" consisting of two parts has been introduced by Davis + Geck (Wayne, NJ, USA) (Fig. 1.54 b). The relatively elastic inner member (polyglyconate) is approximated prior to full closure so that the pedicle can be grasped. Subsequently, the rigid outer member (polyglycolic acid) is pushed over the inner member and thus the clip completely and firmly locked. Each clip is mounted into a complete tip of the forceps, which is disposable, whereas handle and shaft are reusable parts.

The new Hem-lock-clip by Linvatec Weck (Largo, FL, USA) shows some principal improvements. The locking ends provides excellent tissue penetration and the fixation at the tissue is improved due to the concave-convex shape of the branches. This clip is nonabsorbable, which lowers its value. Further testing of these clips is necessary before final clinical application. As all metals more or less interfere with imaging procedures such as CT and MRI, clips made from synthetic material are preferable.

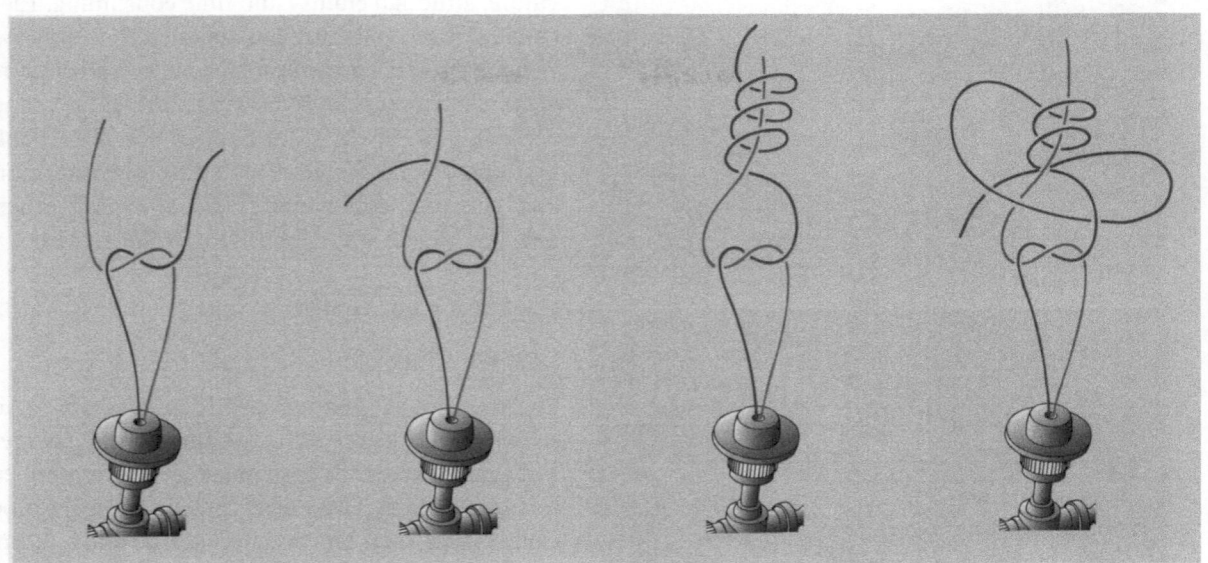

a

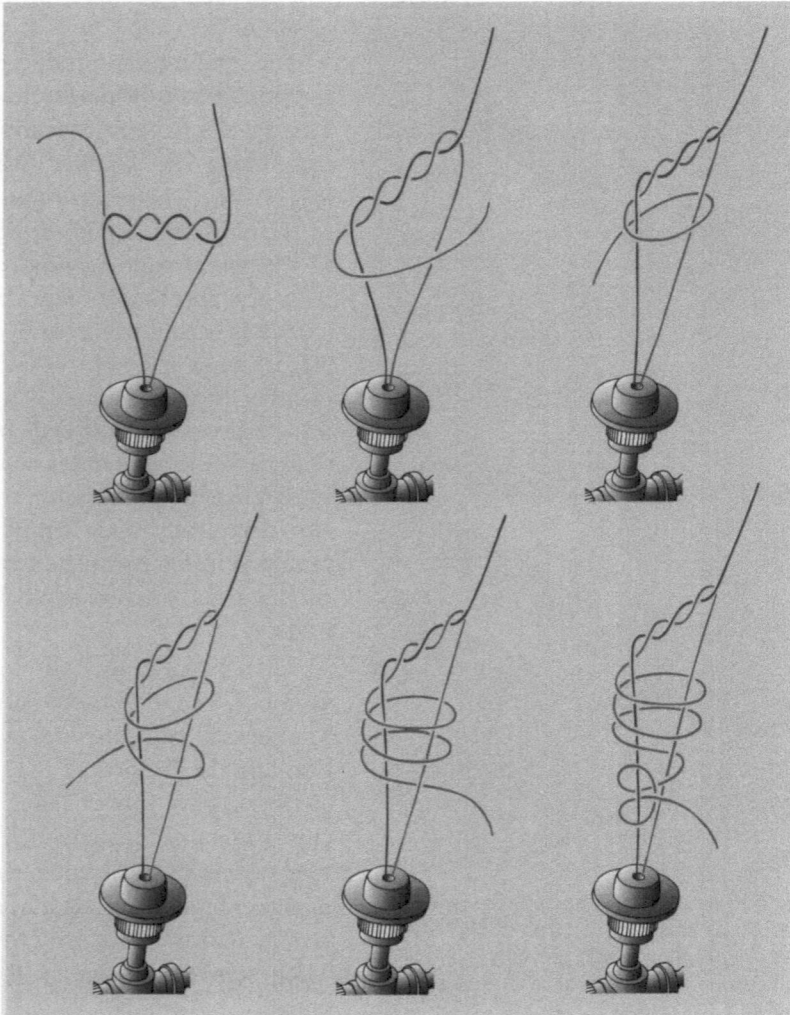

b

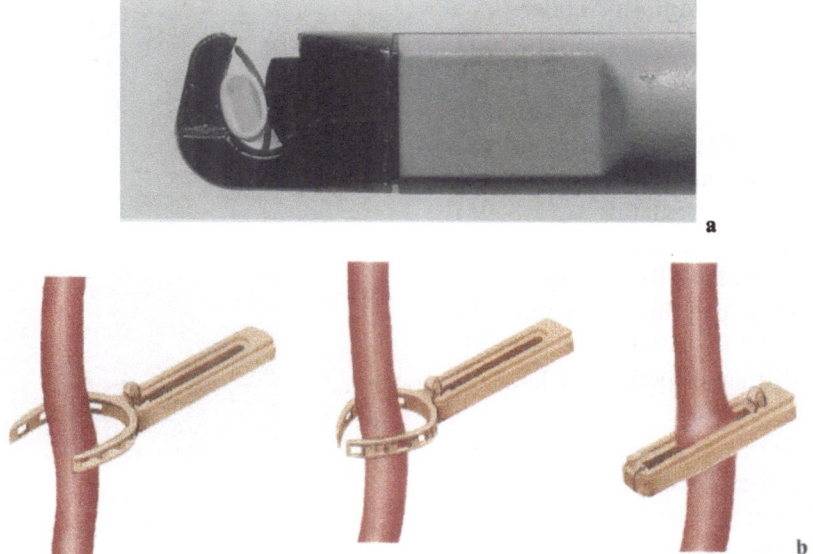

Fig. 1.54. a The rectangle hook-like orientation of the arc-shaped clips and the applier improves control of the actual clipping process (Origin). **b** A new absorbable "lapro clip" (Davis+Geck) consists of two parts that are subsequently applied to the pedicle

Clips for Tissue Approximation

Devices which can be used for tissue approximation by clips include the endohernia staplers of Ethicon (Cincinnati, OH, USA) and USSC. Although their efficacy in endoscopic hernia repair with mesh has been proven, the long-term effects caused by these clips to the surrounding tissue are still unclear. However, there is no comparable fast and reliable fixation system available other than these staplers. The articulating function, in particular, considerably enhances the applicability (Fig. 1.55). Their functioning principle is almost identical: the U-shaped clamp is deformed to a closed square. The only alternative is interrupted sutures, which are more reliable, but it takes considerably longer to apply single interrupted sutures than to apply a single clip.

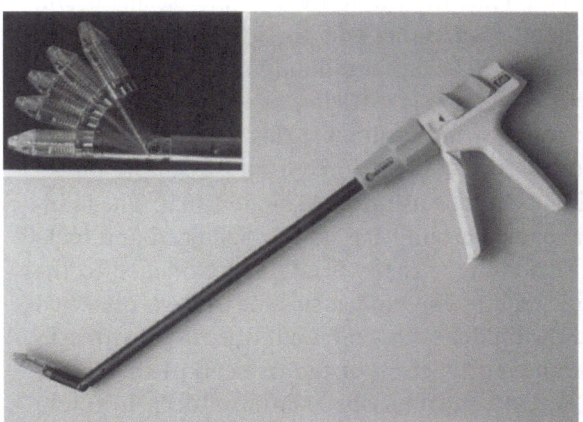

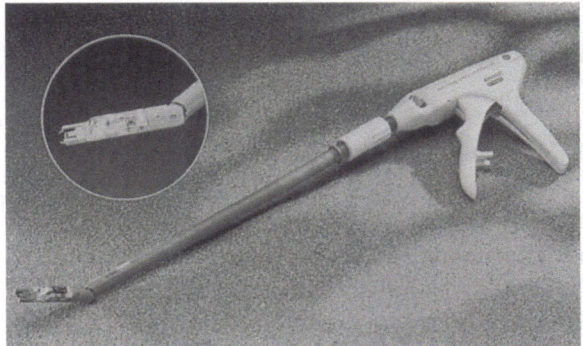

Fig. 1.55a, b. The articulating function of the staplers for tissue approximation considerably enhances their applicability. Ethicon (Cincinnati, OH, USA) (**a**); USSC (**b**)

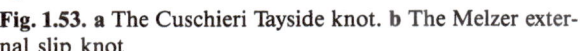

Fig. 1.53. a The Cuschieri Tayside knot. **b** The Melzer external slip knot

Endo-Gastrointestinal-Anastomosis Stapler (Endo GIA)

Staplers have been improved and are now available in different lengths and equipped with different size clips (Fig. 1.56a). The height of the clips ranges from 2.5 to 4.8 mm. The articulating tip (±50°) and the CO_2-powered drive of the USSC staplers are of considerable advantage for accurate positioning end exectution of the procedure. In thoracoscopic surgery the Endo GIA* is an excellent tool for removal of small peripheral lung tumours (Fig. 1.56b).

Particular endoscopic procedures such as sigmoid resection allow the use of transanal "end-to-end anastomosis" with circular staplers. A newly developed flexible stapler has been recently introduced by the company Bieffe (Milan, Italy). Its outstanding feature is the length of approximately 100 cm. Thus the Bieffe EEA stapler seems useful for hemi-colectomies and possible for oesophageal dissection. The intra-abdominal manipulation of the stapler anvil is difficult, as is the performance of a purse-string suture. For this reason we have developed special anvil forceps and a simple purse-string technique using cable binders [85]. The binder is passed around the bowel, tightened and locked. When the tissue is firmly approximated to the stapler rod by the binder, surplus tissue is dissected and the binder's free end is cut off with scissors. To ease the introduction of the free end of the binder we have designed an open slit introducer. In future this binder may also be useful for temporary occlusion or trans-section of organs (hemi-nephrectomy) and, if absorbable, for ligature of major vessels.

Multifunctional Instruments

Change of instruments during endoscopic surgery is time consuming and disrupts dissection considerably. Bleeding often obscures the operative field when an insulated coagulating instrument has to be inserted or clip applied. It is also the main reason for conversion to open surgery, as demonstrated by a multicentre study performed by the major European centres [48]. The solution to this problem is obtained by multifunction instruments which combine dissection, haemostasis, suction and irriga-

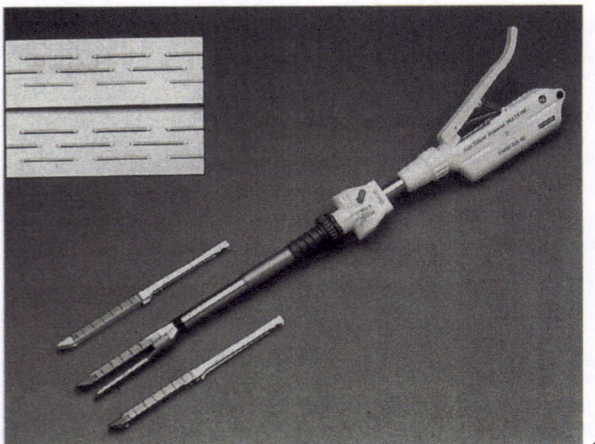

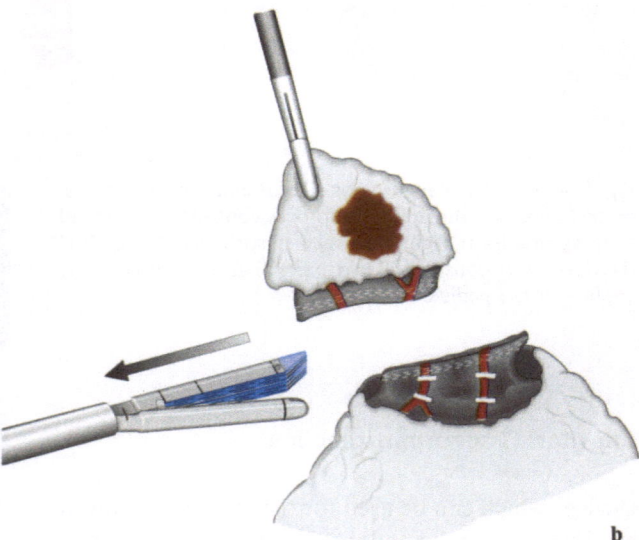

Fig. 1.56. a Endoscopic gastrointestinal staplers (Endo GIA*, Ethicon and USSC) are available in different lengths (30 and 60 mm) equipped with different size clips, from 2.5 to 4.8 mm. The articulating tip (±50°) and the CO_2 pressure drive of the USSC staplers are of considerable advantage for accurate execution of the tissue approximation. **b** The Endo GIA* is an excellent tool for removal of small peripheral lung tumours in thoracoscopic surgery. (From: Endoscopic Surgery Allied Technologies 1 (1993) 301, Thieme Verlag, Stuttgart) 301

tion. However, there are technological limitations in view of the restricted diameter of the access port. An example of a useful multifunctional instrument is the combination, suction-irrigation device by Wolf. It is described in Vol. 1, Chap. 2, and has been modified since. This instrument can be used for dissection, and if bleeding occurs, the function-

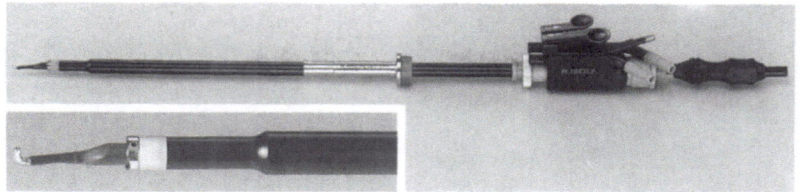

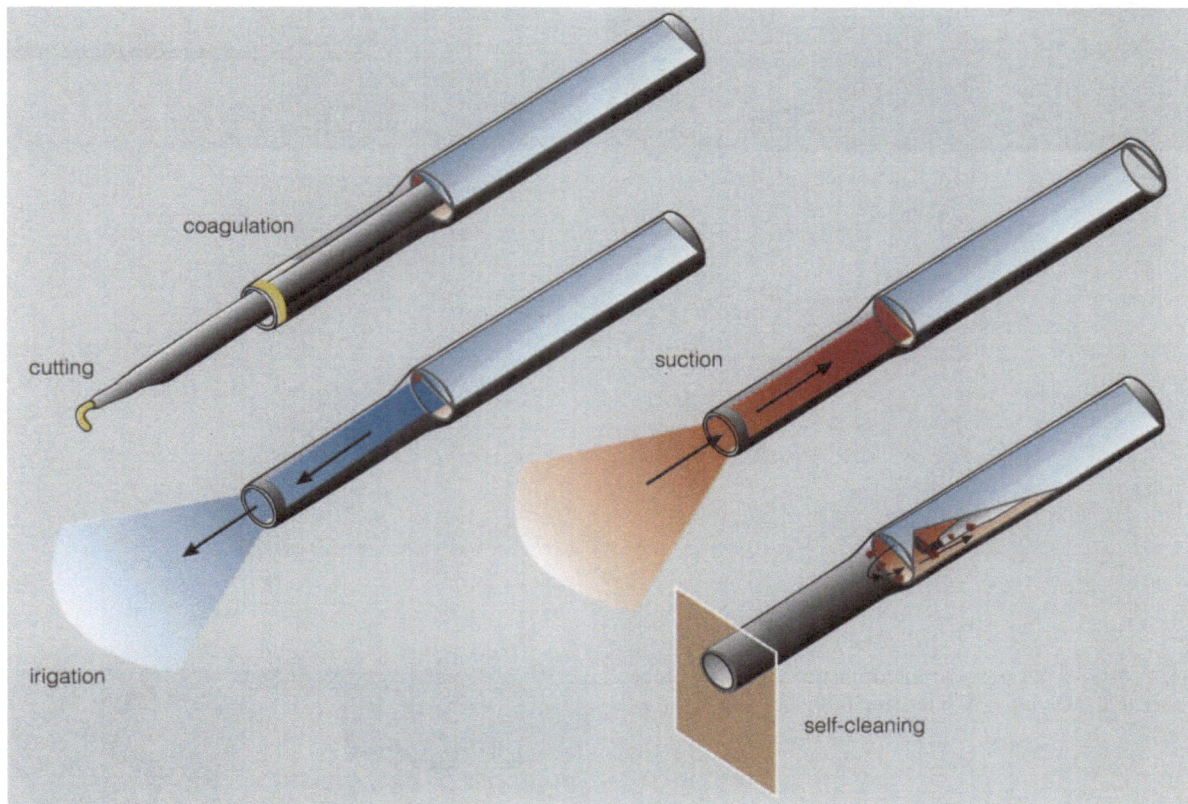

al tip of an inserted instrument is withdrawn and the channel can be used for suction and irrigation and the tip for monopolar coagulation (Fig. 1.57a, b). Other, similar instruments are available, but they are less sophisticated and partly or completely disposable. Figure 1.57c−e shows a variety of multifunctional suction probes.

A removable hook electrode (developed in Tübingen, Germany, in 1990) is incorporated with a suction probe. After withdrawing the probe, the tip allows aspiration as well as proper coagulation because the surface of the tip is enlarged. The suction channel can also be used for introduction of additional probes, including laser fibres. Retractable hooks are available from Access (Plymouth, MA,

Fig. 1.57. a The combination suction-irrigation device (Wolf) facilitates dissection, and in the event of bleeding partial withdrawal of the functional tip of an inserted instrument exposes the channel for suction and irrigation and the tip for monopolar coagulation. **b** Irrigation is obtained via a separate channel, thus cleaning of the main channel is possible during the operation

USA) and as a disposable item from Ethicon and Lapromed. These simple combinations are useful for regular procedures. The more exacting mobilization of bowel, stomach, uterus or prostate requires adequate multifunctional instruments.

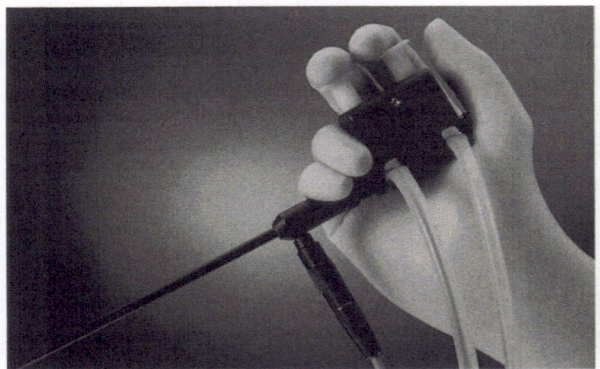

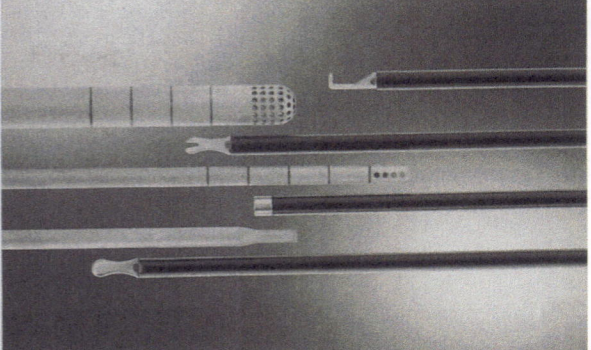

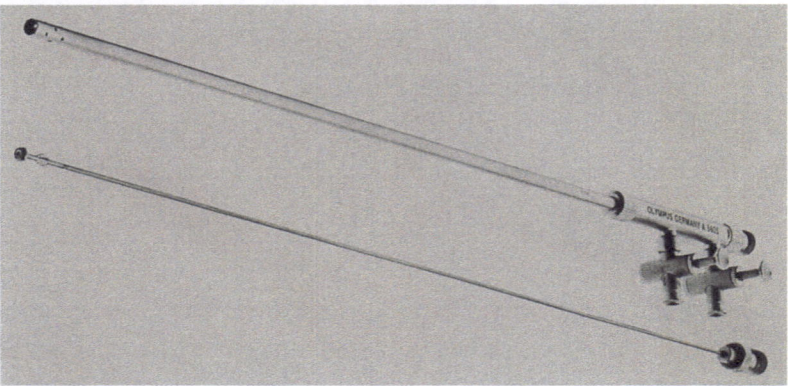

Fig. 1.57. c−e A variety of multifunctional suction probes (Storz (**c, d**), Olympus Winter&Ibe (**e**))

Fig. 1.58. a, b Retrieval bags that employ elastic opening ▶ wires facilitate gathering of the specimen (USSC, Endomedix). **c** The extraction of filled retrieval bags and gallbladders is often difficult due to the ballooning effect while pulling out the bag through the abdominal wall. **d** The "Bergetrokar" (Bühler) facilitates the extraction of specimens such as gallbladder. **e** The Dundee bag (Cameron Balloons). It is made from rib-stop nylon and shaped like a sausage. The specimen can be pulled into the bag; the free end is then drawn out of the abdomen and the contents gathered

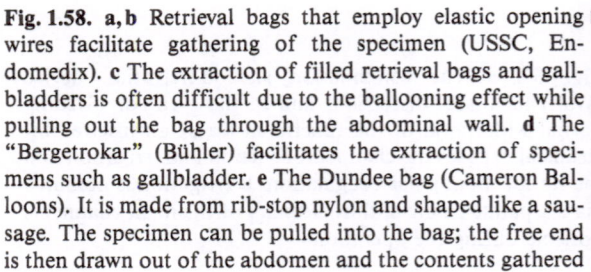

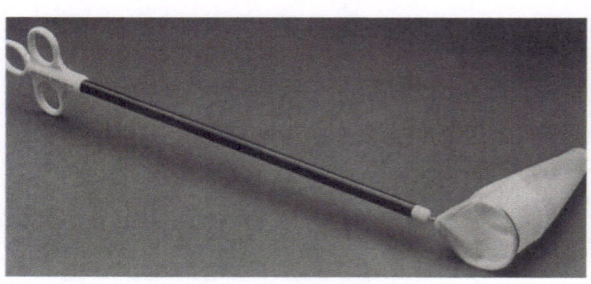

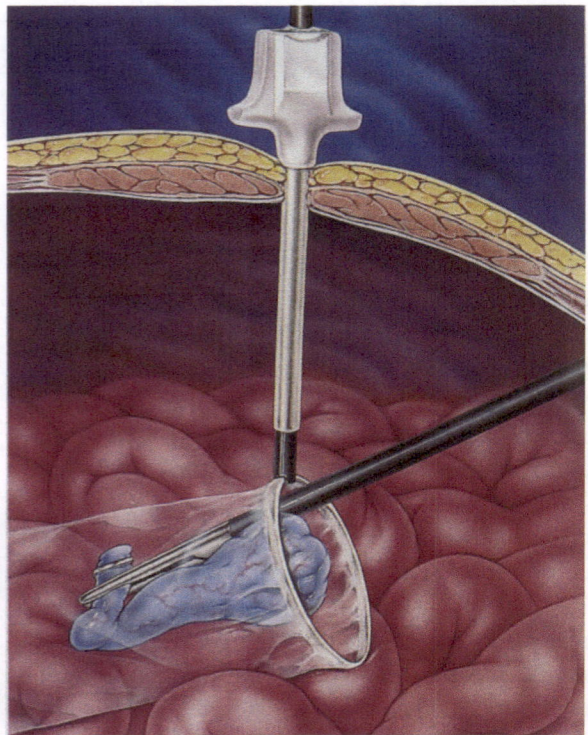

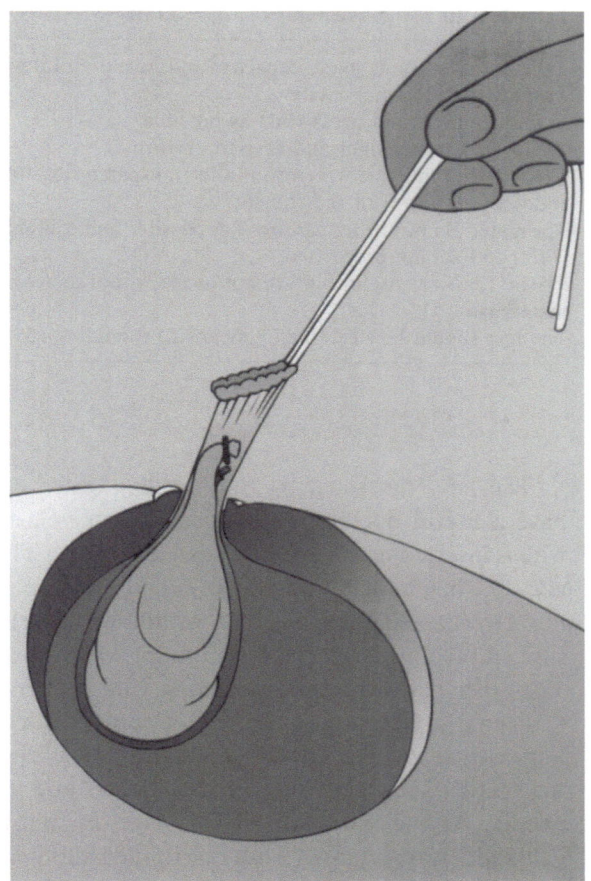

c

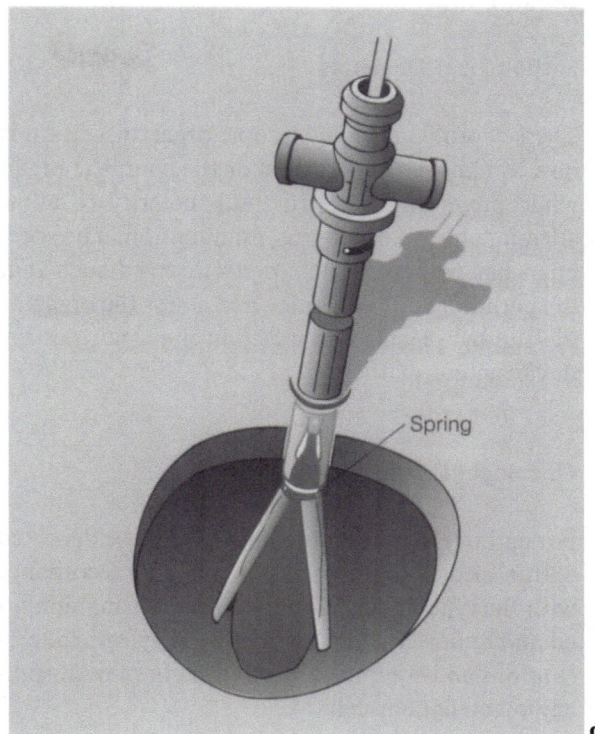

Spring

d

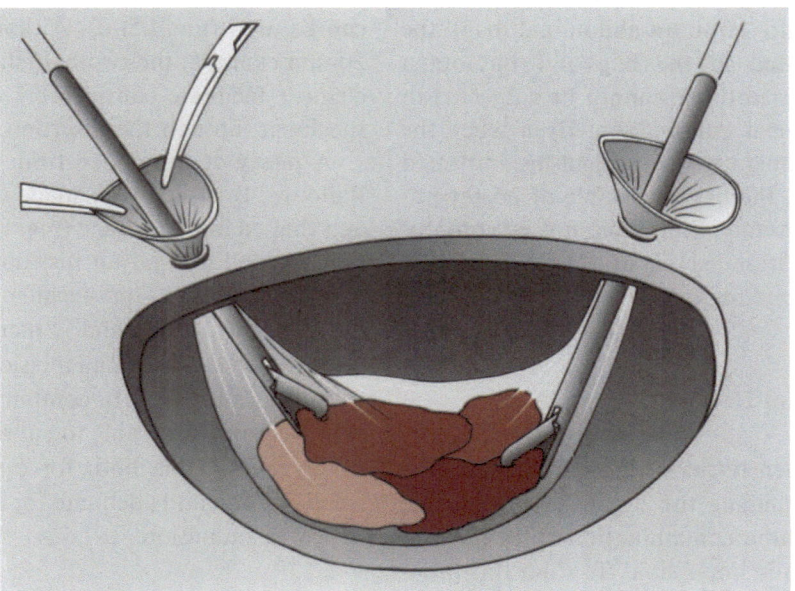

e

Organ Extraction

Pathological Demands

The key problem of endoscopic organ dissection is how to remove the specimen or the complete organ while preserving the structural integrity to allow adequate histopathological examination. The specimen has to be complete or transsected such that the pathologist can examine and assess the organ or the tumour. Hence, transsection must not destroy the structure of the organ.

Oncologic Demands

For curative purposes the tumour must be dissected with a clear margin of intact tissue in accordance with the type of tumour. If a tumour is manipulated and removed within the body cavity, special precautions and equipment are needed to prevent spillage of malignant cells.

Current Morcelators

Several devices have become available based on motor driven morcellation and mincing of tissue. The organ is put into an intra-abdominal bag, the morcelator inserted in the bag and the organ minced. The minced tissue cannot be subjected to reliable pathological examination. Even when the pathological preoperative assessment has indicated a benign process, the basic principle of postoperative histological examination must not be compromised. Fragmentation itself is useful in some situations, e.g. for stone removal.

Retrieval Bags and Devices

Organ or specimen retrieval through a small incision without damaging the organ and losing the contents and without contamination of the abdominal wall is virtually impossible. To solve this problem various retrieval bags have been designed (Table 1.4).

Table 1.4. Important features of retrieval bags

Easy insertion, adequate capacity and ready unfolding within the abdominal cavity.
The opening should be as wide as possible.
The closure water tight and easy to perform.
The material must be waterproof and transparent to allow endoscopic control of the content.
The material must be as tear proof as possible and equipped with good sliding properties.
Plastic films are useful but are not as tear proof as woven materials.
The bag should be steerable by means of a guiding rod.

The bags marketed by Endomedix, USSC etc. have a useful opening mechanism. A superelastic wire is inserted in the opening edge of the bag. This gives the bag both guiding facility and a wide opening. However, the bag must be withdrawn for closure and sealing, which can lead to loss of content. The other bags without an opening wire (Ethicon, Cincinnati, OH, USA; Dexide; Cabot Medical, Langhorne, PA, USA) are simple and appropriate for smaller specimens such as gallbladder and appendix. As the extraction of full bags, as well as gallbladders, is often difficult due to the ballooning effect (Fig. 1.58a) when the bag is pulled through the abdominal wall, the "Bergetrokar" (Bühler) can be used (Fig. 1.58d). Although it is a massive 20-mm cannula, the two half shells of the retrieval element facilitate considerably the passage of the specimen through the insertion.

A newly designed bag from Dundee (Cameron Balloons; Bristol, UK) is made from rib-stop nylon and shaped like a sausage (Fig. 1.58e). One end can be tightened around an instrument and the other end is wide open. The specimen can be pulled into the bag and the free end is then drawn out of the abdomen through a small incision, according to the size of the specimen. In combination with a simple slicer the surgeon is able to cut the organ into slices which are suitable both for extraction through a small incision and adequate for reliable histopathological examination.

References

1. Jakobeus (1910) Über die Möglichkeit, die Zystoskopie bei Untersuchung seröser Höhlung anzuwenden. Münch Med Wochenschr 57:2090–2092
2. Wittmoser R, Pfau F (1953) Technik der endoskopischen Farbenphotographie. Photogr Wissensch 2(2)
3. Semm K (1984) Operationslehre für endoskopische Abdominal-Chirurgie. Schattauer, Stuttgart
4. Buess G (ed) (1990) Endoskopie. Von der Diagnostik bis zur neuen Chirurgie. Deutscher Ärzte-Verlag, Cologne
5. Cuschieri A, Berci G (eds) (1990) Laparoscopic biliary surgery. Blackwell Scientific, Oxford
6. Melzer A, Buess G, Cuschieri A (1992) Instruments for endoscopic surgery. In: Cuschieri A, Buess G, Perrisat J (eds) Operative manual of endoscopic surgery. Springer, Berlin Heidelberg New York
7. Melzer A, Schurr MO, Kunert W et al (1993) Intelligent surgical instrument system ISIS. Concept and preliminary experimental application of prototypes. Endosc Surg Allied Technol 1:165–170
8. Becker H, Melzer A, Schurr MO, Buess G (1993) 3-D techniques in endoscopic surgery. Endosc Surg Allied Technol 1:40–46
9. Bouchet A (1990) Geschichte der Chirurgie vom Ende des 18. Jahrhunderts bis zur Gegenwart. In: Illustrierte Geschichte der Medizin, vol. 5, Andreas & Andreas, Salzburg, pp 2471–2537
10. Davis CJ (1992) A history of endoscopic surgery. Surg Lap Endosc 2:16–23
11. Melzer A, Buess G, Mentges B et al (1991) The developmental principles of minimal invasive surgery. 1st European conference on biomedical engineering. Nice
12. Melzer A (1993) Medicus and Technicus (editorial). Endosc Surg Allied Technol 1:63–64
13. Buess G (1993) Why this journal? (Editorial). Endosc Surg Allied Technol 1:1–2
14. Bertalanfy L (1974) The history and status of general systems theory. In: Couger JD, Knapp RW (eds) System analysis and techniques. Wiley, New York
15. Menz W, Buess G (1993) Potential applications of microsystem engineering in minimal invasive surgery. Endosc Surg Allied Technol 1:171–180
16. Omata S, Terunuma Y (1991) Development of new tactile sensors for detecting hardness and/or softness on an object like the human hand. Transducer's 91, San Francisco
17. Perez CA, Weed HR (1991) Optimization of the relationship between pulse width, pulse frequency and sensation thresholds for vibrotactile information transfer. Annu Int Conf IEEE 13(4)
18. Melzer A (1993) Quality standards of the reliability and applicability of instruments for endoscopic surgery. 1st European congress on endoscopic surgery, Cologne
19. Arbeitskreis für Krankenhaushygiene (1992) Infektionsprophylaxe in der endoskopischen Chirurgie. Hyg Med 17:378–380
20. Hingst J, Steinmann N (1993) Infectiological aspects. International Hospital Hygiene Association, 2nd meeting, Heidelberg
21. Bornef J (1982) Hygiene. Thieme, Stuttgart, pp 435–445
22. Janssen DW, Schneider PM (1993) Overview of ethylene oxide alternative sterilization technologies. Zentralbl Steril 1:16–32
23. Jacobs P, Kowatsch R (1993) Sterrad sterilization system: a new technology for instrument sterilization. Endosc Surg Allied Technol 1:57–58
24. Jewett DJ, Heinson P, Bennet C et al (1992) Blood-containing aerosols generated by surgical techniques: a possible infectious hazard. Am Ind Hyg Assoc 53:228–231
25. Association of Operating Room Standards and Recommended Practises for Perioperative Nursing (1987) Recommended practices for sterilization and desinfection. AORN 45:440
26. Committee on Infection Control in the Handling of Endoscopic Equipment (1980) Guidelines for preparation of laparoscopic instrumentation. AORN 32:65
27. Marshburn PB, Rutala WA, Wannamaker NS, Hulka JF (1991) Gas and steam sterilization of assembled versus disassembled laparoscopic equipment. Microbiologic studies. Reprod Med 36:483–487
28. Ebel B (1990) Biokompatibilität von Implantatwerkstoffen. Bericht 4776. Kernforschungszentrum, Karlsruhe, Germany
29. Wamsteker K (1989) Documentation in laparoscopic surgery. Baillieres Clin Obstet Gynaecol 3(3):625–647
30. Cuschieri A, Berci G (eds) (1990) Laparoscopic cholangiography. In: Cuschieri A, Berci G (eds) Laparoscopic biliary surgery. Blackwell Scientific, Oxford, pp 116–131
31. Greeg RD (1988) The case for selective cholangiography. Am J Surg 155:540–544
32. Pasquale MD, Nauta RJ (1989) Selective versus routine use of intraoperative cholangiography. Arch Surg 124:1041–1042
33. Operating manual for C-Arm series 9400 (1992) OEC diasonics, 384 Wright Brothers Drive, Salt Lake City, Utah 84116, USA
34. Miles WFA, Paterson-Brown S, Garden OJ (1992) Laparoscopic contact hepatic ultrasonography. Br J Surg 79:419–420
35. Ohta Y, Fujiwara K, Sato Y, Niwa H, Oka H (1983) New ultrasound laparoscope for diagnostic of intra-abdominal diseases. Gastrointest Endosc 29:289–294
36. Weir J, Abrahams PH (1992) An Imaging atlas of humam anatomy. Wolfe, London
37. Loughlin KR, Brooks DC (1992) The use of a doppler probe to facilitate laparoscopic varicocele ligation. Obstet Gynecol 174:326–328
38. Loughlin KR, Brooks DC (1992) The use of a Doppler Probe in Laparoscopic Surgery. Lap Endosc Surg 2:191–194
39. Lange T (1993) State of the art of video techniques for endoscopic surgery. Endosc Surg Allied Technol 1:29–35
40. Zobel J (1993) Basics of three-dimensional endoscopic vision. Endosc Surg Allied Technol 1:36–39
41. Lattwein G, Kremer RW (1990) Photo-, Film- und Videodokumentation mit dem starren Endoskop. In: Buess G (ed) Endoskopie. Von der Diagnostik zur neuen Chirurgie. Ärzteverlag, Cologne, pp 208–216

42. Semm K (1992) Intrafasziale Hysterektomie. WISAP, Sauerlach, Germany, p 112

43. Ott D (1991) Laparoscopic hypothermia. J Surg 1: 183–186

44. Ison KT, Matuszewski M, Copcoat MJ (1993) Intraperitoneal temperature monitoring in laparoscopy. Society for Minimally Invasive Therapy, 5th international meeting, Orlando

45. Morin C, Berta C, Rene A (1993) Modification of the body temperature during the operative laparoscopy. Society for Minimally Invasive Therapy, 5th international meeting, Orlando

46. Ott DE (1991) Correction of laparoscopic insufflation hypothermia. J Lap Surg 1:183–186

47. Laparoscopic insufflators. Health Devices 21:183

48. Cuschieri A, Dubois F, Mouiel J, Mouret P, Becker H, Buess G, Trede M, Troidl H (1991) The European experience with laparoscopic cholecystectomy. Am J Surg 161:385–387

49. Farin G (1992) Principles of high-frequency surgery. Erbe Elektromedizin, Tübingen

50. Mecke H (1992) Intraabdominale Verwachsungslösung. Hippokrates, Stuttgart

51. Reidenbach H-D, Theiss R, Holder KW (1986) Experimentelle Studie zur flüssigkeitsunterstützten bipolaren Hochfrequentotomie parenchymatöser Organe. Biomed Tech (Berlin) 31:66–67

52. Farin G (1994) Argon Gas Coagulation. Endosc Surg Allied Techn 2:71–77

53. Grund KE, Storek D, Farin G (1994) Endoscopic argon-gas-coagulation. First clinical experiences. Endosc Surg Allied Technol 2:42–46

54. Rusch VW, Schmidt R, Shoji Y, Fujimura Y (1990) Use of the argon beam electrocoagulator for performing pulmonary wedge resection. Soc Thorac Surg 49: 287–291

55. Dunham CM, Cornwell EE, Mitello P (1991) The role of the argon beam coagulator in splenic salvage. Surg Gynecol Obstet 173:179–181

56. Farin G (1993) Pneumatically controlled bipolar cutting instrument. Endosc Surg Allied Technol 1:97–101

57. Storch BH, Rutgers EJ, Gortzak E, Zoetmueller PA (1991) The impact of CUSA ultrasonic dissection device on major liver resection. Neth J Surg 43:99–101

58. Putnam CHW (1983) Techniques of ultrasonic dissection in resection of the liver. Surg Gynecol Obstet 157:47

59. Amaral JF, Chrostek (1993) 5 mm Ultrasonically activated scalpel. Society for Minimally Invasive Therapy, 5th international meeting, Orlando

60. Cuschieri A, Berci G (1990) Laparoscopic treatment of common duct stones. In: Cuschieri A, Berci G (eds) Laparoscopic biliary surgery. Blackwell Scientific, Oxford, pp 155–169

61. Mentges B, Buess G, Melzer A, Schäfer D, Becker HD (1991) Results of laparoscopic cholecystectomy. In: Mosby year book on lithotripsy and related techniques for gallstone treatment. Mosby, St Louis, pp 183–190

62. Nathanson L, Shimi S, Cuschieri A (1991) Laparoscopic cholecystectomy: the Dundee technique. Br J Surg 78:155–159

63. Cuschieri A (1991) Minimal access surgery and the future of interventional laparoscopy. Am J Surg 161:104–407

64. Berci G, Sackier JM, Paz-Parlow M (1991) New ideas and improved instrumentation for laparoscopic cholecystectomy. Surg Endosc 5:1–3

65. Schaller G, Manegold BC, Künkel M (1992) Optical access to the abdominal cavity. Video, World congress on endoscopic surgery, Bordeaux

66. Klemm B, Salm R, Wanninger J (1993) More safety in the access to the abdominal cavity by looking through the peritoneum at the structures behind it. Society for Minimally Invasive Therapy, 5th international meeting, Orlando

67. Melzer A, Weiss U, Roth K, Loeffler M, Buess G (1993) Visually controlled trocar insertion by means of the "optical scalpel". Endosc Surg Allied Technol 1:239–242

68. Oshinsky GS, Smith AD (1992) Laparoscopic needles and trocars: an overview of design and complications. J Lap Surg 2:117–125

69. Netzhat FR, Silfen SL, Evans D, Netzhat C (1991) Comparison of direct insertion of disposable and standard reusable laparoscopic trocars and previous pneumoperitoneum with Veress needle. Obstet Genecol 78:148–149

70. Hasson HM (1971) Modified instrument and method for laparoscopy. Am J Obstet Gynaecol 110:886–887

71. Reich H, McGlynn (1990) Short self-retaining trocar sleeves for laparoscopic surgery. Am J Obstet Gynaecol 162:453–454

72. Loeffler M, Trispel S (1993) Technological principles of curved instruments and flexible cannulae. Endosc Surg Allied Technol 1:365–370

73. Cuschieri A, Shimi S, Banting S, Van Velpen G, Dunkley P (1993) Coaxial Curved Instrumentation for Minimal Access Surgery. Endosc Surg Allied Technol 1:303–305

74. Périssat J (1992) Laparoscopic cholecystectomy. In: Cuschieri A, Buess G, Périssat J (eds) Operative manual of endoscopic surgery. Springer, Berlin Heidelberg New York, pp 209–232

75. Cuschieri A (1991) Variable curvature shape-memory spatula for laparoscopic surgery. Surg Endosc 5:179–171

76. Stöckel D, Melzer A (1993) New developments in superelastic instrumentation for minimally invasive surgery, medical data meeting. American College of Surgeons, San Francisco

77. Duerig T, Melton K, Cayman M, Stöckel D (eds) (1990) Engineering aspects of shape memory alloy. Butterworth-Heineman, London

78. Lirici MM, Melzer A, Reuthebuch O, Buess G (1993) Experimental development in colorectal surgery. Endosc Surg Allied Technol 1:20–25

79. Schurr MO, Melzer A, Dautzenberg P, Neisius B, Trapp R, Buess G (1993) Development of steerable instruments for minimal invasive surgery in modular conception. Acta Chir Belg

80. Melzer A, Schurr MO, Kunert W, Buess G et al (1993) Intelligent surgical instrument system. Concept and preliminary experimental application of components and prototypes. Endosc Surg Allied Technol 1:165–170

81. Köhler GW (1981) Typenbuch der Manipulatoren. Thiemig, Stuttgart
82. Szabo Z (1994) Analysis of movements during endoscopic suturing. Endosc Surg Allied Technol 2:55–61
83. Melzer A, Schurr MO, Lirici MM, Klemm B, Stöckel D, Buess G (1994) Future trends in endoscopic suturing. Endosc Surg Allied Technol 2:78–82
84. Andrews SM, Lewis JL (1994) Laparoscopic knot substitutes. Endosc Surg Allied Technol 2:62–65
85. Lirici MM, Buess G, Melzer A, Weinreich S, Becker HD (1993) Experimental results of colon resection with the Tübingen procedure. Br Y Surg (in press)

2 Video Technology for Minimally Invasive Surgery

T. Lange and G. Buess

Video technology has become an indispensable aid in endoscopic surgery since the video monitor and the endoscopic camera are the only visual interface between the surgical team and the inside of the body during surgery. The video monitor enables the team both to monitor the handling of surgical instruments and to observe anatomical and pathological structures. Improvements in asepsis, a less tiring working posture and excellent support for training are among the additional advantages video technique has brought to endoscopic surgery.

However, the importance of an efficient visual interface to the operative field often seems to be underestimated:

- Video cameras and video systems on the market today which are advertised as suitable for endoscopy are in fact often only simple adaptations of semiprofessional or professional equipment. Developments anticipating the future demands of endoscopic surgery are noticeably missing.
- Because of a lack in technical know-how in hospitals, not enough use is being made of the options available using professional video equipment. For these reasons, a short overview of the video cassette recording and camera systems currently in medical use, a comparison of their performance, and the outlook for useful future technologies is presented.

Fundamentals

Television Standards

Television broadcasting standards exist in which parameters such as definition and picture frequency have been set up. Worldwide there are two groups of systems: the CCIR standard (Comité Consultatif International des Radiocommunications) in Europe, Africa, Australia, parts of Asia and South America, and the NTSC standard (National Television System Committee) in North and Central America and Japan (Table 2.1).

The NTSC standard shows considerable deficiencies with regard to colour transfer: even a slight displacement of the phase angle of the colour signal causes disagreeable colour casts, especially with skin tones. The PAL system combats this shortcoming by changing over the modulation axis of the colour signal line by line (which is why it is called *phase alternating line*). The same happens with the SECAM (*sequentiel couleur à memoire*) system. The difference is, however, that the two colour difference signals here are not transmitted simultaneously, but one after the other (sequentially). The signal transmitted first is temporarily stored and reproduced with a time delay.

RGB Signal for Optimal Intraoperative Monitor Image

The RGB signal is composed of three separate signals corresponding to the voltages of the colours red, green und blue (Fig. 2.1).

Table 2.1. Television broadcasting standards

	PAL	SECAM	NTSC
Number of lines	625	625	525
Visible lines, maximum	575	575	486
Field frequency (cps)	50	50	60
Frames per second	25	25	30

cps, cycles per second; PAL, phase alternating line; SECAM, *sequentiel couleur à memoire*; NTSC, National Television System Committee

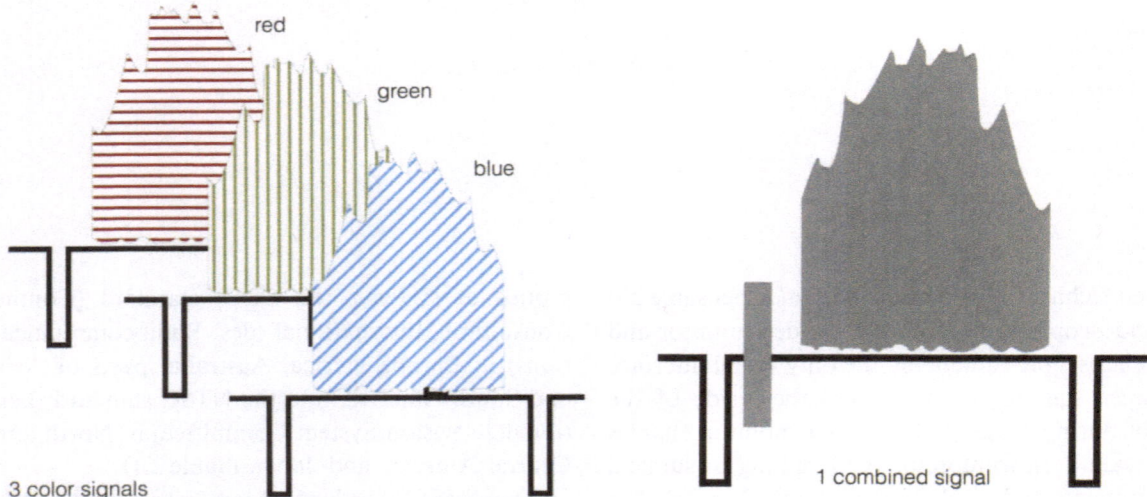

Fig. 2.1. Red, green, blue (*RGB*) signal (three colour signals)

Fig. 2.2. Composite signal (one combined signal)

With a high resolution RGB camera together with an RGB monitor the optimum of image quality during endoscopic operations can be achieved.

The luminance value results from the addition of the RGB values: $Y = R + G + B$. Professional three-chip cameras produce these signals with one chip for each of these colours. In single-chip cameras the electrical information is divided into three separate voltages for red, green und blue by means of a stripe filter behind the image sensor.

The RGB signal has not been encoded at this point for one of the various recording formats (e. g. VHS, SVHS, U-matic, Betacam SP) or colour transmission standards (e. g. PAL, NTSC, SECAM); that is, it does not show the quality impairments of these signal transformations. Furthermore, its bandwidth is not restricted either.

For these reasons, the RGB signal is the best signal a camera can produce. It can be fed directly into an RGB monitor, where it is led without any further encoding to the three cathodes of the tube. These again compose the monitor picture out of red, green and blue pixels. Only for later tape recording is the RGB signal transformed into a luminance signal Y and two colour difference signals U and V, out of which the specific signals for tape recording are produced.

Composite and Component Signal Processing

Composite Signal

When colour television was first introduced in the USA and Europe, compatibility to black and white TV was important. Therefore the signal carrying the colour information (chrominance) was modulated over the signal carrying the brightness information (luminance) and combined in one single "composite signal" (Fig. 2.2).

Furthermore, the bandwidth of the signal had to be restricted. With this signal processing standard, colour reproduction is often problematic: interference between the luminance and chrominance information cause cross-luminance and cross-colour distortions (interference patterns). Because colour signal oscillation is within the range of visibility, a wandering line (line jitter) appears especially at pronounced colour boundaries together with flickering and noise in large coloured areas.

These effects are further intensified by interlaced scanning. When copying video material recorded with composite signals and processing it during electronic editing, quality becomes impaired very soon and gets worse with every generation of copies.

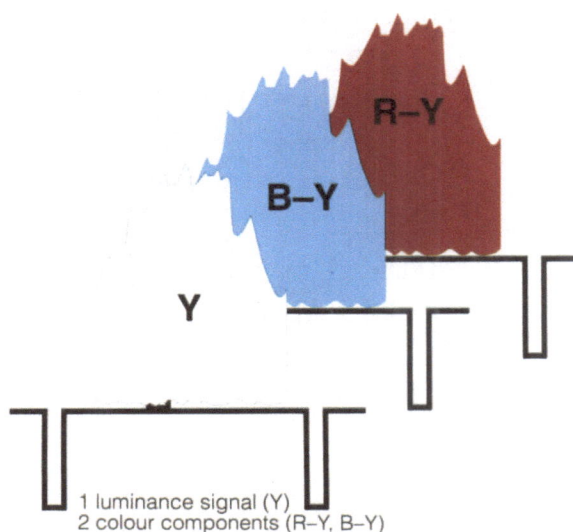

Fig. 2.3. Component signal. One luminance signal (*Y*) and two colour components (*R-Y, B-Y*)

Table 2.2. Video standards and their signal processing

Composite signal	Component signal
VHS	Betacam (Y-U-V)
U-matic low-band	Betacam SP (Y-U-V)
U-matic high-band	M II (Y-U-V)
U-matic high-band SP	D1 (Y-U-V)
D2	SVHS (Y/C)
D3 (Y-U-V)	Hi 8 (Y/C)
	HDTV

See text for abbreviations

Component Signal

Modern professional recording systems use component signal processing (Fig. 2.3). Here, the luminance signal (Y) and two colour difference signals (U and V) are recorded on three independent video channels. (See Table 2.2 for a comparison of composite and component signals).

Component recording systems are attractive because of their high colour fidelity and detail reproduction, and because they show no visible loss of quality even after three or four generations of copies. As a result of component signal technology, these systems are free of cross-luminance and cross-colour distortions. Because of their high bandwidth and low quality loss in copying, component recordings, even after repeated editing, are of broadcast quality.

Interlaced scanning

The European PAL television picture frequency standard is 25 pictures per second. In order to avoid severe flickering, which is tiring to the viewer, each picture is divided into two fields for interlaced scanning, thus achieving a field frequency of 50 fields per second. With interlaced scanning, the lines are not shown one after the other. Instead, lines 1, 3, 5, 7, 9 ... of field 1 are followed by lines 2, 4, 6, 8, 10 ... of field 2. The human eye can then no longer distinguish between the fields − with the exception of the problems of colour representation. Here, interlaced scanning intensifies flickering and jitter at pronounced colour boundaries and in large coloured areas.

Recording Systems for Magnetic Tape

U-Matic

In the early 1970s the U-matic system was developed. This uses a 3/4″ magnetic chromium dioxide tape and a helical scan recording system. It was the professional standard for more than 20 years and is still in use all over the world. The U-matic system can only process composite signals as they were used when colour TV was first introduced. It combines the brightness (luminance) and colour (chrominance) picture information into a single signal.

A particularly important problem is that the recorded U-matic video material has a poor multigeneration performance. Because of the low writing speed of the U-matic system (10.7 m/s) the colour information in the video signal has to be restricted in bandwidth on the colour intercarrier ("colour-under" technology).

The first generation of the U-matic low-band system was modified and the U-matic high-band and U-matic high-band superior performance (SP) systems developed.

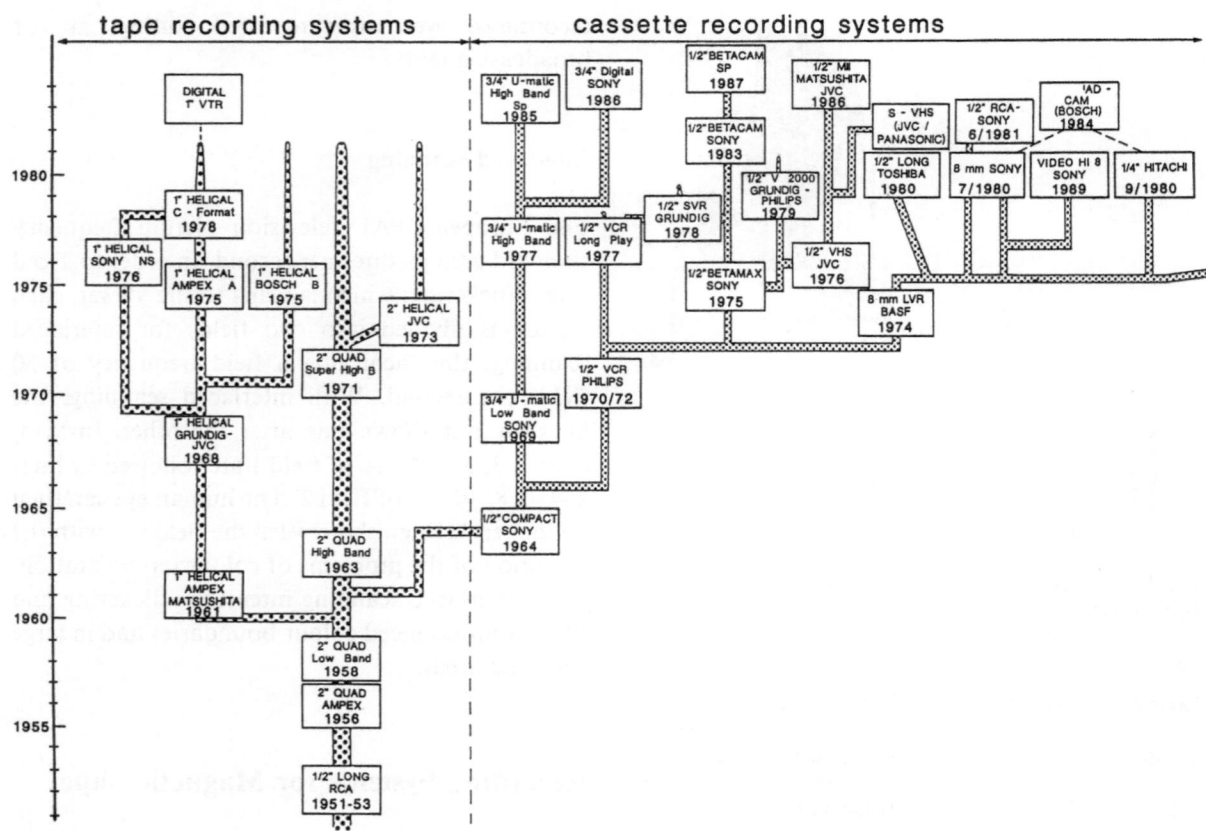

Fig. 2.4. Family tree of video systems

Table 2.3. System parameters of the U-matic system in 3/4″ tape format

	Low-band	High-band	High-band SP
Video band width (mcps)	3.0	3.5	3.8
Colour intercarrier (mcps)	0.688	0.923	0.924

mcps, Megacycles per second

Because of these disadvantages, the U-matic system is in decline, and is being replaced in science and industry with either Super-VHS for low end requirements, or component tape recording systems – Betacam SP (Sony) and M II (Panasonic) – for high end requirements (Fig. 2.4; Table 2.3).

Consumer and Semiprofessional Systems

Modern systems in the consumer and semiprofessional sector are VHS and Super VHS (SVHS; 1/2″ cassette format), and Video 8 and Video Hi 8. (The Video 2000 system and Beta-max have nearly disappeared from the market.) These systems are not compatible with each other, except for VHS, which is upwardly compatible to SVHS.

VHS and Video 8

The VHS system uses a composite signal as does the U-matic system (one common signal for chrominance and luminance). It also stores the colour information using "colour-under" technology. Tape speed is only 4.87 m/s.

Table 2.4. System parameters of semiprofessional video standards

	VHS	Video 8	SVHS	Video Hi 8
Luminance (mcps)	4.3	4.8	6.2	6.7
Chrominance (mcps)	0.627	0.732	0.627	0.732
Frequency range (mcps)	0.6	0.5	1.6	2.0
Horizontal resolution (lines)	250	260	400	400

mcps, Megacycles per second

The Video-8 standard (Sony), a small video recording format, was developed especially for compact camcorders in the consumer sector. The disadvantages of VHS and Video 8 are insufficient resolution and colour fidelity and the great loss of quality in the composite signals during copying and cutting.

SVHS and Video Hi 8

The SVHS standard (JVC/Panasonic) and Hi 8 (Sony) represent an improvement in picture quality, together with a better colour performance and reduced quality impairment after copying.

The increase in horizontal resolution in SVHS was achieved by increasing the mean frequency modulation (FM) carrier frequency from 4.3 to 6.2 mcps, and by enlarging the frequency range from 1 to 1.6 mcps. The recording of the video signal is effected using separate components for the luminance signal (Y) and the chroma signal (C) (Fig. 2.5). Thus, with original material of good quality, one can obtain three generations of copies with acceptable picture quality. With the Video Hi 8 standard (Sony) recording technology was improved using separate Y/C signals and new metal evaporated (ME) tapes.

Advanced SVHS Systems

The so-called professional SVHS systems (JVC, Panasonic) offer higher picture quality and better multi-generation performance by means of high

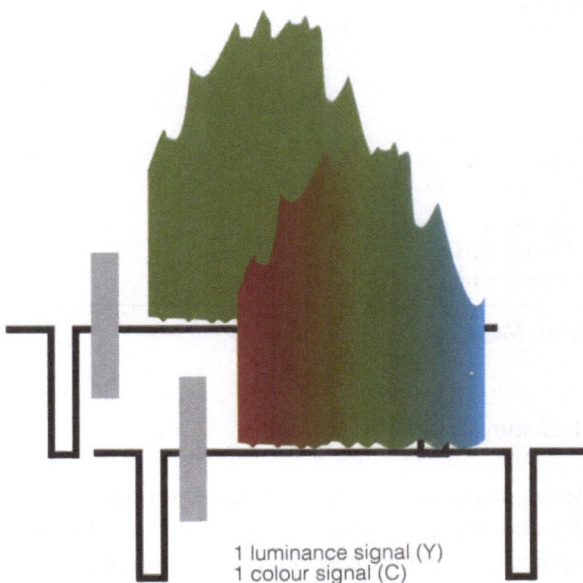

1 luminance signal (Y)
1 colour signal (C)

Fig. 2.5. Super VHS signal. One luminance signal (Y) and one colour signal (C)

quality video heads, a chroma enhancer, an increased chroma bandwidth, and drop-out compensation (a distorted signal resulting from a damaged part of the tape is replaced by a repetition of the last failure-free line held in memory). Integrated time base correctors (TBC) also enhance picture stability, minimize "jitter" and make it possible to adjust the colour. These systems can be usefully employed for documentation and low-budget productions in research and teaching.

Professional Component Recording Systems

For productions in broadcast quality the component recording systems Betacam SP and M II have been established as the new standards (Table 2.5). An outstanding picture quality and excellent multi-generation performance is provided by these systems. They separate the picture information into three component signals. The use of a component recording system only makes sense, however, if a high quality three chip camera is used in combination.

Table 2.5. Parameters of the component tape recording systems Betacam SP and M II

	Betacam SP	M II
Luminance channel		
Video bandwidth	5.5	5.5
Frequency range	2.0	1.8
Chrominance channels		
Chroma carrier	6.1	6.4
Frequency range	1.7	2.0

mcps, Megacycles per second

Betacam (Sony)

Betacam technology records the luminance signal (Y) and the chrominance signals (U and V) in a segmented form on two independent parallel video channels using two video heads. At the same time, chrominance information is transformed into compressed component signals and is stored using compressed time division multiplex (CTDM) technology. In combination with the even more effective 1/2″ metallized tapes, this technology has now been developed into Betacam SP.

M II (Panasonic)

The M II system also records component signals: the colour information (U and V) is compressed using the chrominance time compression multiplexing (CTCM) technique and stored sequentially on a chroma channel (c) together with an additional colour synchronization signal (chroma burst).

Future Systems

The new video technologies which are being developed today will be of value for scientific film and documentation only if they can hold their own on the market and can be offered at a reasonable price. Most notable among these are digital video magnetic tape recording systems and high definition television (HDTV).

Digital Recording Systems

The most remarkable features of the digital storing and processing of video signals on magnetic tape are the excellent picture quality and the outstanding multigeneration performance (6.5 mcps bandwidth, more than 20 generations without appreciable loss). Factors causing interference, such as the deterioration of the signal-to-noise ratio (S/N ratio), moiré effects and drop-outs, are to a large degree eliminated. Digital video tape recording (VTR) systems are especially suitable for high-tech postproduction because the considerable quality impairments of analog systems due to numerous generations of copies can be avoided.

In 1985, a world standard was established for digital video recording, the 4-2-2 standard. With the D1 system, a component encoding of the analog RGB signal into a luminance signal with 5.75 mcps and two colour difference signals (U and V) with 2.75 mcps each is made. For digitization the Y signal is scanned with a sampling frequency of 13.5 mcps, the U and V signals with 6.75 mcps each (4-2-2 system).

The D2 system, in contrast, digitizes composite signals. Hence, D1 and D2 recorders can be easily integrated into existing analog component or composite studio environments.

The D3 system, from the Japanese broadcasting organization NHK, is the first complete digital system, beginning with the camera, the VTR and the program assembly switcher to the broadcast studio.

The latest development is a digital Betacam system introduced by Sony which is compatible to the analog Betacam system. With bit rates reduction (BRR) techniques, the video information is reduced without compromise to the image quality. With the traditional picture format of 4:3, a resolution of 540 TV lines (or a bandwidth of 6.9 mcps) is achieved. With a wide picture format (16:9 for PALPLUS or HDTV), the resolution is 405 TV lines.

High Definition Video Systems

Early in the 1970s, the development of a high-resolution television system, HDTV began. The objectives were a substantial improvement of picture resolution and avoidance of cross-colour distortions

Table 2.6. High-definition television and high-definition video systems in the picture format 16:9

System	Japan (NHK/Sony)	Europe (Eureka 95)	USA
Number of lines	1125	1250	1050
Visible lines (92%)	1035	1150	966
Pixels per line	1831	2035	1709
Total number of pixels	1895085	2340250	1650894
Field frequency (cps)	60	50	59.94
Video band width (mcps)			
Luminance channel	20	20	20
Chrominance channels	7	7	7

cps, Cycles per second; mcps, megacycles per second

through the use of component signals. A wide picture format of 16:9 fills the complete field of vision at the recommended viewing distance of twice the height of the picture. This creates a new quality of telepresence and encourages the eye of the viewer to wander around in the scene.

Owing to a resolution which is eight times higher, large size projection corresponding to the capacity of the human eye to resolve detail has become a reality. Nothing more remains to be desired with regard to sharpness.

The introduction of HDTV as a television standard has still to be implemented. There are still transmission problems and as yet no technical solutions for flat, large-size monitors for the consumer living room. Three systems versions from Japan, Europe and the USA are currently under discussion. However, because of the demand for compatibility with existing PAL, NTSC and SECAM standards, it is not very likely that a global standard format will be established (Table 2.6).

A complete equipment line exists already for both the Japanese and the European systems, including camera, VTR and laser disk systems, electronic editing systems, control monitors and equipment for large-size projection.

Fierce debate has broken out concerning the establishment of compatible intermediate stages and transmission standards of European analog HDTV. The alternatives are: a further development of the PAL standard (e.g. PALPLUS, a downwardly compatible PAL system in the 16.9 wide screen format with separate luminance and chrominance signals) or satellite transmission standards (e.g. D2-MAC and HD-MAC).

Further optimization of the existing PAL system was achieved by reducing the large-area flicker on the receiver using image stores which pass on the received 50 fields to the picture tube at double frequency (100 cps). In the USA, preliminary decisions have recently been taken to establish a modern, totally digital HDTV standard. This will certainly have an effect on the further technical development of European HDTV. In the meantime, the engineers developing HDTV are concentrating on applications for science and advertising.

In October 1993, we introduced high-definition camera and recording equipment to endoscopic surgery. In collaboration with Broadcast Television Systems (BTS), the developer of European HDTV, and Richard Wolf GmbH the HDTV camera has now been adapted to take a circular rod lense. The resulting image represents a quantum leap forward from today's video standards, with the endoscopic picture covering 85% of the normal HDTV format. Resolution is remarkably high, showing all detail sharply and precisely. For the first time, working posture is genuinely relaxed and working distance from the 30-inch monitor is optimal.

Owing to the excellent light sensitivity of the camera, no lighting problems occurred during our testing; furthermore, the outstanding picture definition gave a remarkably improved depth perception. Further development will now concentrate on optimizing the handling, size and weight of the system.

Cameras

As far as recording systems are concerned, professional technology is only necessary for post-production, i. e. for the production of scientific or educational films. In contrast, only cameras and monitors are of direct relevance to the quality of the visual image used during endoscopic surgery.

Charge-Coupled Device Camera

The tube cameras which were still widely used a few years ago, have now been replaced by chip cameras with charge-coupled semiconductor elements (charge-coupled device, CCD cameras). Among the advantages of CCD cameras are:

- Stronger light differentials (scene contrasts) can be handled without blooming effects.
- A higher sensitivity to light.
- Less weight with greater mechanical reliability.
- Improved electronic stability.

CCD Chip Technology

A charge-coupled semiconductor functions thus: the photoelectric charge resulting from the incoming light (or photon current) is transmitted from the image area into a coupled storage. This is then scanned at a defined clock frequency. Interline transfer (IT) technology adds a vertical smear to the image during the transfer of the charge packets from the image area to the storage area. This effect has been considerably reduced by the "on-chip lens" technology. Frame-transfer (FT) technology, with its higher sensitivity to light, completely prevents smear by operating a shutter during the shift of charge packets, thus preventing incoming light from contaminating the next picture. Frame interline transfer (FIT) technology is a combination of the two techniques, with additional storage, faster scanning, and a further improvement to image quality.

RGB Signals

Colour separation in single-chip cameras is achieved by adding a stripe filter to the optical beam. Each of these filter stripes only accepts a defined colour (red, green, blue = additive colour combination principle). The luminance signal (Y) and the chrominance signals (U and V) are generated from the output voltages for R, G, or B with the help of a matrix switcher. These are again encoded into composite and SVHS signals. Some single-chip cameras supply an output for the RGB signal. This, however, cannot be compared to the quality of an RGB signal from a three-chip camera.

Three-chip cameras supply a separate CCD chip for each of the red, green and blue image parts as an image sensor. A colour separation system consisting of prisms and dichroic filters separates the image into the basic R, G, and B components. The three chips generate the output voltages corresponding to chrominance, colour saturation, and luminance. This RGB signal is fed, without any further encoding, over three separate lines into an RGB monitor, where it is led directly to the three cathodes of the tube. This direct, uncoded signal, separated according to R, G, and B components is a substantial improvement with regard to picture quality and colour fidelity.

With one of the best RGB three-chip cameras and an RGB monitor the increase in detail information is so great that it can only be described as a new quality of seeing. For critical assessments (e. g. unclear anatomical or pathological structures) this difference can be of decisive importance.

The New Endoscopic Cameras: An Evaluation

Of the many endoscopic cameras on the market today, we will briefly introduce and evaluate nine new systems, some of which were only available to us as prototypes at the time of testing (end of 1992). Systems are defined by noticeably different concepts. For comparison purposes, a Sony DXC 750 P adapted for endoscopic use by our MIC research group in Tuebingen was used as a reference, owing to its excellent image quality.

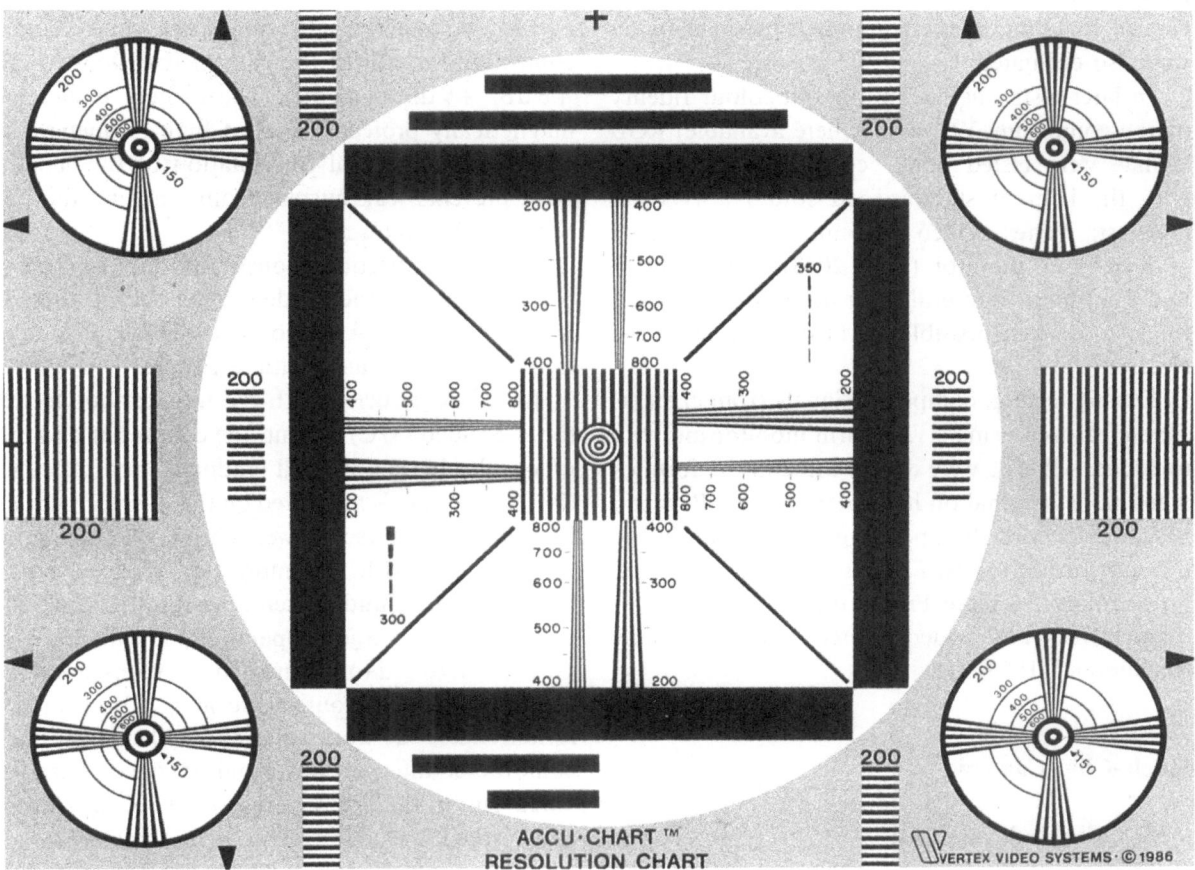

Fig. 2.6. Resolution chart. Horizontal resolution is the number of distinct vertical lines that can be seen in a picture. For vertical resolution the number of horizontal lines must be counted

A number of new technical features – especially digital video signal processing and new types of automatic exposure – are now being integrated into many endocameras.

With digital signal processing, the analog video information is translated into binary code by digital capture and enhancement circuits. With all video information translated into a stream of digital values, the signal can be manipulated by filtering, noise reduction, image enhancement and data compression, all without adding extra noise.

Today, electronic shutters are often used to control the readout speed of charge packets on the image sensor (CCD). An alternative technique regulates the sensitivity of the pixels on the CCD directly. With either method, automatic exposure can be achieved without increasing the electronic gain, and without penalty of additional picture noise associated with extra gain. Furthermore, automatic exposure can be provided without the need for controlling the light source with the video signal. As a result, image quality and operational safety are further enhanced.

The performance of single-chip cameras, especially, has greatly improved in the last 2 years. However, if surgery is being documented for later inclusion in larger film or video productions, three-chip cameras with interface to professional post-production equipment is still a better option.

In our test, all cameras were critically assessed in the operating theatre (for example, in transanal surgery, with its associated high level of light absorption). Here, light sensitivity (necessary minimum illumination), noise associated with raised electronic gain, and colour reproduction were important. The ease of handling of the equipment by the surgeon was also evaluated.

In later tests, the resolution and colour fidelity of the composite, Y/C and (where available) RGB signals were tested under controlled conditions, with the help of standardized studio test charts (Teletest; Vertex Video Systems; Fig. 2.6) on a 19-inch Sony monitor (PVM 2043). Noise, smear and blooming were evaluated at various gain settings, and, where possible, at various settings of the electronic shutter.

During testing, composite signals from cameras were measured using a waveform monitor and vectorscope. All tests were documented in the form of a component signal on high-performance Betacam SP tape. In both the operating theatre and during the standardized tests, FBAS signals were digitized on a Polaroid Freeze Frame recorder, exposed as diapositives, and video-printed with the Sony Mavigraph UP 5000 P.

Single-Chip Cameras

Wolf CCD Endocam 5501

The new Richard Wolf model (Wolf; Knittlingen, Germany) has a small, light-weight head, complete with a finger-tip button to control a VCR or printer (Fig. 2.7). A 1/2-inch interline transfer CCD with colour mosaic filter can operate under a minimum illumination of 3 lux. With digital signal technology the chroma and luminance signals are processed separately. Digital edge enhancement and aperture accentuation are used in this camera. The control unit is used to activate the automatic white balance control and to adjust the gain in fixd steps (0 dB, +6 dB, +9 dB, +12 dB). The camera is electromagnetically protected against high frequency interference; additional BF isolation of the camera head prevents leak current from reaching the patient via the endoscope.

Output connections consist of only one composite video and one S video (Y/C) output; there is no RGB output. A video-controlled light source must be used for automatic exposure.

In tests conducted with the monitor connected to the S video (Y/C) output, the colour bar and the grey-scale charts were well graduated and differentiated. The signals measured on the waveform monitor and the vectorscope were correct. These results corresponded with the impression we received in the clinical test, undertaken during a transanal endoscopic microsurgery operation, in which good graduation of red tones and generally very good reproduction of all colours was evident. Using a resolution chart, 420 horizontal and 350 vertical lines could be counted on our monitor. A comparative videoprint of the Y/C signal showed 400 horizontal and vertical lines. However, due to a conscious accentuation of the aperture, the image does not look as sharp as it might: visible flaring, especially along black/white borders, combined with a noticeable increase in noise even at low (+6 dB) or medium (+9 dB) gain levels, mean that the image looks too soft, despite the good detail definition.

Fig. 2.7. Wolf CCD Endocam 5501

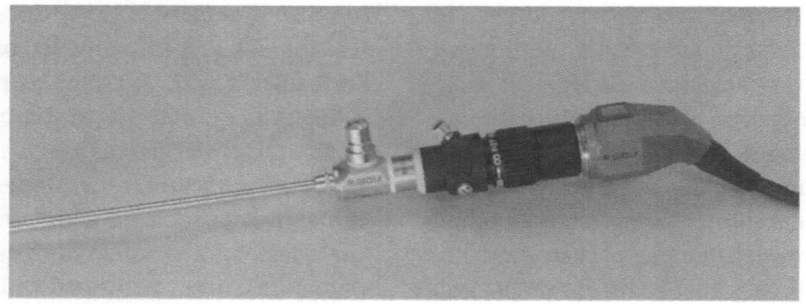

Stryker 594 Medical Video Camera

The Stryker 594, (Stryker Endoscopy; San Jose, CA, USA), an analog single-chip camera, has a small, light-weight camera head with a mechanism for universal lens adaptation. At the camera processor the Auto White balance function is started. The result tends to be somewhat too red, but it can be corrected by an additional colour adjustment regulator.

A remote control unit may be connected to operate a video recorder or printer. After removing the camera cable, internal colour bars for monitor calibration appear on the monitor screen.

An auto shutter that can also be switched to a fixed speed gives automatic exposure control between 1/60 and 1/10000 s. Gain amplification can be chosen between 0 dB (standard mode), +9 dB (mode II) and +18 dB (mode I).

The resolution was measured with 400 horizontal and vertical TV lines. Already in standard mode (0 dB) noise was remarkable. It did, however, not increase very much (as expected) when amplifying the gain with +9 dB and +18 dB. Image contrast was very low: in our test with the grey-scale chart black fields appeared as average grey tones.

Storz Endocam PAL

The Storz Endocam PAL (Storz; Tuttlingen, Germany) a light, medium-sized camera, is easy to handle (Fig. 2.8). The fast and reliable white balance control is situated on the control unit (camera processor). It can be toggled between manual and automatic use. Exposure is regulated by the variation of the CCD shutter speed, in fixed steps between 1/60 and 1/10000 s. An additional automatic gain control with a range of −4 dB to +14 dB is used for fine regulation between shutter speed steps. An LED indicator displays the current shutter speed.

There is a good range of outputs: one composite, two S video (Y/C), as well as an RGB output with its superior image quality on the monitor. There is also a genlock input for external synchronization and a keyboard input for an optional character generator.

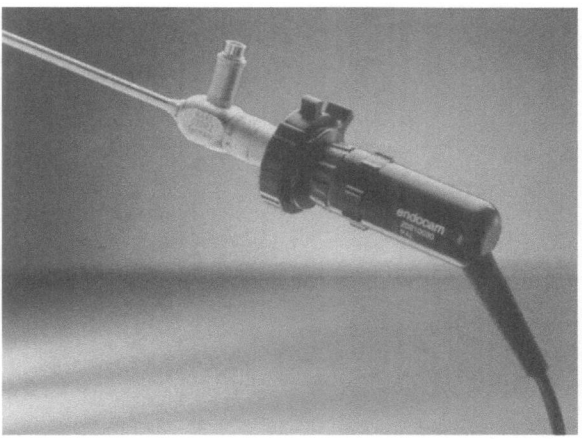

Fig. 2.8. Storz Endocam PAL

The 1/2-inch chip in this camera achieves a resolution of 350 horizontal lines and 400 vertical lines, using the RGB output and a Sony PVM 2043 monitor. The colour bars and the grey scale from the test charts appear finely graduated on the monitor. Serious noise, smear or blooming were not a problem. On the waveform monitor, no deviations from the standard signal were observed. Nevertheless, the image appears too bright, and the contrast along black/white interfaces was not as clear as might be desired.

AVT Horn MC 1009/F

The AVT Horn MC 1009/F (AVT Horn; Aalen, Germany) is a single-chip Sony camera adapted for endoscopy (Fig. 2.9). It uses analog signal processing and regulates exposure with shutter and gain controls, both of which have automatic and manual modes.

The chip is a 1/2-inch interline transfer hyper HAD CDD from Sony capable of dealing, with a minimum illumination of 4.5 lux at F 1.2 when the automatic gain control is on. The S/N ratio is over 46 dB.

The camera head is light weight but at a length of 12 cm somewhat large. Even after only a short period of operation it became rather hot. The operating elements − two regulating potentiometers and six DIP switches − are small and are embedded in the camera head.

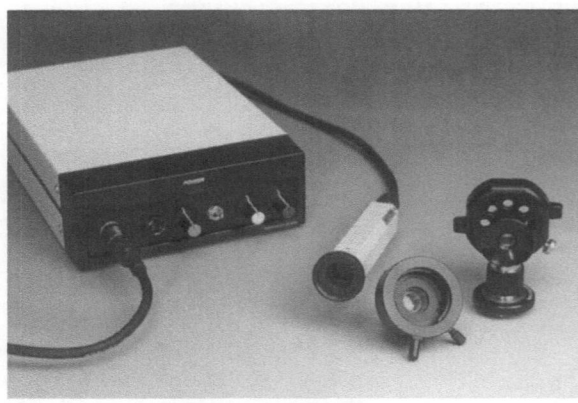

Fig. 2.9. AVT Horn MC 1009/F

The white balance can either be adjusted manually, using the two potentiometers for red and blue correction, or automatically in a novel continuous mode, which we found to be of little practical value. Two DIP switches allow a choice between fixed values of 5600 °K (daylight) or 3200 °K (artificial light).

An automatic shutter control (called "CCD iris") operates in fixed steps between 1/50 and 1/1000 s. The minimum and maximum values can also be manually selected and used as fixed shutter speeds. The automatic gain control ranges from 0 dB to +12 dB.

The camera showed good colour registration on our monitor, with good reaction times for the automatic shutter. However, with the shutter in manual mode, the automatic gain control showed very long reaction times (in some cases more than 1 s, under low light conditions). On the resolution chart, the composite signal of the camera provided both 400 horizontal and vertical lines. (The alternative version of this camera – the MC 1009/S, which includes a S Video (Y/C) signal – was not available to us at the time of testing.)

MP Video Medicam 900

The Medicam 900 is an integrated imaging system from MP Video (Hopkinton, MA, USA). It combines camera, monitor, light source, insufflator, tank and remote control into one solidly constructed, compact and practical wheeled unit. This unit also includes the isolation transformer. However, a lockable compartment proved not to be deep enough to take a professional S video recorder.

The camera head is light weight, small and ergonomic. Two programmable, fingertip buttons allow the user – in combination with an optional remote control unit – to activate peripheral devices such as a VCR or video printer. A picture-in-picture function can also be activated by finger tip. This allows two separate images to share the monitor screen during dual camera procedures (for example, during laparoscopic choledochoscopy or combined resections of the rectosigmoid colon). The cable provided is designed to be easily interchangeable in the operating theatre.

The camera uses a new Panasonic chip, offering a S/N ratio of 48 dB. The analog signal processing circuits of the camera interface with the Medicam 900 light source by means of a control circuit capable of optimizing the output of both units. By measuring the illumination level at the camera's CCD chip prior to setting the automatic gain control, the Medicam 900 is able to increase the intensity of the light source in preference to raising the electronic gain (electronic gain is associated with increase in noise). Thus, automatic gain is only used if the maximum 250 W from the light source proves insufficient. To use the automatic gain, function called "boost circuit" must be activated; however, in this mode, serious picture noise becomes visible. A disadvantage of the light source is that the bulb can be damaged when connecting a Storz light cable.

The main exposure control mechanism is an automatic shutter which constantly alters its speed in response to illumination requirements. MP Video claims that this is a continuous, stepless shutter system. Nevertheless, a perceptible "stepping" effect was clearly observed. This turned out to be due to the changing light levels of the light source operating in automatic mode. The effect did not occur when operating the light source in manual mode.

A "small scope" function can be chosen to maintain adequate automatic exposure if the picture fills only a part of the camera's field.

The image displayed by the Medicam 900 camera is clear, of good contrast, and of high definition. Four hundred horizontal and 450 vertical lines were counted. Colour registration was very good and the measured signals showed the correct values. Visible noise showed only when activating the "boost circuit" in light conditions so low as to be very unlikely to occur in normal endoscopy.

The camera provides two composite, two S video (Y/C) and one RGB output. The Medicam 900 system shows that high image quality can also be achieved with analog signal processing, if high quality components are combined with intelligent system integration.

Circon Micro Digital-1

The latest prototype from Circon (Santa Barbara, CA, USA), the Circon Micro Digital-1 (Fig. 2.10) uses 24-bit digital circuitry for signal processing. This offers good image quality, even at high levels of electronic gain. Flaring, washout and "jitters" are eliminated by digital filtering and image enhancement. A field replacement cable is easy to change in the operating theatre.

The small, lightweight head of the camera has two fingertip control buttons for automatic gain (in three steps from 0 to +12 dB), freeze frame, VCR and printer control.

At the control unit, an automatic single-or-continuous white balance control is offered. Freeze frame display and toggling between manual and automatic exposure are also possible. For automatic exposure an electronic shutter with fixed steps between 1/60 and 1/15700 s is used. This elimi-

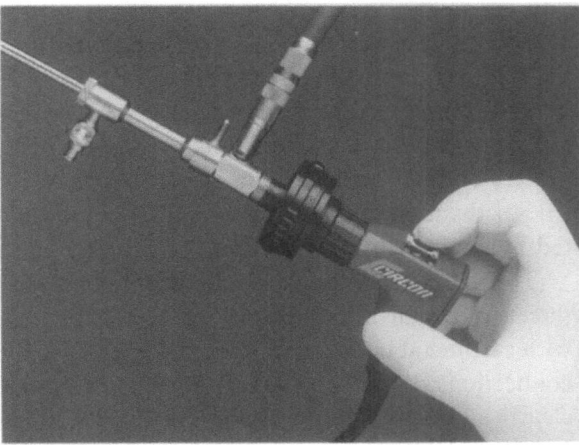

Fig. 2.10. Circon Micro Digital-1

nates the need for sophisticated video-controlled light sources.

An illumination value of only 1 lux (AGC on), or 5 lux (AGC off) can be achieved without compromise to image quality. An LED readout on the control unit displays information about lighting conditions. Camera-generated colour bars for preoperative monitor calibration are also supplied. Multiple output connections are provided: two composite video, two S video (Y/C) and RGB. The prototype we tested showed a high-contrast, brilliantly clear and sharp image on the monitor.

Surprisingly, only 400 lines of vertical and horizontal resolution could be counted. The excellent separation (contour definition) between adjacent black and white areas, due to the digital signal processing, gave the impression of very high definition (although this is not to be compared with the significantly superior definition of three-chip cameras). Moreover, picture quality is fully maintained, even if the gain is increased maximally to +12 dB; no visible noise occurs. The S/N ratio at 56 dB is very good.

Less satisfactory was the testing of the camera with our colour bars and grey-scale charts. Here, the image appeared too bright, with too little differentiation both in the highlights and in the colour range between magenta and red. This observation was substantiated on the waveform monitor and on the vectorscope: the internal colour-bar signal had a luminance of 30% above standard. These measurements corresponded to our impressions during the clinical test: although the exposure seemed to be correct, there were fewer graduations in the red range than with other, similar cameras. After having informed the developers, Circon told us "... a revision of the camera circuitry has eliminated this problem. The full range of contrast is now restored."

Another observation during clinical testing was a serious "blooming" effect when light was too strong for the automatic shutter control compensation. After reducing the light intensity to the minimum practical level (as advised by Circon), these effects disappeared at once, and the camera gave hightlights which were sharply defined, if not very differentiated.

Circon is working on both a three-chip camera with digital signal processing and on a solution for noninterlaced monitor display of digital video signals. Detailed and reliable information about these interesting developments was, however, not available at the time of writing.

Lemke MC 404 Digital 2

We evaluated the new Lemke digital camera model (Lemke; Gröbenzell, Germany) in a prototype version (Fig. 2.11). The cameras of this company have long been on the marked under such names as Storz, Martin and Wisap.

All the electronics (with the exception of the CCD chip) were designed by Lemke and are integrated into a very compact camera body. The CCD signal is digitized ($3 \times 8 = 24$ bits) without further preamplification, immediately it comes from the 1/2-inch Sony chip. For this reason, an excellent S/N ratio of 55 dB is achieved, which, in combination with an ability to work in minimal illuminations of $1-3$ lux without increased gain, offers a noise-free image in all areas of endoscopic application.

Instead of an electronic shutter controlling the readout rate of the charge packets from the chip in fixed, recognizable steps, the MC 404 is equipped with continuous digital control of the chip sensitivity. This eliminates shutter effects. It operates by using a control signal to adjust the operating voltage of the picture elements on the chip, raising and lowering their threshold (zero) level to suit the ambient lighting.

The separated luminance and chrominance (Y and C) signals are digitally processed, using 8 bits for each.

The light measurement fields on the chip are adjustable by software between integral and spot metering.

After the camera is switched on, a digital system check is automatically carried out, including a test of the camera cable and a check of the colour memory.

When performing a white balance, the correct distance between lens and white test area is controlled by dialogue boxes on the monitor. Menus in these dialogue boxes may be accessed in any of four languages. The colour value is then permanently stored. The electronics are so stable as to be almost indestructible – even by a short-circuit of all poles. They are also well shielded from high-frequency interference. Any damage to the camera cable is displayed as a warning on the monitor, and the cable can be exchanged at any time in the operating theatre, without the use of tools.

The camera head is small and light and has an ergonomic focusing lever, operated with the thumb. This is even adjustable for left-handers. A practical express coupling for the ocular facilitates the sterile changing of the circular rod lens system, without the need for a new camera covering.

In the monitor test, the camera shows a resolution of 450 to 500 horizontal and vertical lines – unsurpassed among the single-chip cameras. The colours are finely tuned, especially in the all-important red range.

Thanks to well thought-out integration with a high-quality monitor system, picture quality and operating convenience are excellent. Instead of having a conventional cable junction, the flat, compact camera body is latched into a compartment on the side of the monitor. The picture signal is transmitted by contacts on the back of the camera.

The 43-cm monitor (a model with a 51-cm screen diagonal is under development), complete with cast metal body and a potential compensation connection, offers surprisingly high performance, clearly surpassing even the Siony PVM 2043. The Venetian effects, which often occur due to the misalignment of the lines of the two separately scann-

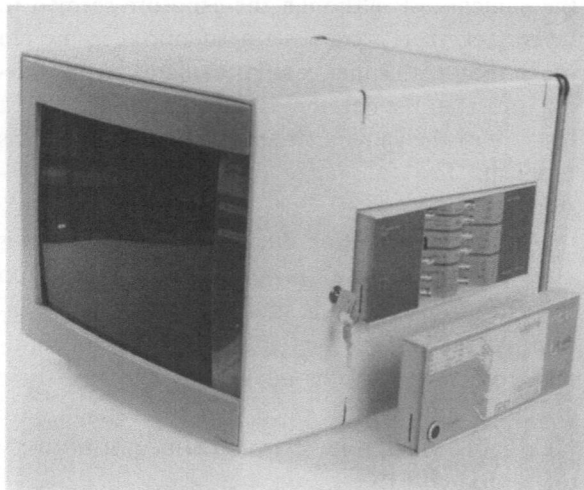

Fig. 2.11. Lemke MC 404 Digital 2

ed fields of an interlaced picture, are completely missing. Colours are finely tuned. In pictures from an S video signal (Y/C), the oscillation of the colour carrier (flickering along colour limits, for example at the colour bars) observed on all other monitors is filtered out, such that the picture quality corresponds to that of an RGB signal.

The built-in Phillips tubes with black-level stabilization and tinted glass screen offer a brilliant, high-contrast image, even in surroundings with high ambient light. A compensating circuit balances changes in tube performance due to age.

There is one composite, one S-video (Y/C) and one RGB in- and output as well as a data connection for image processing and documentation, remote control, and a rapid diagnostic routine for servicing. In the future, telephone diagnosis using an integrated modem is planned.

An new light source, controlled digitally by the camera, rounds off the new system. The light is, in fact, not controlled by the video signal, but by the same digital control signal which adjusts the chip's sensitivity. The metal oxide-vaporized mirror lamp (of only 75 W) is said to be 300% as efficient as other light sources and was certainly found in practice to be fully sufficient for all endoscopic applications.

At least for the present, the Lemke MC 404 prototype takes a leading position among single-chip cameras with regard to performance, ergonomics, and system integration.

Three-Chip Cameras

Stryker 784 Medical Video Camera

The Stryker 784 is a new model based on analog signal processing (Fig. 2.12). The camera head has average dimensions for a three-chip camera but is not too heavy and is easy to handle. An adaptation mechanism facilitates the connection of all kinds of circular rod lenses. At the camera processor there is an automatic white balance function, which in our test, however, tended to show too much red. With an additional colour adjustment regulator this could be corrected easily. When the camera cable is disconnected, the processor displays colour bars for monitor calibration.

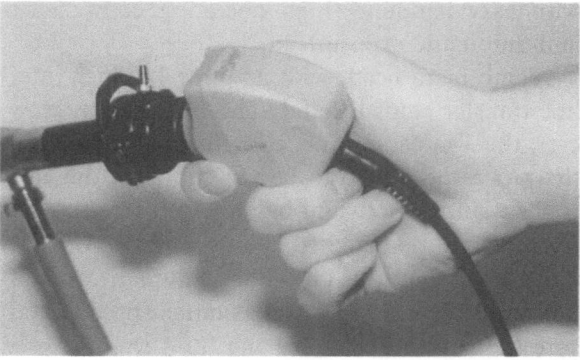

Fig. 2.12. Stryker 784 Medical Video Camera

The resolution values (>800 TV lines horizontally, 450 TV lines vertically) indicated by the manufacturer could not be tested because our Sony monitor PVM 2043 only shows a maximum of 600 lines. In fact, surprisingly, a resolution of 600 horizontal TV lines and 400 vertical TV lines could be measured with the resolution chart.

Colour representation was correct and well graduated; image control and edge accentuation, however, appeared too low and a slight flaring along black/white borders was visible.

Discrete noise in the standard mode (0 dB) increased noticeably in mode I (gain amplification of +9 dB). With a S/N ratio of 60 dB, as claimed by Stryker, the noise should be far less remarkable. Probably the excellent S/N ratio value and the extremely low minimum illuminance of 1,5 lux (without gain amplification) is due to a preamplification of the signal directly after the chips with the disadvantage of a certain increase in noise.

Only two composite and two S video outputs are provided. RGB and component outputs are missing. It is difficult to understand why Stryker engineers encode the internal RGB signal to composite and S video outputs, but do not offer the superior RGB signal to the user.

Storz Tricam 9070 BP

The new version of this camera, the Storz Tricam 9070 BP (Fig. 2.13), that we tested is a high-performance three-chip camera in which the severe problems of the older Tricam 9070 P have been overcome. Furthermore, it combines this performance with easy handling, high operating convenience, and automatic exposure.

The camera head, with its three 1/2-inch interline transfer chips is handy and lightweight. However, the 3-m cable connecting the camera head to the processor proved to be too short for our use.

The automatic white balance and internal colour bars are operated from the camera processor. Exposure is controlled by either automatic or manual adjustment of the CCD shutter speed. Exposure is fine-tuned between the fixed shutter-speed steps with an integrated automatic gain control (range: 0-+18 dB). A keyboard for character generation is an optional attachment.

Sufficient connections to monitors and recorders are all available – one RGB, one S video (Y/C) and one composite. However, a YUV component signal output for professional recording systems such as Betacam SP or M II is missing. This seems an unacceptable omission on a top of the range camera such as the Tricam 9070.

Using the resolution chart, the RGB signal from the camera displayed a brilliant and well-defined image, with 550 horizontal and 500 vertical lines on our monitor. The colour bar and grey scale test charts appeared correct on our monitor, but the vectorscope and the waveform monitor showed incorrect colour luminance levels (the yellow level in the composite signal, in particular, was too high). In correspondence with this, the clinical test indicated that the composite signal had too much yellow and too little red, and the RGB signal a little too much red. Storz engineers offered to make improvements in collaboration with us, and to test them under clinical conditions.

Sony DXC 750 P

Despite the weight and dimensions of its head (600 g, 70×75×113 mm) we use the Sony DXC 750 P (Fig. 2.14) with its three 2/3-inch interline transfer chips in our Tuebingen research group for top-quality documentation. However, it is not only for reasons of size and weight that this camera cannot be considered as part of a standard solution: the film plane had to be adjusted in order to mount adapted photographic lenses of fixed focal lengths of 35 and 55 mm and connect them to the circular rod lense optic. Moreover, this camera requires the continuous attention of a technician during its operation. This rather special solution is included here, however, because it represents the state-of-the-art with respect to picture quality and thus serves as an excellent reference. The camera processor offers manual control of many functions: white and black balance, gain in fixed steps of +0, +9, or +18 dB or continuously, detail compensation, selection of shutter speeds between 1/30 and 1/10000 s, and master pedestal control. A gamma correction circuit and a linear matrix circuit can be used to influence the luminance characteristics and

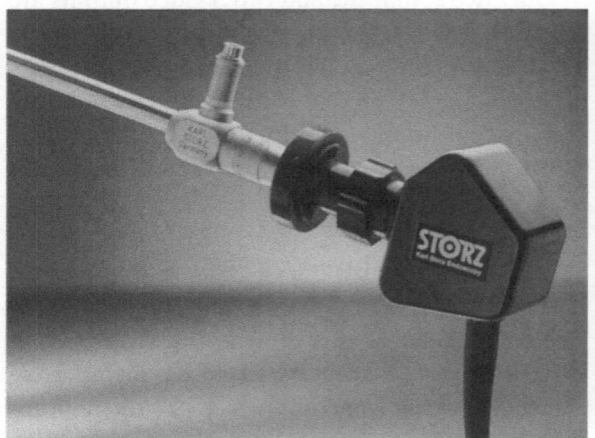

Fig. 2.13. Storz Tricam 9070 BP

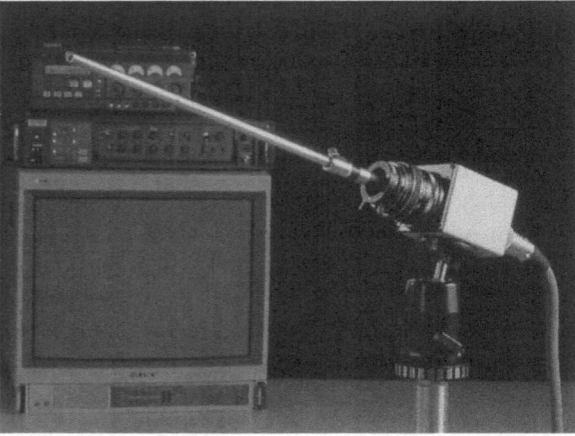

Fig. 2.14. Sony DXC 750 P

the colour rendering. However, all these functions (with the exception of the black or white colour balance) can only be operated manually. Because automatic exposure is missing, the video level has to be fine-tuned continuously (and manually!) during surgery, by a nonsterile technican, in order to obtain high-quality recordings.

Minimum illumination is 25 lux at F 1.4 and +18 dB: this means that the camera requires much more light than all the single-chip cameras. We have found, however, that strong standard light sources, combined with a fluid cable, provide enough light for almost all minimally invasive operations, without the need to increase the electronic gain. Nevertheless, in the rare cases in which extra gain is required, this results in significant noise and the noticeable reduction of the otherwise superior image quality.

All the necessary outputs, including those for professional video recording systems, are provided: two composite, one S video (Y/C) and two RGB. One of the RGB outputs can be switched to provide the YUV component signal required for systems such as Betacam SP or M II. The camera can be genlocked externally if the synchronized use of more than one camera at a time is required.

Internal colour bars for monitor calibration and an LED to indicate low light conditions are also offered. A keypad to generate characters is included.

With our monitor connected to the RGB output, the resolution chart showed 600 lines, both horizontally and vertically. This defines the Sony DXC 750 P as offering the finest picture available for endoscopic used. Both the colour reproduction and the grey-scale signal were perfect in the monitor test and on the waveform monitor and vectorscope (Table 2.7 see p. 88, 89).

Future Prospects

In the next few years a transition from analog to digital video processing is to be expected. Affordable digital video systems compatible to analog component equipment will increasingly be used in professional production studios. These new techniques will also be integrated into equipment for use in endoscopic surgery.

In addition to increased resolution and excellent multi-generation performance, the benefits will be a more efficient interface to computer based image processing and documentation. The possibility of a noninterlaced monitor picture representation with high frequency (>72 cycles per second) and even new picture formats with higher definitions due to digital signal processing is an interesting open question.

Intermediate stages on the way to HDTV will bring with them improvement still compatible to today's video standards; with the introduction of Palplus in 1995 the picture format will change to 16:9.

An important task will be the integration of camera and video functions into an microprocessor-controlled central control panel for surgeons and technicians in a future endoscopic operating theatre.

Table 2.7. Comparison of camera parameters

	Single-chip cameras				
	Wolf CCD Endocam 5501	Stryker 594 Medical Video Camera	Storz Endocam PAL	AVT Horn MC 1009/F	MP Video Medicam 900
Image sensor	1/2″ Interline transfer CCD chip (Matsushita)	1/2″ CCD	1/2″ Interline transfer CCD	1/2″ Interline transfer Hyper HAD CCD (Sony)	1/2″ CCD
CCD resolution	681 (H) × 582 (V) lines	681 (H) × 582 (V)	752 (H) × 582 (V) lines	752 (H) × 582 (V) lines	1 lux (boost on)
Minimum illuminance	3 lux at f 1.4 (+ 12 dB gain)	3 lux	3 lux at f 1.4	4.5 lux at f : 1.2 (AGC on)	
Signal/Noise ratio	>46 dB	46 dB	50 dB	>46 dB	48 dB
TV resolution (information given by manufacturers)	430 TV lines horizontally 410 TV lines vertically	>500 TV lines horizontally	>400 TV lines (horizontally)	460 TV lines	>500 TV lines
TV resolution (our measurements on Sony monitor PVM 2043)	420 TV lines horizontally 400 TV lines vertically	400 TV lines horizontally and vertically	350 TV lines horizontally 400 lines vertically	400 TV lines horizontally and vertically	400 TV lines horizontally 450 TV lines vertically
Automatic shutter control	No	1/60 − 1/10000 s in fixed steps	1/60 − 1/10000 s in fixed steps	1/25 − 1/1000 s in fixed steps	Continuously
Automatic gain control	No; manual gain control low + 6 dB mid + 9 dB high + 12 dB	No; manual gain control standard 0 dB, II + 9 dB, I + 18 dB	− 4 dB- + 14 dB	0 dB- + 12 dB	Yes ("boost circuit")
Automatic white balance	From halogen to hti or xenon light	Yes	Range: 2200 K − 6500 K	No; manual or continuous white balance control	Yes
Output	1 Composite 1 S video (Y/C)	2 Composite 2 S video	1 Composite 2 S video (Y/C) 1 RGB	1 Composite	2 Composite 2 S video (Y/C) 1 RGB
Dimensions of camera head	2.7 × 5.0 cm (RM-mount) 2.8 × 10.0 cm (c-mount)	70 × 50 × 45 mm (incl. lens)	2.8 × 6.8 cm	12.0 × 2.2 × 2.2 cm	3.7 cm (dia), 4.8 cm long
Weight of the camera head (g)	60 (RW-mount) 120 (c-mount)	55	113	95	84

Single-chip cameras		Three-chip cameras		
Circon Micro Digital-1	Lemke MC 404 Digital 2	Stryker 784 Medical Video Camera	Storz Tricam 9070 BP	Sony DXC 750 P
1/2″ CCD	1/2″ Lens-on-chip CCD (Matsushita)	3 × 1/2″ Hyper-HAD-CCD	3 × 1/2″ Interline transfer CCD chips	3 × 2/3″ Interline transfer chips
410 000 pixel	682 lines/ 480 000 pixel	752 (H) × 582 (V)	752 (H) × 582 (V) lines	786 (H) × 581 (V) lines
5 lux (0 dB) 1 lux (+ 12 db)	1 – 3 lux (no gain)	1.5 lux (standard mode, no gain)	6 lux at 1.4 (auto mode)	25 lux at f 1.4 (+ 18 dB)
56 dB	55 dB	> 60 dB	52 dB	58 dB
No information	510 TV lines	> 800 TV lines horizontally 450 TV lines vertically	> 600 TV lines	700 TV lines
400 TV lines horizontally and vertically	450 – 500 TV lines horizontally and vertically	600 TV lines horizontally 400 TV lines vertically	550 TV lines horizontally 500 TV lines vertically	600 TV lines horizontally and vertically
1/60 – 1/15 700 s in fixed steps	No; continuous control of CCD sensitivity 1 : 16 000	Yes; manual and automatic mode	1/30 – 1/10 000 s in fixed steps	No; manual shutter control from 1/25 – 1/10 000 s
No; manual gain control low + 3 dB mid + 6 dB high + 12 dB	Up to + 100% of the normal signal	Manual gain control + 9 dB (mode I)	+ 18 dB maximum	No; manual gain control + 9 dB + 18 dB and manual fine tuning
Range: 0 K – 6900 K	All light sources: monitor menu with colour value memory	2800 K – 6500 K	2200 K – 8600 K	Automatic and manual black and white controls
2 Composite 2 S video (Y/C) 1 RGB	1 Composite 1 S video (Y/C) 1 RGB	2 Composite 2 S video	1 Composite 1 S video (Y/C) 1 RGB	3 Composite 1 S video (V/C) 2 RGB (1 switchable as YUV component signal)
8.9 × 2.1 × 3.8 cm	6.0 × 2.2 × 2.2	103 × 56 × 45 mm (incl. lens)	4.3 × 5.7 × 3.6 cm	7.0 × 7.5 × 11.3 cm
90 incl. optic	59	No information	230	600, without cable and lens

Suggested Reading

1. Buess G, Faust U, Feinauer B (1990) Endoskopie – von der Diagnostik bis zur neuen Chirurgie. Deutscher Ärzte-Verlag, Cologne
2. BTS Broadcast Television Systems (1991) „3. Darmstädter Fernsehtage '91 – ein technisch-wissenschaftliches Symposium"
3. Bücken R (1992) NAB '92: Digitale HDTV-Premiere. Medien Bull 9
4. Bücken R (1992) Die Produktionstechnik für HDTV. Kameramann 7:24–33
5. Bücken R (1992) Industrie wirft HD-MAC nicht weg. Kameramann 4
6. Clason WE (1975) Elsevier's dictionary of television and video recording. Elsevier, Amsterdam
7. Fuchs C (1992) Europäische HDTV-Übertragungsnorm schon tot? Ein Gespräch mit C.E.R.I.S.E.-Mitarbeiter Jean-Paul Thorn. Kameramann 7:66–68
8. Hilgeford U (1992) Schrägspur-Medium. Grundlegendes zur analogen Videotechnik. c't Magazin für Computertechnik 10
9. Hübscher H et al (1989) Elektrotechnik Fachbildung, Kommunikationselektronik 2, Radio-/Fernseh-/Funktechnik. Westermann, Brunswick
10. Johnson P A guide to CCD sensors. BTS GmbH, Darmstadt
11. Kammann U (1992) 16:9 steigt auf – D2-MAC stürzt ab. Interview mit Albrecht Ziemer, dem Technischen Direktor des ZDF. Kameramann 8:128–148
12. Kling B (1992) Post-Produktion für PALplus-Demovideo. Kameramann 6:94–95
13. Luther AC (1991) Digital video in the PC environment. McGraw-Hill, New York
14. Millerson G (1987) Video production handbook. Focal, London
15. Müller AH (1992) Der elektronische Schnitt. HV & F Heiko Sven Hausemann, Hamburg
16. Rabiger M (1989) Directing – film techniques and aesthetics. Focal, Boston
17. Sheldon I (1991) The evolution of CCD imagers. Sony Broadcast and Communications, Basingstoke
18. Tektronix (1990) Signal measurements – PAL systems. Tektronix, Beaverton
19. van Appeldoorn W (1992) HDTV in aller Munde. Kameramann 4
20. Webers J (1991) Handbuch der Film- und Videotechnik: die Aufnahme, Speicherung und Wiedergabe audio-visueller Programme. Franzis, Munich
21. Westendorff T (1985) Video-Grundlagen. Einführung in die Fernsehtechnik. elrad 10–12, 1984 and 1–3 1985
22. Whelan JM, Jackson DW (1992) Videoarthroscopy: review and state of the art. Arthroscopy 8(3):311–319

Appendix: Camera producers

Richard Wolf GmbH
Pforzheimer Str. 32
Postfach 40
75438 Knittlingen
Germany

Stryker Endoscopy
210 Baypointe Parkway
San Jose, California 95134
USA

Karl Storz GmbH & Co.
Mittelstr. 8
78532 Tuttlingen
Germany

AVT Horn
Langertstr. 76
73431 Aalen

MP Video
Kirschner Medical Corporation
63 South St., Hopkinton
MA 01748
USA

Circon Corporation
460 Ward Drive
Santa Barbara, California 93111
USA

Lemke GmbH
Danziger Str. 21
82194 Gröbenzell
Germany

Sony Corporation
Tokyo
Japan

3 Anaesthetic Management in Endoscopic Surgery

B. M. KOTTLER and G. LENZ

Introduction

The techniques of endoscopic surgery have ushered a revolution in traditional surgery. Many operations which previously entailed substantial stress to patients can now be carried out endoscopically with minimal discomfort. This has led to more extensive use of endoscopic surgery, not least in risk patients. The endoscopic technique has the following advantages over open surgical procedures: less perioperative stress for the patient, minimal postoperative discomfort due to small incisions, in most cases only moderate postoperative pain, superior cosmetic results, short hospitalization times, performance on an outpatient or short-stay basis, shortened return to normal activity and savings in costs [6, 10, 15].

The principles of anaesthetic management for endoscopic surgery focusing on laparoscopic and thoracoscopic procedures using CO_2 gas insufflation will be discussed in this chapter.

General Considerations

Endoscopic surgery is widely referred to [8] as minimally invasive surgery (MIS). With regard to anaesthesia for MIS, a statement by Shanta and Harden is valid not only for laparoscopy but also for many endoscopic techniques: "Laparoscopic surgery is not a benign procedure. It is associated with minor and major complications, including death" [36]. Serious problems, which cannot always be treated successfully, include gas embolism and cardiovascular collapse [19, 36]. Therefore maximum perioperative anaesthetic patient care is advisable despite the alleged "minimal" surgical nature of many endoscopic procedures.

There is no special anaesthesia for endoscopic operations. Thus every patient who has to undergo an endoscopic operation should be treated in accordance with generally recognized anaesthetic procedures. In principle if the patient is able to undergo anaesthesia, he can be treated by endoscopic surgery. However, this should not preclude a discussion of the advantages and disadvantages of endoscopic or open surgery between the surgeon and the anaesthetist in individual cases.

If the patient has a history of retinal haemorrhage, laparoscopy should only be considered with great reservation. Case reports of visual impairment following laparoscopy support the assumption that pneumoperitoneum and the Trendelenburg position may contribute to a potentially harmful increase in retinal venous pressure [38]. Laparoscopy must also be regarded as relatively or absolutely contraindicated in patients with ventriculoperitoneal or peritoneovenous shunts. If a ventriculoperitoneal shunt (part of which is tunnelled into the subcutaneous tissues before its entry into the abdomen) has only been set up a short time previously, there may be ventilatory impairment due to massive subcutaneous emphysema during laparoscopy [35]. Elective laparoscopic surgery should therefore be delayed until the tract has fibrosed and sealed. Peritoneovenous catheters such as Denver shunt have a valve which opens at a pressure differential of $2 \, cmH_2O$. This is associated with a high risk of air or CO_2 embolism, and therefore laparoscopy is absolutely contraindicated [35].

Minor gynaecologic operations of short duration such as diagnostic pelvic laparoscopy or clip sterilization are frequently performed safely under general anaesthesia with mask ventilation or even with local infiltration anaesthesia in the periumbilical region where the trocar will be introduced [15, 44]. Kenefick et al. found that despite spontaneous ventilation via a mask only moderate hypercarbia developed under 2% – 3% isoflurane in oxygen and 65% nitrous oxide in women undergoing laparoscopy for investigation of infertility [21]. Significant acidosis or cardiac arrhythmia were also absent.

In principle, laparoscopic operations can also be carried out under spinal or epidural anaesthesia [36]. However, this does not appear to be a real alternative and should be reserved for occasional cases. Prerequisites include no prior respiratory or cardiac disease and good patient compliance during the operation and cooperation from the surgeon. Deep intraoperative sedation should be avoided, since the patient must be able to react to the raised CO_2 due to artificial CO_2 pneumoperitoneum with an increase of the respiratory minute volume and maintenance of normocarbia. Despite blockade of appropriate nerve segments (T2−L1), patient discomfort such as nausea and vomiting have to be coped with intraoperatively. Irritation and pain in the area innervated by the phrenic nerve (cervical segments 3−5, infraclavicular area, shoulder, neck) are also common [36] because of insufflation of the peritoneal cavity with CO_2 [36]. Spinal or epidural anaesthesia will not block this cervical spinal segment-mediated pain.

Considering the advantages and disadvantages of various methods of anaesthesia in laparoscopy, general anaesthesia with tracheal intubation and controlled ventilation is the best choice in most cases, especially if the upper abdomen is the target of surgical intervention and the operation is expected to last long. This is corroborated in particular by the following advantages over other techniques: better control of the cardiorespiratory state, simple maintenance of an adequate pCO_2 during controlled ventilation, no risk of aspiration, possibility of complete muscle relaxation and easy positioning of the patient in deep head-down tilt or other positions not easily tolerated by conscious patients [15].

With thoracoscopic methods, single-lung anaesthesia is required in most instances. This can only be effected under general anaesthesia with double-lumen endobronchial intubation [16].

Endoluminal rectal surgical procedures can be performed after consultation with the surgeon under regional anaesthesia (e.g., lumbar subarachnoid or epidural nerve block). The decision in favour of a specific method of anaesthesia should take into consideration the expected duration of the operation and the required patient positioning. If a prone position is necessary or a long procedure is expected, general anaesthesia should be planned from the start. If uncontrolled coughing or movement of the patient or general agitation occur under regional anaesthesia, it may be necessary to continue the operation under general anaesthesia. It is therefore advisable to point this out to the patient when the physician administers premedication.

No recommendations can be made with regard to the choice of anaesthetic for general anaesthesia. In many cases, inhalation anaesthesia [21] or a balanced anaesthesia, e.g. with volatile anaesthetics, opiates and nondepolarizing muscle relaxants [15, 19], is very suitable. Total intravenous anaesthetic techniques e.g. using, for example, propofol-fentanyl-vecuronium have also been employed successfully [34]. The question is still open as to whether these really have any material advantages over volatile anaesthetics. However, it is possible that they more likely comply with the stipulations of the anaesthetist that the patient should recover from the anaesthesia as quickly as possible after endoscopic surgery, especially when using short-acting drugs. The use of nitrous oxide during laparoscopy is controversial because of concerns regarding its contribution to bowel distension, to the increased postoperative nausea and (in the case of intentional or unintentional bowel perforation with subsequent release of volatile bowel gas) the possibility of concentrations in the peritoneal cavity high enough to support combustion of bowel gas [6, 31, 39]. However, in a study involving 50 patients undergoing elective laparoscopic cholecystectomy, Taylor et al. found no significant differences between the groups receiving isoflurane in an air/oxygen mixture or with 70% nitrous oxide in oxygen with respect to operative conditions, bowel distension and the incidence of postoperative nausea or vomiting [39]. Thus, use of nitrous oxide does not have to be dispensed with in laparoscopic cholecystectomy [21, 39].

Perioperative use of analgesics, including morphine and fentanyl, can cause spasm of the sphincter of Oddi. However, there is no reason to regard opiates, for example, as being contraindicated on this account. The incidence of spasm may be decreased by administration of small incremental doses (titration) until the desired analgesic effect is attained. If difficulties nevertheless arise in imaging contrast flow into the duodenum during intraoperative cholangiography in the course of laparoscopic cholecystectomy, the spasm of the sphincter of Oddi can be easily abolished by intravenous administration of 1.0 mg glucagon [15].

Divergent views are expressed on the question as to whether endoscopic surgery should be restricted to patients without impaired cardiovascular and respiratory function. There is no general answer to this question and it must be emphasized that each patient should be assessed on an individual basis considering, in particular, the following factors: underlying cardiac or pulmonary disease, endoscopic technique, expected duration of the procedure and intraoperative positioning. Furthermore, it must be taken into consideration that the different endoscopic procedures may have dissimilar impact on the cardiovascular and respiratory state. Patients at cardiac risk are alleged to be stressed only minimally by most endoluminal rectal surgical interventions. On the other hand, patients compromised by cardiovascular conditions may respond unpredictably to haemodynamic changes induced by laparoscopic or thoracoscopic procedures.

Nevertheless, bearing in mind that appropriate invasive monitoring will be required for effective management [15], patients with cardiac or respiratory risks should not be generally excluded from endoscopic surgery. Intraoperative surveillance and maintenance of adequate oxygenation, perfusion and stable heart rate are frequently difficult. They are a challenge to the anaesthetist. With experienced and skilled surgical and anaesthetic staff, extensive perioperative monitoring of vital parameters and choice of noncardiodepressant and short-acting drugs, patients at risk can also be anaesthetized with a high margin of safety. However, the anaesthetist should be prepared to recommend instant conversion to an open technique if haemodynamic, oxygenation, or ventilation difficulties occur during the endoscopic procedure [6].

Monitoring

Standard intraoperative patient monitoring comprises continuous evaluation of the patient's oxygenation, ventilation, circulation and temperature. It is essential to monitor vital signs continuously, especially in laparoscopic and thoracoscopic procedures. Minor or major complications may occur suddenly and unexpectedly.

Oxygenation is best assessed by means of pulse oximetry. Easy methods of checking ventilation include observation of chest wall excursions and auscultation of bilateral respiratory sounds. It is prudent to repeat lung auscultation during each change of position, after insufflation of the peritoneal cavity with CO_2, during all periods in which a fall in oxygen saturation is detected, and after extubation [36]. Particularly in thoracic procedures involving the lower mediastinum, there is an increased risk of unilateral or bilateral pneumothorax and pneumomediastinum. During laparoscopy, properly placed endotracheal tubes may inadvertently move deeper and enter the main bronchial stem. This may occur, for example, if the patient is in the steep Trendelenburg position and the hilus of the lung is displaced upwards [36].

End-tidal CO_2 analysis (ETCO$_2$) is essential. It is inevitable that ETCO$_2$ will rise rapidly during laparoscopy with CO_2 pneumoperitoneum. This results from mechanical impairment of ventilation in consequence of CO_2-induced abdominal distension and systemic absorption of CO_2 from the peritoneal cavity [15]. Controlled hyperventilation with small tidal volumes will easily restore adequate ETCO$_2$ levels. Large tidal volumes should be avoided because this causes undesirable movements of the liver and gallbladder [36]. During laparoscopic cholecystectomy, ETCO$_2$ almost always accurately reflects changing arterial CO_2 levels [25, 28]. ΔCO_2 (PaCO$_2$ − ETCO$_2$) should therefore be within normal limits, with median values between 2 and 4.5 mmHg in adults [11]; ETCO$_2$ can be used to adapt ventilation reliably. However, if there is any doubt, arterial blood gas analysis should be performed immediately. A greater difference between PaCO$_2$ and ETCO$_2$ can be expected during thoracoscopic procedures. While ventilation of the upper lung is discontinued, there is a right-left shunt through the upper lung with an increase in

$PaCO_2$ and ΔCO_2 difference respectively [11]. However, this $PaCO_2 - ETCO_2$ difference may not be any greater than the original, combined two-lung ΔCO_2 [11]. For calculation of ΔCO_2 and appropriate adjustment of ventilation by means of repeated blood gas measurements during thoracoscopy, indwelling arterial cannulation is necessary.

To ensure the adequacy of circulatory function, the following parameters should be determined: electrocardiogram (ECG), blood pressure measurement and pulse plethysmography or oximetry. The five-lead ECG will enable ST segment measurement and early detection of myocardial ischaemia [18, 36]. Besides this, noninvasive impedance cardiography, which enables stroke volume and cardiac output to be calculated, has been successfully performed in patients undergoing laparoscopy [19, 23]. Depending on the individual patient's condition and the endoscopic procedure, additional invasive monitoring techniques (e.g. arterial cannulation, central venous catheter, pulmonary arterial monitoring) should be considered.

Patient Positioning

Frequent intraoperative changes in the position of the patient are characteristic for endoscopic surgery. Primary patient positioning in a supine, prone, lateral decubitus, lithotomy, Trendelenburg or reverse Trendelenburg position depends on the area of surgery. Additional positioning variants are possible by tilting the operating table during the operation.

It is essential that the patient cannot slip off the operating table in any conceivable position. Shanta et al. described a case in which the upper body, including the neck and head, of a patient slid off the operating table during laparoscopic cholecystectomy when the patient was put into reverse Trendelenburg position with rotation to the left [36]. Any patient should therefore be secured to the operating table using two belts (knee and chest). The chest belt should allow respiratory movements of the chest [36].

Positioning for endoscopic surgery may often result in difficult and tedious access to the patient's head and endotracheal tube. Use of nonkinking

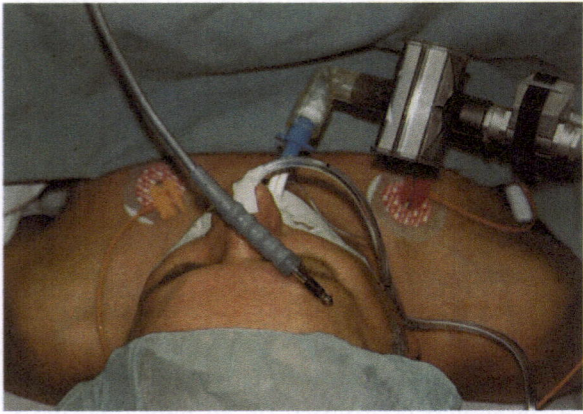

Fig. 3.1. Video equipment cable: a possible hazardous source of eye injury during endoscopic procedures

(e.g. reinforced) endotracheal tubes is to be recommended. Care is also needed to protect the eyes from drying out and from direct trauma [12]. Video equipment cables crossing over the region of head can cause severe eye injuries in inadvertent disconnections or by accidentally dropped cable ends. Protective measures such as eyeshields therefore appear to be mandatory (Fig. 3.1).

Despite all precautionary measures, there is a residual risk of nervous or tissue damage due to intraoperative positioning in individual cases. The following factors can increase this risk: occlusive arterial disease, diabetic neuropathy, exaggerated and long-lasting positioning (e.g. steep reverse Trendelenburg position), hypotension, intraoperative hypothermia, obesity, vasoconstriction and prolonged surgical procedures [20, 29, 42].

A lower limb neuropathy after laparoscopic operations is a multifactorial process. Nerve damage, venous thrombosis, compartment syndrome or a combination of these three clinical conditions must be considered in the differential diagnosis. Restraining belts placed across the upper thighs or just below the knees in conjunction with steep reverse Trendelenburg's position during laparoscopic cholecystectomy were the putative causes of lower limb neuropathies (meralgia paresthetica, peroneal neuropathy) in two obese patients [20].

According to data presented by Warner and Martin on 198461 consecutive Mayo Clinic surgical/anaesthetic lithotomy patients operated on between 1957 and 1991, the incidence of persistent lower limb nerve injury is approximately 1 : 3675 [42]. Intra-abdominal CO_2 insufflation causes an increase of up to 78% in femoral venous pressure in most patients, and therefore promotes venous stasis and deep vein thrombosis [1]. Compartment syndrome is defined as a symptom complex caused by elevated pressure of tissue fluid in a closed osseofascial compartment of the limb, with consecutive decrease of blood circulation to the myoneural components [29]. Possible mechanisms include decreased leg perfusion by elevation of the limb above the heart, excessive local pressure from improper placement of the legs in the holders, external pressure from equipment or staff, and compression of pelvic vessels [29]. Compartment syndrome requiring surgical fasciotomy occurred with a probability of 1 : 39692 in the retrospective lithotomy position survey of Warner and Martin [42].

Endoluminal rectal surgery must often be performed in the prone position. Careful positioning with special regard to the head and neck can diminish severe neurovascular disturbance. Above all, maintenance of a neutral cervical position and avoidance of obstruction to the cerebral arterial inflow and venous outflow are essential protective measures. Numerous case reports are available showing severe injuries due to the prone position, e.g. eye trauma following direct pressure [12], lingual and buccal nerve neuropathy [43], and even quadraplegia in a patient with cervical spondylosis [9]. Patients with severe carotid artery stenosis, poor intracranial compliance, and cervical spondylosis appear to be unsuitable candidates for intraoperative prone positioning [9, 26].

Ensuring a correct intraoperative patient position is a joint task of the surgeon and anaesthetist. From the viewpoint of the anaesthetist, measures to prevent positioning injuries should be concentrated on very meticulous positioning and fixation of the patient. Endangered parts of the body should be cushioned well. Improper patient position may sometimes be detected by pulse oximetry [17], for example, if the radial pulse disappears after abduction of the arm during positioning (hyperabduction syndrome). Figure 3.2 shows body regions which are especially prone to nervous or tissue damage. The intraoperative anaesthetic management should aim, above all, to maintain constant temperature

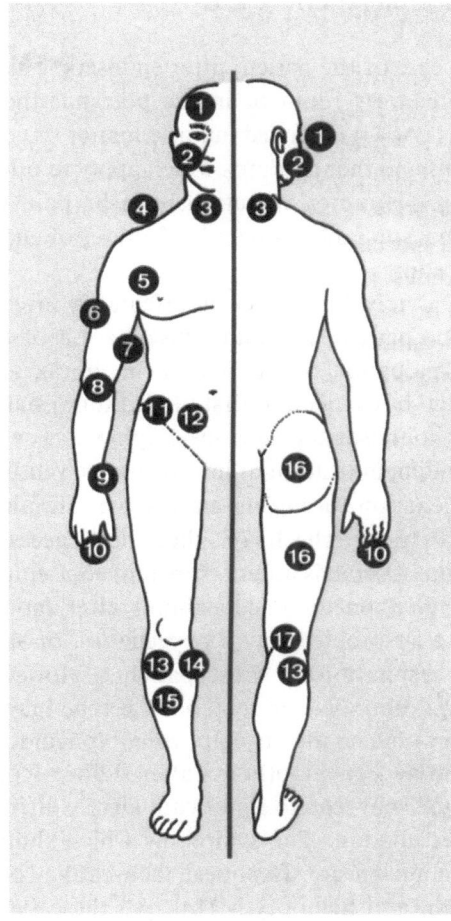

Fig. 3.2. Body regions especially prone to nervous or tissue damage. *1*, eye; *2*, buccal, facial, hypoglossal and trigeminal nerve; *3*, neck; *4*, accessory nerve; *5*, brachial plexus; *6*, radial nerve; *7*, median and ulnar nerve; *8*, ulnar nerve; *9*, median nerve; *10*, fingers; *11*, lateral femoral cutaneous nerve; *12*, femoral nerve; *13*, common peroneal nerve; *14*, saphenous nerve; *15*, superficial and deep peroneal nerve; *16*, siciatic nerve; *17*, tibial and common peroneal nerve

(normothermia or only slight hypothermia) and blood pressure (normotension). If a steep reverse Trendelenburg position is necessary for laparoscopy in obese patients, it is recommended that the body weight be supported by additional foot boards [20]. One can then avoid the weight of the patient being mainly concentrated on the lower limb straps. Venous stasis during laparoscopy may be counteracted by pneumatic compressive stockings [1]. Unfortunately, any occlusive bandages may promote compartment syndrome [29].

Postanaesthetic Care

The care of the patient after endoscopic surgery in the recovery room or in the postanaesthesia care unit (PACU) is carried out as a matter of course according to the standards which apply to other operations. However, attention is to be paid to some typical special postoperative features of endoscopic procedures.

On arrival in PACU, an orientative investigation of the patient, including auscultation of the lung and palpation of the abdomen, thorax and neck should be carried out first of all. Abnormal respiratory sounds, subcutaneous emphysema or a corresponding indication of intraoperative ventilation or oxygenation problems necessitate an immediate chest X-ray check of the chest necessary. If pneumothorax is absent, subcutaneous emphysema and even pneumomediastinum after laparoscopy cause no problems with oxygenation or spontaneous respiration in most patients. However, if a pneumothorax is present, a chest tube may be necessary. Subcutaneous emphysema, pneumomediastinum and pneumothorax after thoracoscopic procedures may lead to significant airway difficulty after extubation. The symptoms which should alert the clinician are dyspnoea, tachycardia, persistent cough, and hemoptysis [14]. All these symptoms, including the X-ray appearance, may become manifest for the first time at the end of the operation after extubation. If this is the case, a tracheal rupture must be ruled out or verified by flexible bronchoscopy. Tracheal tears due to the use of double-lumen endobronchial tubes are a rare but recognized complication. This is also the case with the newer, disposable polyvinylchloride tubes, which were only initially thought to be safer than the red rubber tubes [14]. Frequently treatment entails surgical suture closure of the tracheal injury.

Ventilation should be monitored by pulse oximetry in the PACU. Postoperative respiratory function is likely to be less impaired and its recovery improved after laparoscopy compared to open surgical techniques. Putensen-Himmer et al. [34] found that forced vital capacity and forced expiratory volume in 1 s were significantly greater in the laparoscopy than in the laparotomy group at 6, 24 and 72 h after cholecystectomy operation. Further, higher arterial O_2 tensions were observed in the

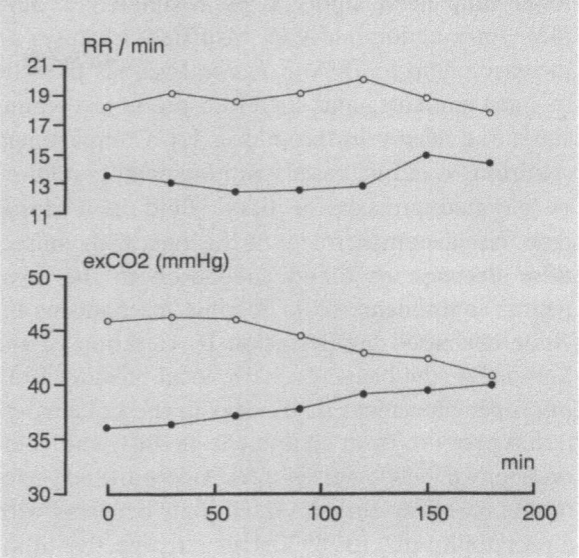

Fig. 3.3. The effect of CO_2 in the peritoneal cavity on postoperative spontaneous respiration (*RR*, respiratory rate; *exCO2*, endexpiratory carbon dioxide) in patients undergoing laparoscopic cholecystectomy (*open circles*) or laparotomy for cholecystectomy (*solid circles*). (From [40])

laparoscopic cholecystectomy group. Nevertheless, the remaining CO_2 after laparoscopy has important implications for postoperative spontaneous respiration in the immediate postoperative period in PACU. For up to 3 h, the respiratory rate is increased to eliminate residual CO_2 [40]. Patients in whom the laparoscopic technique has been used also show a significantly raised expiratory CO_2 in the first three postoperative hours as compared to open cholecystectomy (Fig. 3.3). This may not be a problem for the patient with normal respiratory function. Oxygen saturation will not be affected in spite of high expiratory CO_2. However, if methods or drugs such as opiates, which are capable of decreasing CO_2 response, are used residual CO_2 elimination will take longer. This is highly relevant in patients with underlying cardiac and pulmonary diseases such as heart failure, hypotension and emphysema [40].

Inadvertent blood vessel (aorta, iliac artery, iliac vein) injury can occur during all laparoscopic procedures. This may not be noticed during the operation [33]. It is therefore very important to check all patients in PACU for clinical signs of hypotension and bleeding. Moreover, hematocrit measurement should be considered if there is any doubt. Oza et al. [33] reported a case of a 35-year-old woman who underwent an uneventful laparoscopic sterilization. In the recovery room, the patient developed progressive hypotension over 1 h and a significant fall in hematocrit. Emergency relaparotomy revealed a puncture wound on the right lateral aspect of the aorta, midway between the right renal artery and the origin of the inferior mesenteric artery [33].

After laparoscopic surgery, many patients suffer from nausea and vomiting. Risk factors are obesity, gender (female), young age, history of prior nausea and vomiting following anaesthesia, uncontrolled pain and ambulation [13]. Small doses of droperidol (up to 20 µg/kg) are prophylactic and can be administered after induction of anaesthesia, at least in patients who are known to be at increased risk. Even doses of droperidol as low as 5 µg/kg may be effective [13]. Severe side effects of droperidol such as sedation, extrapyramidal symptoms, dysphoric reactions and psychosis should not be a problem as long as small doses are used.

There is no reason for withholding potent analgesics such as opiates in postoperative pain management if they are required — although endoscopic procedures cause little pain because of small incisions. Upper body muscle pains in the neck and shoulder and stiffness are common after laparoscopy [37] and most patients require more than 3 days recovery time before they can resume normal activity. Nonsteroid anti-inflammatory drugs also have an effective analgesic potency and minimize the incidence of nausea and vomiting [32]. They may be superior to opiates because somnolence and respiratory depression are absent and the length of the PACU stay can be decreased.

Laparoscopy

After induction of anaesthesia, a nasogastric or orogastric tube (Salem sump catheter) is inserted to reduce the risk of injury by a Verres needle or the trocar to the stomach and to facilitate laparoscopy [15]. Bladder catheterization is often considered necessary in laparoscopic procedures. However, if the patients are instructed to empty their bladders shortly before operation, bladder catheters can be

safely dispensed with during laparoscopic cholecystectomy [30]. Because of the extremely low incidence of gas embolism during laparoscopy, ultrasonographic techniques (Doppler) are not recommended for gas detection [41].

Intraperitoneal CO_2 insufflation should be performed slowly and the resulting intra-abdominal pressure should not be higher than 12–15 mmHg [36]. CO_2 is normally absorbed rapidly via the splanchnic vessels and intravascular entry of small amounts of CO_2 will therefore not cause cardiovascular disturbance because it is highly soluble in blood [15]. However, it must be stressed that high intra-abdominal pressures or anaesthetic techniques that reduce splanchnic blood flow may diminish CO_2 absorption and increase the likelihood of symptomatic CO_2 embolism.

During laparoscopic surgical interventions, the Trendelenburg position (e.g. gynaecological laparoscopy), steep reverse Trendelenburg position (e.g. laparoscopic cholecystectomy) or lateral tilt may be required [5, 15, 36]. With Trendelenburg tilt and CO_2 pneumoperitoneum, haemodynamic changes include a reduction in stroke volume and in cardiac index and increase of total peripheral resistance, blood pressure and central venous pressure [15, 19, 23, 36]. During reverse Trendelenburg position, decreased venous return may be in part responsible for the fall in blood pressure frequently noticed. The effect of intraoperative positioning and pneumoperitoneum on venous return and blood pressure is largely dependent on the patient's individual intravascular volume status prior to CO_2 insufflation [15]. Anaesthetic considerations and management of special complications are summarized in Table 3.1.

Cardiovascular collapse during induction of CO_2 pneumoperitoneum or initial trocar insertion may be due to bleeding, CO_2 embolism or pneumothorax. During laparoscopy, intra-abdominal structures, including blood vessels, may be unintentionally injured and intraoperative haemorrhage may follow.

Clinical signs of venous CO_2 embolism may be present immediately in most cases, but delayed onset in the postoperative period is also possible [27]. If intravenous embolism of large amounts of CO_2 occurs, a dramatic fall in blood pressure, dysrhythmia, cyanosis and pulmonary oedema may be no-

Table 3.1. Complications during laparoscopic surgery and anaesthetic management

Complication	Symptoms	Therapy
Bleeding	Hypotension, tachycardia	Surgical treatment, volume replacement
Cardiac dysrhythmia	Absence of normal preoperative cardiac rhythm	Exclude CO_2 embolism, hypercarbia, hypoxia, hypotension, cardiac ischaemia, light anaesthesia and pneumothorax
CO_2 embolism	Decrease of cardiac output, cardiac collapse, mill wheel or other heart murmurs, cyanosis, pulmonary oedema	Change position to left lateral with head down (Durant position), immediate deflation of pneumoperitoneum, cardiopulmonary resuscitation, insertion of a central venous catheter for gas aspiration; consider emergency cardiopulmonary bypass if available
Hypercarbia	Increasing $ETCO_2$	Adjustment of adequate ventilation; exclude CO_2 embolism, pneumothorax and subcutaneous emphysema; reduce intra-abdominal pressure
Hypertension	Increase in blood pressure above preoperative values	Exclude or treat hypercarbia by adjustment of adequate ventilation
Hypotension	Decrease in blood pressure below preoperative values	Exclude bleeding, CO_2 embolism, pneumothorax, vasovagal reflex and intravenous fluid deficit; decrease high insufflating pressure; head down position, volume replacement and vasopressor in case of orthostatic collapse
Pneumothorax	Lung auscultation: no respiratory sounds, sudden fall in oxygenation, tachycardia	Check endotracheal tube, chest drainage, reduce intra-abdominal pressure
Subcutaneous emphysema	Palpation of chest, axillae and/or neck reveals subcutaneous crepitus	Exclude pneumothorax by auscultation of respiratory sounds, decrease insufflation pressure, consider cessation of nitrous oxide, chest X-ray in the PACU
Vasovagal reflex	Hypotension, bradycardia	Interrupt laparoscopy, immediate deflation of pneumoperitoneum, atropine i.v., volume replacement

ticed [15]. $ETCO_2$ may at first increase abruptly, with large amounts of CO_2 embolism, followed by a sudden decrease if right ventricular failure (gas lock or acute pulmonary hypertension) develops [15]. If there is excessive bleeding during laparoscopy owing to injury of blood vessels, CO_2 may attain easy intravascular access and this should alert the anaesthesiologist to the possibility of CO_2 embolism [15].

Unilateral or bilateral pneumothorax is a well-known complication during laparoscopy [4, 36]. It may be caused by trauma to the peritoneal lining of the diaphragm by expanding gas or may be due to the presence of congenital diaphragmatic defects [36].

Hypotension often develops when a reverse Trendelenburg position is adopted. Adequate hydration to replace expected preoperative fluid defi-

cit before this manoeuvre will diminish or abolish hypotensive circulatory impairment [27].

In subcutaneous emphysema, concomitant pneumothorax should always be considered. In most cases, this can be ruled out by auscultation of equal and bilateral respiratory sounds. If nitrous oxide is used for general anaesthesia, it should be discontinued in the presence of subcutaneous crepitus for reasons of safety. Subcutaneous emphysema alone is generally asymptomatic and does not affect oxygenation [35, 36], but hypercarbia and an increase in peak respiratory pressure more pronounced than would be expected from peritoneal CO_2 insufflation alone is often noticed [35, 36].

Thoracoscopy

All patients undergoing thoracoscopic surgery should be monitored by ECG, continuous arterial and central venous blood pressure measurement, pulse oximetry, capnography/capnometry ($ETCO_2$) and repeated blood gas analysis. Insertion of a Swan-Ganz catheter should be considered for patients at cardiovascular and/or pulmonary risk.

If a mediastinal approach is used for a thoracoscopic operation (e.g. endoscopic microsurgical dissection of the oesophagus), a conventional single-lumen endotracheal tube can be used. This is also possible in unipuncture or multipuncture thoracoscopic technique because collapse of the lung is achieved by varying the inflow of gas and the insufflation pressure [7]. Owing to the availability of disposable double-lumen tubes and the possibility of checking the position under bronchoscopic control, special tubes, e.g. Univent tube (Fuji Systems Corporation, Tokyo, Japan) with an anterior channel housing a movable blocker and the right- or left-sided polyvinyl double-lumen tube Broncho-Cath (Mallinckrodt, Argyle, NY, USA) are being increasingly employed. If diagnostic thoracoscopy and surgical intervention are to be carried out in one session, use of a double-lumen tube is mandatory. Irrespective of which side the thoracoscopy is to be performed in, a left double-lumen tube should always be used [16]. Right endobronchial tubes are much harder to place correctly and have a greater tendency to move to an inappropriate location intraoperatively [16].

Cardiac and ventilatory impairment may develop during the procedure. Pressures during CO_2 insufflation in the thoracic cavity should not exceed 6.0 mmHg in order to prevent mediastinal shift and a low cardiac output [7]. Mild inotropic cardiac support and adequate volume supply is essential. Hypoxic vasoconstriction of the nonventilated lung may be abolished by vasoactive drugs, which should therefore be used with caution and with the smallest dose necessary [3].

Hypoxaemia should be anticipated (secretions, atelectasis, tube malposition) during one-lung ventilation and must be treated in a stepwise manner. The definition of hypoxaemia during one-lung ventilation may vary between PaO_2 of less than 80 [24] or 60 [16] mmHg and oxygen saturation of less than 95% or 90%, respectively. First-line therapy includes airway aspiration, adjustment of tidal volume, tube repositioning (fiberoptic control). If this fails to improve oxygenation, most authors [16] use the alternating CPAP/PEEP search protocol described by Benumof [2]. By analogy to the recommendations of Benumof, immediate addition of continuous positive airway pressure (CPAP) to the nondependent, nonventilated lung can usually be expected to correct hypoxaemia reliably [16]. If hypoxaemia continues, positive endexpiratory pressure (PEEP) has to be applied to the dependent, ventilated lung through a standard PEEP valve in the anaesthesic circuit [16, 24]. Contrary to the principles of one-lung anaesthesia in the case of hypoxaemia proposed by Benumof, Lewis et al. recommend addition of $5-10 \, cmH_2O$ of PEEP to the dependent ventilated lung initially [24]. This has the advantage of not impeding the thoracoscopic procedure. In 200 noncardiac thoracic surgical procedures, it was shown that hypoxia developed during one-lung ventilation in 57 (28.5%) patients [24]. The addition of $10 \, cmH_2O$ of PEEP probably reopened collapsed alveoli, with a resulting rise in PaO_2 in 40% of cases. In the remaining hypoxic patients, positive airway pressure to the nondependent lung had to be established [24]. If all manoeuvres for correction of hypoxaemia fail, the double-lumen tube must be unclamped.

After the operation, intercostal underwater seal drainage (chest tube) is advisable. Patients with severe preoperative pulmonary or cardiac impairment may require postoperative respiratory support. In a study of more than 40 patients with a history of smoking, a high incidence of cardiovascular disease and poor preoperative status (ASA physical status IV) after thoracoscopic laser ablation of emphysematous bullae, the mean duration of postoperative mechanical ventilation was 9 ± 14 days [16]. In contrast, immediate extubation or at least early weaning after thoracoscopy is possible in healthier patients [22]. In the PACU, a chest X-ray is necessary. Patients should be discharged if adequate and stable ventilation and oxygenation are determined by pulse oximetry or blood gas analysis during breathing of room air.

References

1. Beebe DS, McNevin MP, Belani KG, Letourneau JG, Crain MR, Goodale RL (1992) Evidence of venous stasis after abdominal insufflation for laparoscopic cholecystectomy [Abstract]. Anesthesiology [Suppl 3A] 77: A148

2. Benumof JL (1987) Anesthesia for thoracic surgery. Saunders, Philadelphia, pp 284–285

3. Cheney FW, Colley PS (1980) The effect of cardiac output on arterial blood oxygenation. Anesthesiology 52: 496–503

4. Cheney FW, Posner KL, Caplan RA (1991) Adverse respiratory events infrequently leading to malpractice suits. A closed claims analysis. Anesthesiology 75: 932–939

5. Collins KM, Docherty PW, Plantevin OM (1984) Postoperative morbidity following gynaecological outpatient laparoscopy. A reappraisal of the service. Anaesthesia 39:819–822

6. Cunningham AJ, Brull SJ (1993) Laparoscopic cholecystectomy: anaesthetic implications. Anesth Analg 76: 1120–1133

7. Cuschieri A (1992) General principles of thoracoscopic surgery. In: Cuschieri A, Buess G, Périssat J (eds) Operative manual of endoscopic surgery. Springer, Berlin Heidelberg New York, pp 105–109

8. Cuschieri A, Buess G (1992) Nature and scope of endoscopic surgery. In: Cuschieri A, Buess G, Périssat J (eds) Operative manual of endoscopic surgery. Springer, Berlin Heidelberg New York, pp 9–13

9. Deem S, Shapiro HM, Marshall LF (1991) Quadraplegia in a patient with cervical spondylosis after thoracolumbar surgery in the prone position. Anesthesiology 75:527–528

10. Fisher KS, Reddick EJ, Olsen DO (1991) Laparoscopic cholecystectomy: cost analysis. Surg Lap Endosc 1:77–81

11. Fletcher R (1990) The arterial-end-tidal CO_2 difference during cardiothoracic surgery. J Cardiothorac Anesth 4:105–117

12. Gild WM, Posner KL, Caplan RA, Cheney FW (1992) Eye injuries associated with anesthesia. A closed claims analysis. Anesthesiology 76:204–208

13. Guyton DC (1991) Oral, nasopharyngeal, and gastrointestinal systems. In: Gravenstein N (ed) Manual of complications during anesthesia. Lippincott, Philadelphia, pp 619–662

14. Hasan A, Low DE, Ganado AL, Norton R, Watson DCT (1992) Tracheal rupture with disposable polyvinylchloride double-lumen endotracheal tubes. J Cardiothorac Vasc Anesth 6:208–211

15. Hasnain JU, Matjasko MJ (1991) Practical anesthesia for laparoscopic procedures. In: Zucker KA, Bailey RW, Reddick EJ (eds) Surgical laparoscopy. Quality Medical Publishing, St. Louis, pp 77–86

16. Hasnain JU, Krasna MJ, Barker SJ, Weiman DS, Whitman GJR (1992) Anesthetic considerations for thoracoscopic procedures. J Cardiothorac Vasc Anesth 6: 624–627

17. Hovagim AR, Backus WW, Manecke G, Lagasse R, Sidhu U, Poppers PJ (1989) Pulse oximetry and patient positioning: a report of eight cases. Anesthesiology 71:454–456

18. Hyduke JF, Pineda JJ, Smith CE, Rice TW (1989) Severe intraoperative myocardial ischemia following manipulation of the heart in a patient undergoing esophagogastrectomy. Anesthesiology 71:154–158

19. Johannsen G, Andersen M, Juhl B (1989) The effect of general anaesthesia on the haemodynamic events during laparoscopy with CO_2-insufflation. Acta Anaesthesiol Scand 33:132–136

20. Johnston RV, Lawson NW, Nealon WH (1992) Lower extremity neuropathy after laparoscopic cholecystectomy. Anesthesiology 77:835

21. Kenefick JP, Leader A, Maltby JR, Taylor PJ (1987) Laparoscopy: blood-gas values and minor sequelae associated with three techniques based on isoflurane. Br J Anaesth 59:189–194

22. Krasna M, Flowers JL (1991) Diagnostic thoracoscopy in a patient with a pleural mass. Surg Lap Endosc 1:94–97

23. Lenz RJ, Thomas TA, Wilkins DG (1976) Cardiovascular changes during laparoscopy. Anaesthesia 31:4–12

24. Lewis JW, Serwin JP, Gabriel FS, Bastanfar M, Jacobsen G (1992) The utility of a double-lumen tube for one-lung ventilation in a variety of noncardiac thoracic surgical procedures. J Cardiothorac Vasc Anesth 6:705–710

25. Luiz T, Huber T, Hartung HJ (1992) Veränderungen der Ventilation während laparoskopischer Cholezystektomie. Anaesthesist 41:520–526

26. Mahla ME (1991) Nervous system. In: Gravenstein N (ed) Manual of complications during anesthesia. Lippincott, Philadelphia, pp 383–419

27. Marco AP, Yeo CJ, Rock P (1990) Anesthesia for a patient undergoing laparoscopic cholecystectomy. Anesthesiology 73:1268–1270

28. McKinstry LJ, Perverseff RA, Yip RW (1992) Arterial and end-tidal carbon dioxide in patients undergoing laparoscopic cholecystectomy [Abstract]. Anesthesiology [Suppl 3A] 77:A108

29. Montgomery CJ, Ready LB (1991) Epidural opioid analgesia does not obscure diagnosis of compartment syndrome resulting from prolonged lithotomy position. Anesthesiology 75:541–543

30. Mowschenson PM, Weinstein ME (1992) Why catheterize the bladder for laparoscopic cholecystectomy? J Laparoendosc Surg 2:215–217

31. Neuman GG, Sidebotham G, Negoianu E, Bernstein J, Kopman AF, Hicks RG, West ST, Haring L (1993) Laparoscopy explosion hazards with nitrous oxide. Anesthesiology 78:875–879

32. Oh S, Fabrick J, Pagulayan G (1992) Evaluation of toradol for pain control after laparoscopic cholecystectomy [Abstract]. Anesthesiology [Suppl 3A] 77:A440

33. Oza KN, O'Donnell N, Fisher JB (1992) Aortic laceration: a rare complication of laparoscopy. J Laparoendosc Surg 2:235–237

34. Putensen-Himmer G, Putensen C, Lammer H, Lingnau W, Aigner F, Benzer H (1992) Comparison of postoper-

ative respiratory function after laparoscopy or open laparotomy for cholecystectomy. Anesthesiology 77: 675–680

35. Schwed DA, Edoga JK, McDonnell TE (1992) Ventilatory impairment during laparoscopic cholecystectomy in a patient with a ventriculoperitoneal shunt. J Laparoendosc Surg 2:57–59

36. Shantha TR, Harden J (1991) Laparoscopic cholecystectomy: anesthesia-related complications and guidelines. Surg Lap Endosc 1:173–178

37. Smith I, Ding Y, White PF (1992) Post-laparoscopic myalgias: effect of propofol, succinylcholine, and atracurium [Abstract]. Anesthesiology [Suppl 3A] 77:A951

38. Stow PJ (1986) Retinal haemorrhage following laparoscopy. Anaesthesia 41:965–966

39. Taylor E, Feinstein R, White PF, Soper N (1992) Anesthesia for laparoscopic cholecystectomy. Is nitrous oxide contraindicated? Anesthesiology 76:541–543

40. Tolksdorf W, Strang CM, Schippers E, Simon HB, Truong S (1992) Die Auswirkungen des Kohlendioxid-Pneumoperitoneums zur laparoskopischen Cholezystektomie auf die postoperative Spontanatmung. Anaesthesist 41:199–203

41. Wadhwa RK, McKenzie R, Wadhwa SR, Katz DL, Byers JF (1978) Gas embolism during laparoscopy. Anesthesiology 48:74–76

42. Warner MA, Martin JT (1992) Incidence of lower extremity nerve injury in the lithotomy position [Abstract]. Anesthesiology [Suppl 3A] 77:A1130

43. Winter R, Munro M (1989) Lingual and buccal nerve neuropathy in a patient in the prone position: a case report. Anesthesiology 71:452–454

44. Wurst H, Finsterer U (1990) Pathophysiologische und klinische Aspekte der Laparoskopie. Anästh Intensivmed 31:187–197

4 Right Subtotal Thoracoscopic Oesophagectomy with Lymphadenectomy

A. Cuschieri

Introduction

Blunt transhiatal oesophagectomy first reported by Grey Turner [1] and popularized by Orringer and others for both benign and malignant disease [2–5] carries certain advantages over the two-stage Lewis-Tanner procedure [6, 7] or the three-stage oesophagectomy [8], largely due to the avoidance of a thoracotomy. There are, however, some disadvantages which are inherent to blunt dissection of the oesophagus. These include blood loss and trauma to the azygos vein, bronchi and recurrent laryngeal nerves. The procedure is particularly difficult in large tumours of the middle third of the oesophagus and the risk of damage to mediastinal structures by the blind dissection is increased if there is extramural spread of the tumour. In addition, cardiac arrhythmias are common during the retrocardiac mobilization. Nodal dissection and lymphadenectomy is not possible with blunt transhiatal oesophagectomy, and although this may not affect survival in the majority of patients – since most oesophageal resections are palliative – the excision of involved lymph nodes may indeed affect dysphagia-free survival. The first visually guided technique of endoscopic oesophagectomy was reported by Buess et al. [9] using a specially designed operating mediastinoscope which permits safe perivisceral dissection of the intrathoracic oesophagus. This method is described in Vol. 1, Chap. 12 and is suitable for small tumours, preferably without extensive node involvement since the scope for lymphadenectomy is limited by this approach. The subtotal right thoracoscopic oesophagectomy [10, 11] allows dissection of large thoracic oesophageal tumours and lymphadenectomy that is equivalent in all respects to that achieved by the McKeown procedure. In addition, the dissection of the cervical oesophagus is performed largely through the thoracoscopic route.

Indications and Contraindications in Right Subtotal Thoracoscopic Oesophagectomy

Assuming fitness for surgery, right subtotal thoracoscopic dissection of the oesophagus is indicated for intrathoracic oesophageal tumours (middle and lower third). It is not advisable for tumours involving the gastro-oesophageal junction as these require resection of the upper third of the stomach to ensure distal clearance. This additional gastric resection precludes gastric pull through for the cervical anastomosis. Right subtotal thoracoscopic oesophagectomy is also impossible if the pleural cavity is completely obliterated by dense adhesions (encountered in 8% of patients in our series). Soft, loose areolar adhesions binding the surface of the lungs to the rib cage can be separated with coaxial curved and bayonet instruments, if necessary via a small (5 cm) incision, and do not constitute a contraindication.

Preoperative Work-up and Preparation

The vast majority of these patients are elderly and often have co-existent cardiorespiratory disease. Fitness for surgery is assessed by history and physical examination, 12-lead and exercise electrocardiogram (ECG) and pulmonary function tests. In addition to exclusion of inoperability by nerve involvement (paralysis of the vocal cord or diaphragm), a chest X-ray, liver function tests, and computed tomography (CT) scan of the liver and chest (mediastinum and lung fields) are essential. In some cases, not even CT images indicate for certain whether the oesophageal tumour has invaded the descending thoracic aorta. In these patients operability can only be determined at the time of thoracoscopic dissection. This situation has arisen in three out of the first 23 patients in our series (13%). As the thoracoscopic dissection is performed first, a laparoscopy is essential to exclude involvement of the cardia and adjacent stomach in distal tumours. It is also useful for exclusion of secondary deposits in the liver and peritoneal surfaces. The laparoscopy may be performed at the time of oesophagectomy or beforehand.

Chemoprophylaxis against deep vein thrombosis with subcutaneous heparin is used in all patients, the first dose being administered at the time of induction of anaesthesia. The patients also wear graduated elastic antithrombosis stockings. Two doses of prophylactic antibiotics (cephalosporin or aminoglycoside and metronidazole) are administered, at the time of surgery and 12 h later.

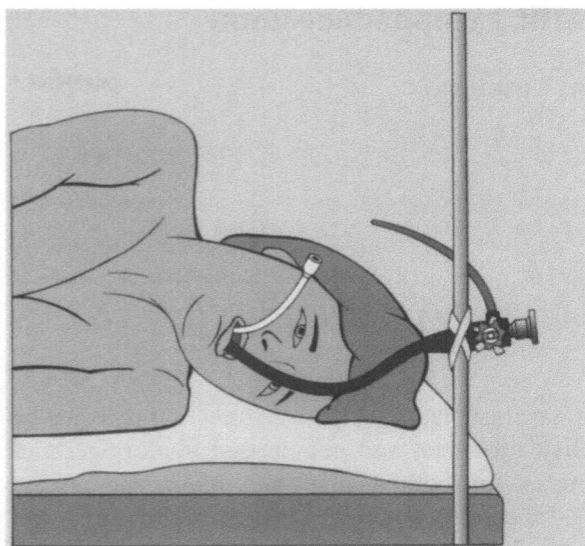

Fig. 4.1. The flexible endoscope after insertion into the oesophagus with its tip proximal to the tumour affixed by its handpiece to a drip stand. This endoscope is used to lift and alter the position of the oesophagus during the dissection

Stages of the Operation

The operation is conducted in two stages. The right thoracoscopic dissection is performed first with the patient in the prone posterolateral position. Once this is completed, the position of the patient is changed for the second stage. This consists of synchronous cervical dissection and mobilization of the stomach by two surgical teams. The second stage is carried out with the patient in the supine position and requires redraping. Although gastric mobilization can be performed endoscopically, we now prefer to do this through a midline incision as with the current technology, laparoscopic mobilization of the stomach adds considerably to the operating time.

Anaesthesia

Expert general endotracheal anaesthesia is required with endobronchial collapse of the right lung (Carlens tube). The urinary bladder is catheterized for estimation of the hourly urine output. Arterial and central venous pressure, ECG, blood gas and end-tidal CO_2 are monitored continuously. A large intravenous cannula for rapid infusion of crystalloids and blood in the event of haemorrhage is essential.

Insertion of Flexible Endoscope

After the patient has been anaesthetized and before he is turned into the posterolateral position, a flexible endoscope is passed into the oesophagus and its end placed just proximal to the upper margin of the tumour. The light is then switched off and the endoscope is affixed by its handpiece with adhesive tape to a drip stand (Fig. 4.1). This endoscope is used to lift the oesophagus during the dissection.

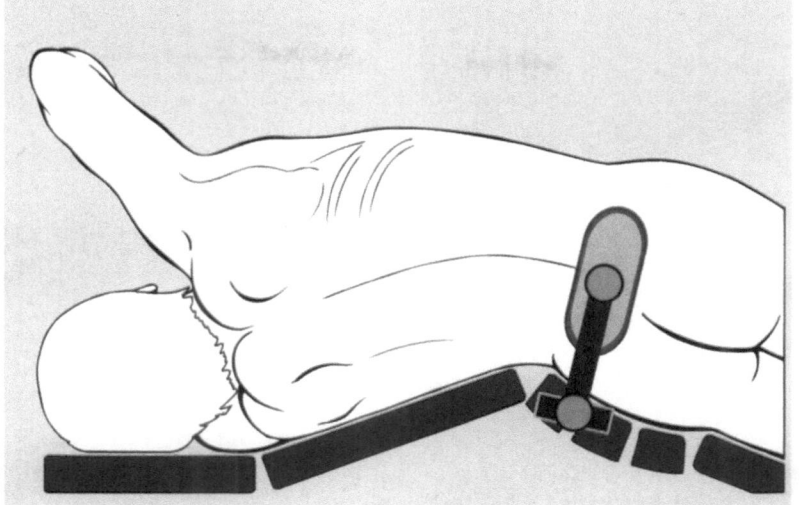

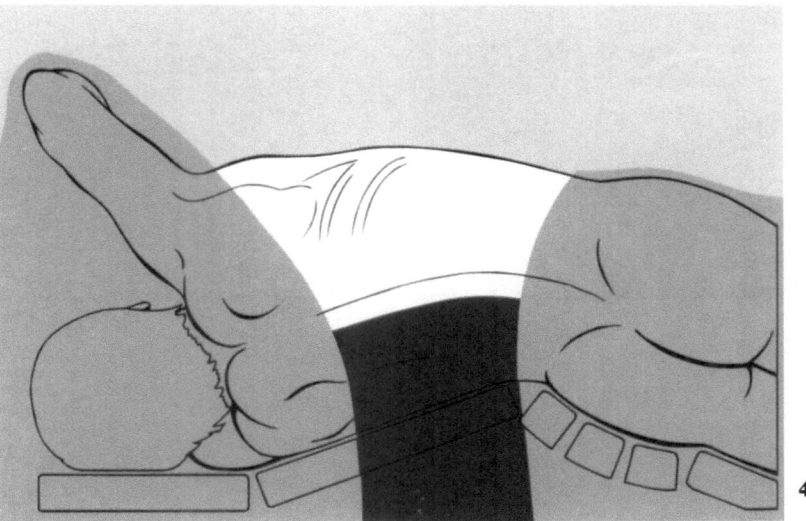

Patient Positioning and Skin Preparation for Right Thoracoscopic Dissection of the Tumour and Oesophagus

Fig. 4.2. Prone posterolateral position for subtotal right thoracoscopic oesophagectomy

Fig. 4.3. Draping for subtotal right thoracoscopic oesophagectomy

The patient is placed in the prone posterolateral position with the right chest cavity upwards (Fig. 4.2). The right arm is kept well abducted on a rest and the ribs are splayed by splitting the operation table or raising the bridge. The patient must be positioned so that the chest is leaning slightly to the left side and the collapsed lung displaced by gravity away from the operative field. Adequate strapping of the patient to the operating table and a back rest are essential to prevent slipping during the course of the operation. The skin of the entire chest wall from shoulder to waist is prepared with medicated soap and then disinfected with the antiseptic of choice. Draping is such as to leave the entire right chest wall from the nipple line anteriorly to the spinous processes posteriorly (Fig. 4.3).

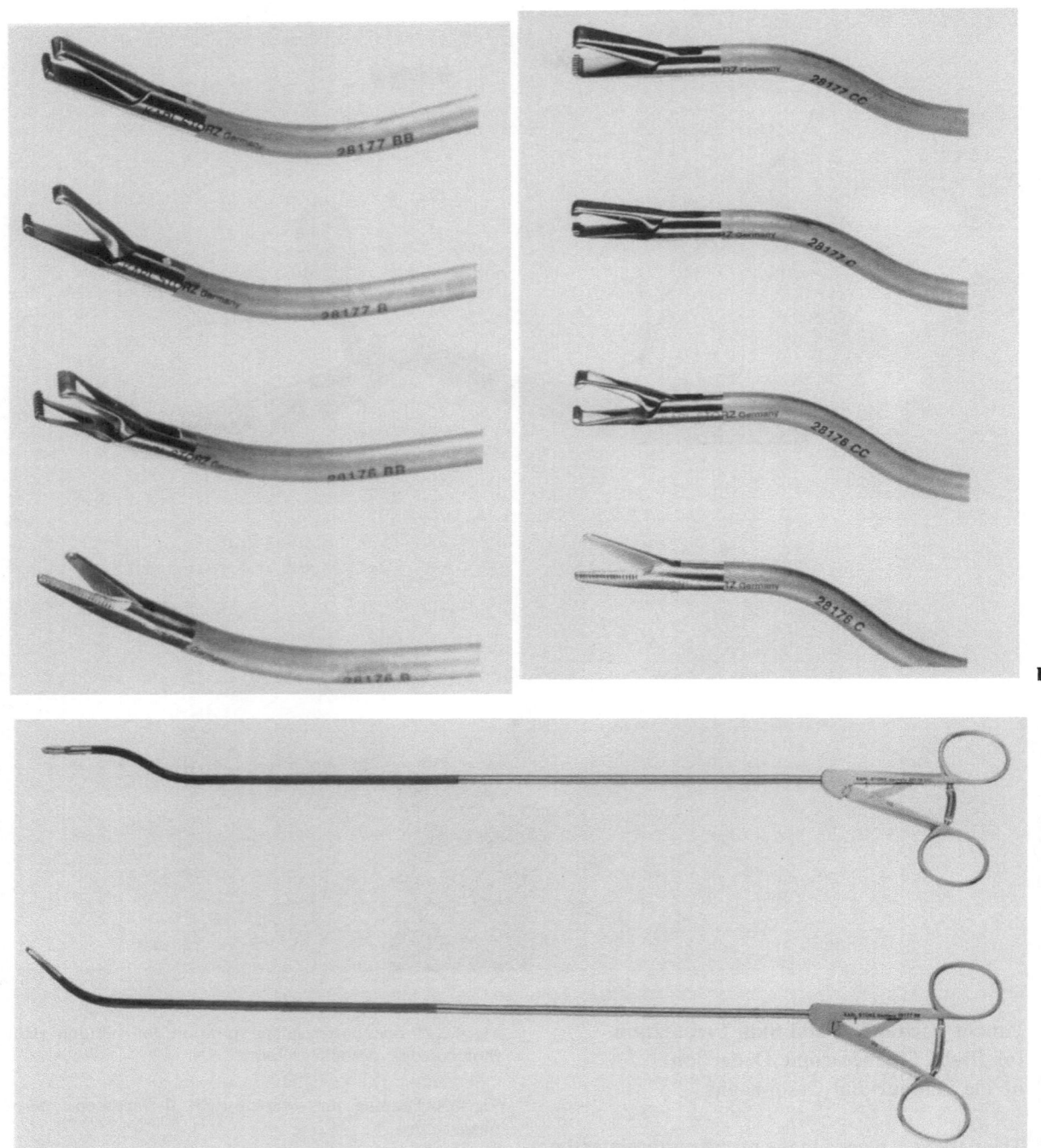

Fig. 4.4a–e. Coaxial curved and bayonet instruments (**a–c**) introduced through reusable metal flexible cannulae (**d, e**) (Storz, Tuttlingen, Germany)

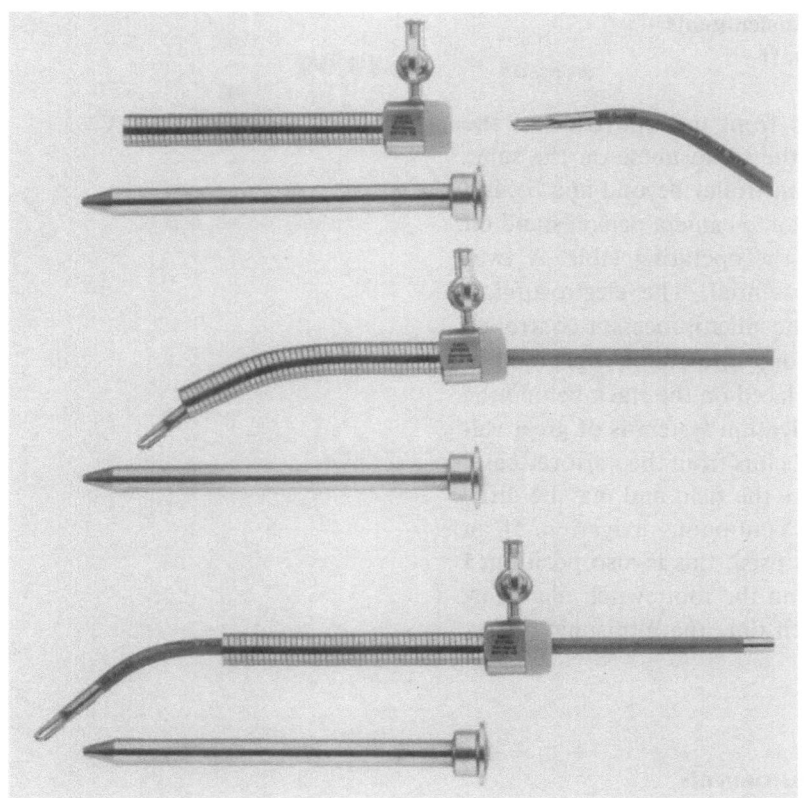

d

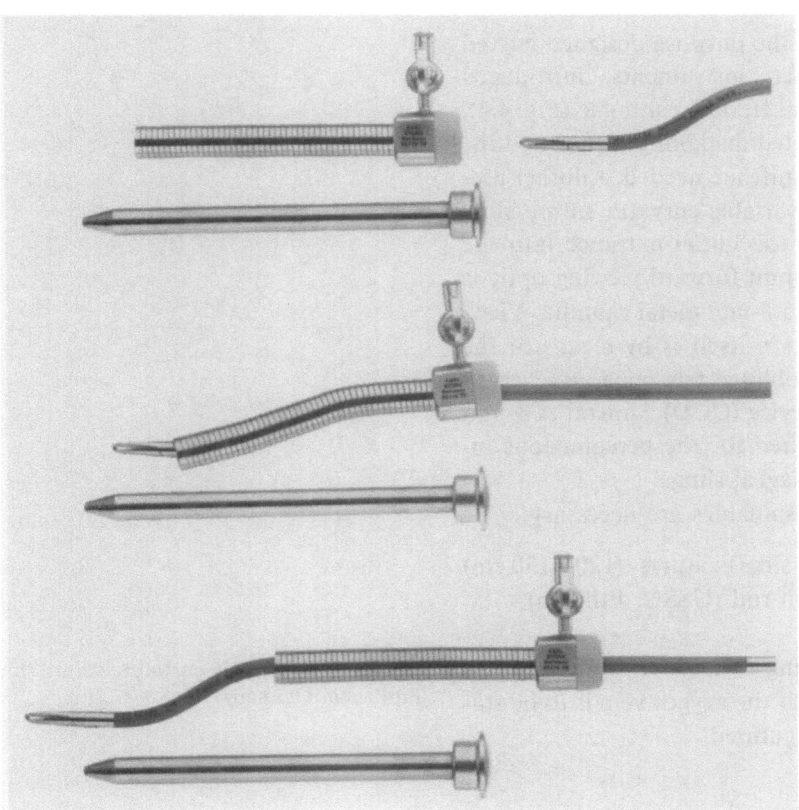

e

Layout of Ancillary Instruments and Positioning of Staff

The surgeon operates from the right side of the operating table with the scrub nurse on the same side and the instrument trolley beyond and behind her. The first assistant and camera person stand on the opposite side of the operating table. A two-monitor display is essential. The electrosurgical unit, preferably of the microprocessor-controlled type, suction irrigation, insufflator, light source and camera unit are placed on the stack behind the surgeon. A pulsed irrigation system is of great value in dispersing blood clots from the aortovertebral gutter as these obscure the field and may be difficult to dislodge with continuous irrigation. If an ultrasonic dissector is used, this is also positioned behind the surgeon and the foot switch placed by the surgeon's feet each time the ultrasonic dissection is needed.

Details of Specific Instruments and Consumables for the Procedure

The author now uses the purpose designed curved coaxial and bayonet instruments introduced through reusable metal flexible cannulae (Fig. 4.4). In addition, an insulated duckbill graspers and the electrosurgical hook knife are needed. Another useful instrument is the variable curvatur suture/sling passer (Fig. 4.5). For the initial entrance into the right chest cavity a 5-mm forward viewing optic is used inside a bevelled 5.5-mm metal cannula. Viewing during the operation itself is by means of the 10-mm 30° forward oblique telescope attached to the charge-coupled device (CCD) camera. A 3-mm needle holder is required for the percutaneous insertion of the oesophageal sling.

The following consumables are necessary:

- Dacron or black silk ligatures (120–150 cm) mounted on a push rod (USSC, Ethicon)
- Metal clips
- Vascular silicon sling
- EndoGIA (USSC) if the azygos vein is to be stapled rather than ligatured.

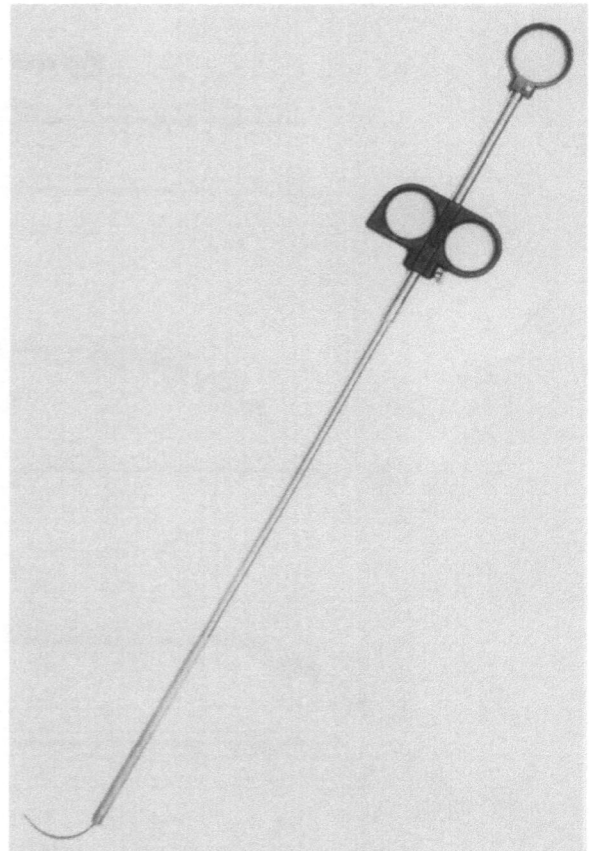

a

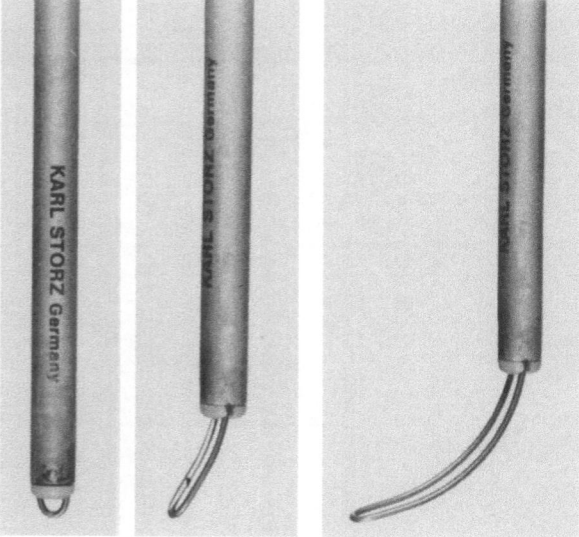

b, c, d

Fig. 4.5a–d. Variable curvature suture/sling passer (Storz, Tuttlingen, Germany)

Open Thoracotomy Tray

It cannot be stressed enough that *all major thoracoscopic dissections require the immediate availability of an open sterile thoracotomy set with vascular clamps*. These instruments are kept covered by a sterile drape on a separate trolley so that they are readily available in the event of sudden severe intrathoracic bleeding. The author has always insisted on this precaution and it has certainly prevented a death on the table when aortic bleeding was encountered during the dissection of a large middle third tumour from the descending thoracic aorta.

Operative Steps of Right Thoracoscopic Oesophagectomy

Types and Placement of Trocar and Cannulae

The types and placement of trocar and cannulae are shown in Fig. 4.6. We now routinely use four cannulae: two flexible (8-mm; p2, p3) and two rigid (11-mm; p1, p4). If the EndoGIA stapler is to be used, the posterior of the latter two cannulae must be 12 mm in size (p4). The siting of the upper two flexible cannulae is just below and 3 cm anterior and 3 cm posterior to the inferior angle of the scapula. The lower two rigid cannulae are inserted two

intercostal spaces further down along the same line as the upper two. It is important that the posterior cannulae are inserted 2 cm anterior to the angle of the ribs for two reasons: to avoid damaging the intercostal nerves and to clear the prominence of the vertebral column.

Safe Entry into the Right Pleural Cavity and Collapse of the Right Lung

The details of safe insertion of thoracic cannulae are outlined in Vol. 1, Chap. 8. The rigid 5.5-mm bevelled metal cannula used for the visually guided entry of the right thoracic cavity is subsequently replaced by a flexible one. For most of the operation, the optic is inserted through the lower anterior port. Sometimes, the right lung has not been collapsed completely. This is most commonly due to faulty positioning of the intrabronchial balloon but can also be encountered in patients with obstructive airways disease with air trapping. In the latter situation further collapse of the lung is obtained by low flow CO_2 insufflation (2 l/min) at a pressure which must not exceed 8 mmHg, otherwise a mediastinal shift with arrhythmias and hypotension may supervene.

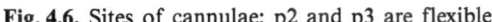

Fig. 4.6. Sites of cannulae; p2 and p3 are flexible

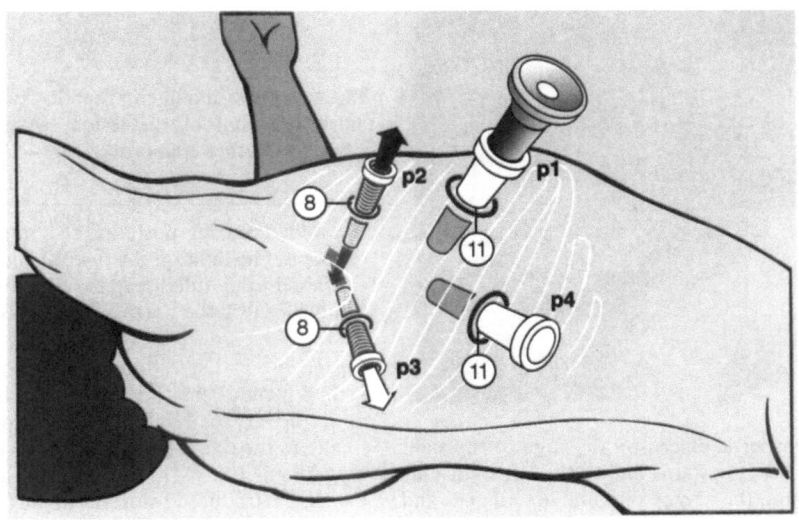

Exposure of the Mediastinum and Assessment of the Tumour and Its Operability

A Duval or Babcock's grasper is placed on the edge of the right upper lobe and this is displaced upwards and to the left by the assistant to display the right mediastinum, the azygos vein, the oesophagus and the tumour (Fig. 4.7). A careful search is made for pleural tumour deposits and if such lesions are encountered, they are excised and sent for immediate frozen section histological examination. We have encountered this once and because of the finding, the oesophagectomy was abandoned and an endoprosthesis inserted. In this patient, the small deposits were not visualized on the preoperative CT scans.

Next, the tumour mobility and attachment to surrounding structures is ascertained in two ways. Two graspers are placed, one on each side of the lesion, and the tumour moved from side to side (Fig. 4.8) to assess lateral and medial fixation of the tumour. Posterior fixation is best ascertained using the flexible endoscope. The light on the instrument is switched on and its tip flexed to its fullest extent (with the necessary torque) to lift the oesophagus just proximal to the tumour out of the aortocardiac gutter (Fig. 4.9). If these manoeuvres indicate that the tumour is mobile, the procedure starts with dissection of the azygos. If lateral or upward mobility

is judged to be restricted, trial mobilization of the tumour constitutes the first step of the operation.

Dissection of the Azygos Vein

If the tumour is mobile, the dissection starts at the level of the azygos vein, irrespective of the tumour site. The mediastinal pleura is divided by the curved

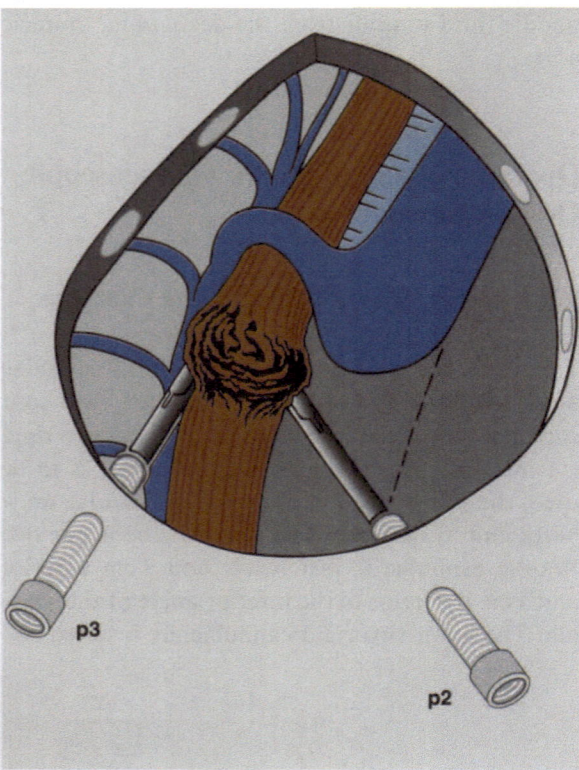

Fig. 4.8. Assessing lateral mobility of the tumour by side to side movement of the lesion by means of two graspers placed on either side (via p2, p3)

→

Fig. 4.9. Assessing posterior fixation using the flexible endoscope. The light on the instrument is switched on and its tip flexed to its fullest extent to lift the oesophagus and the tumour out of the aorto-cardiac gutter

Fig. 4.10 a – c. Dissection of the azygos vein. The mediastinal pleura being divided below the azygos vein (**a**) and above the azygos vein and the incision then extended proximally to the thoracic inlet along the anterior surface of the oesophagus (**b**). **c** The variable curvature superelastic sling passer is introduced below the azygos vein and then encircles it

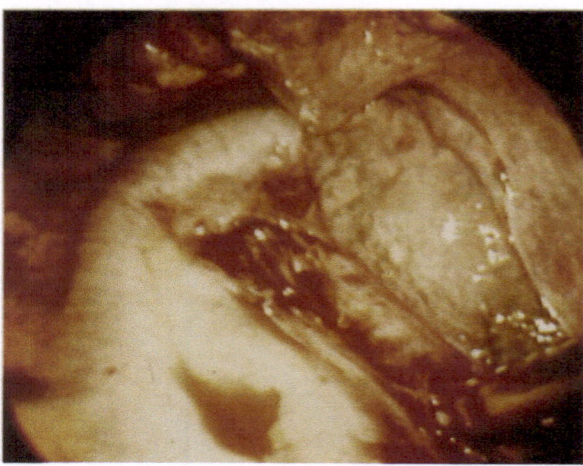

Fig. 4.7. Duval's grasper is placed on the edge of the right upper lobe. This is lifted upwards and to the left to display the right mediastinum, the azygos vein, the oesophagus and the tumour

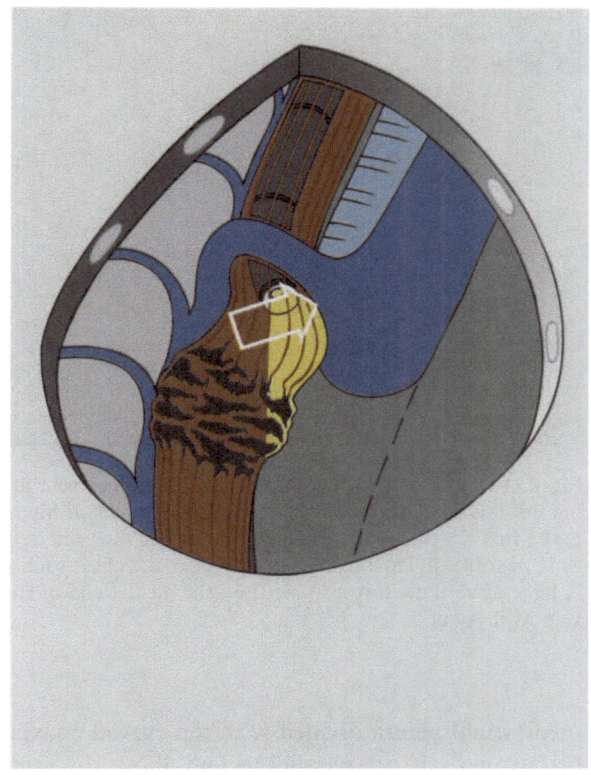

4.9

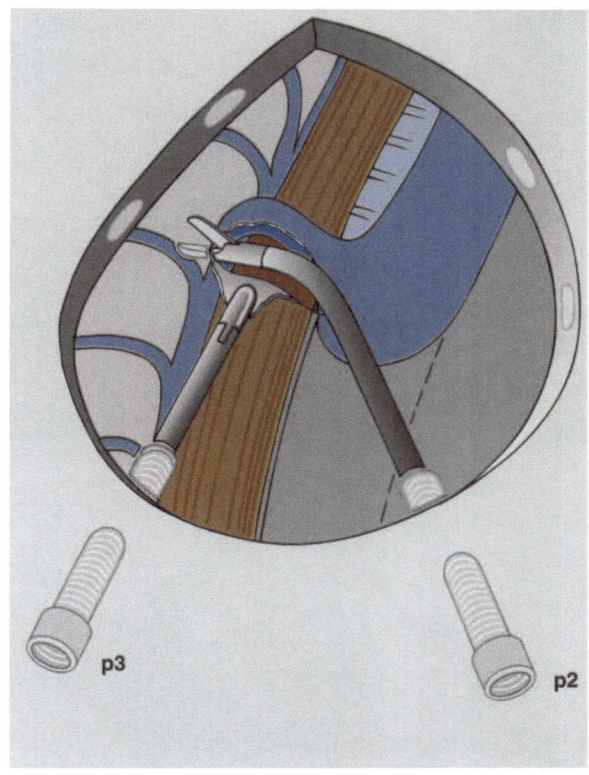

4.10a

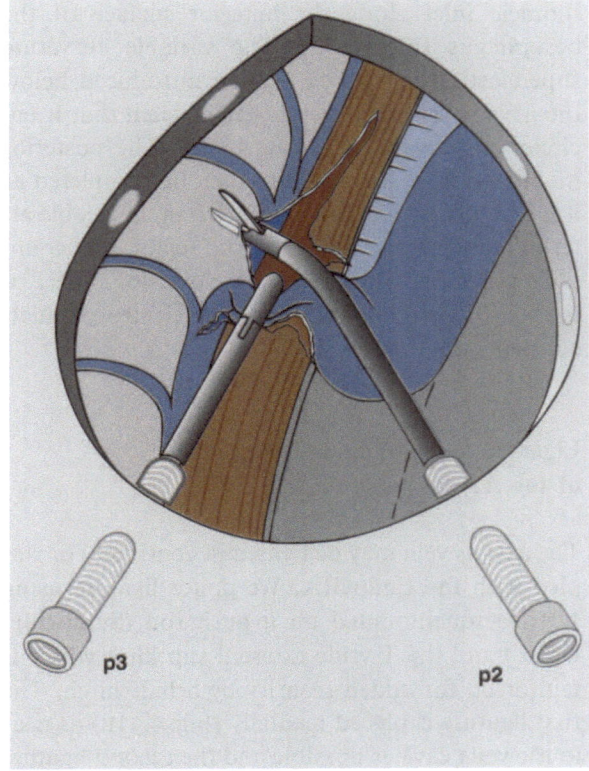

4.10b

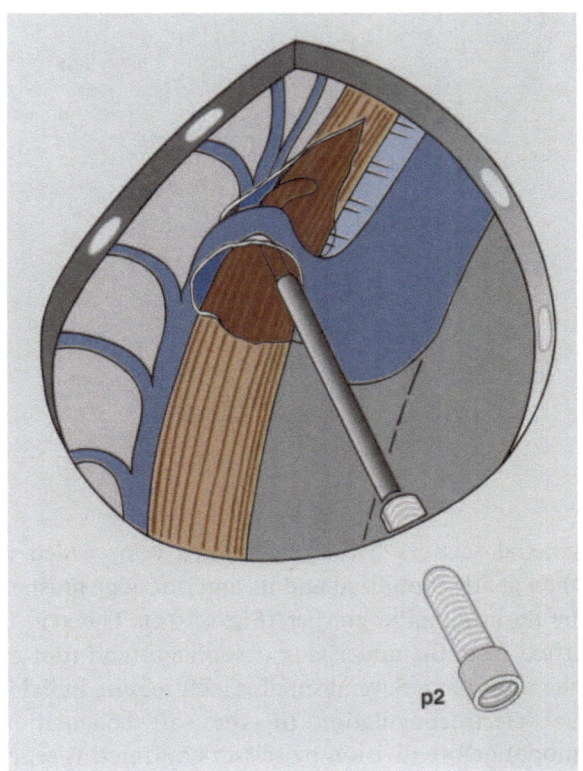

4.10c

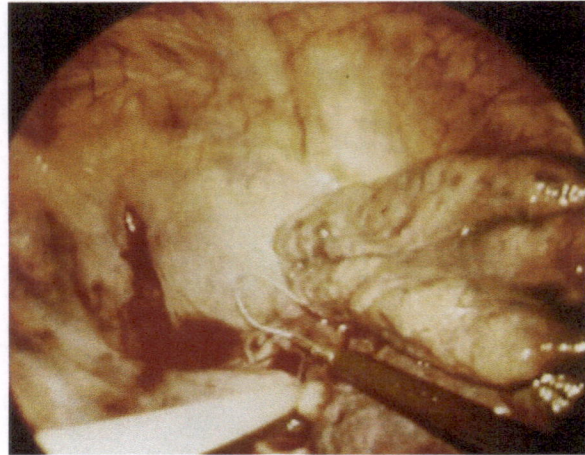

a

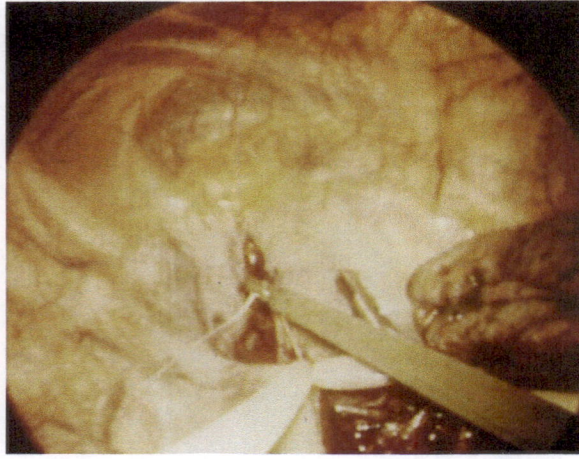

b

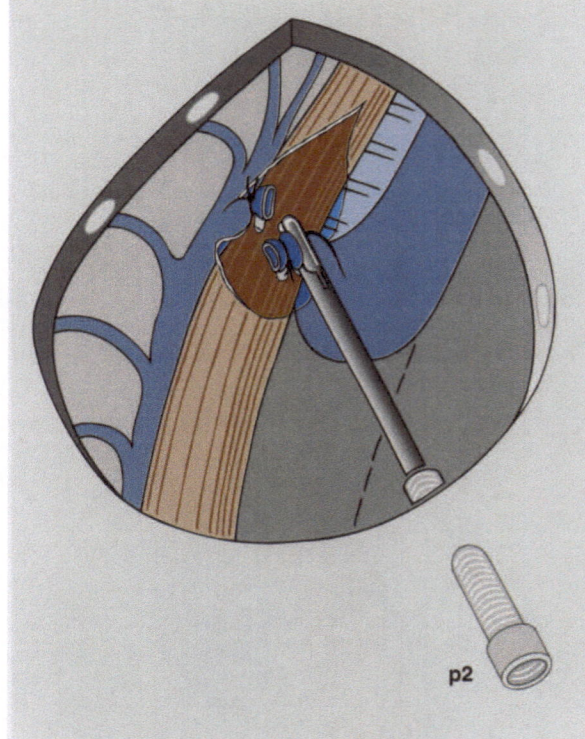

c

Fig. 4.11 a–c. Ligature in continuity of the azygos vein using the Tayside external slip knot reinforced by a half hitch. **a** The first ligature placed medially as near to the vena cava as is possible. **b** The second laterally near the chest wall. **c** A large atraumatic forceps placed on the medial end of the vein as it is cut

mediastinal pleura divided with the curved coaxial or bayonet scissors parallel to and above the vein. This incision is then extended proximally to the thoracic inlet along the anterior surface of the oesophagus (Fig. 4.10 b). The variable curvature superelastic sling passer is then introduced below the azygos vein and then extruded such that it encircles the azygos vein (Fig. 4.10 c). The posterior mobilization of the vein can then be completed as it is held up by the sling passer. Often, a sizeable arterial branch from the intercostal region is encountered on the lateral side of the posterior aspect of the vein. This should be clipped or electrocoagulated, depending on its size.

Ligature or Stapling and Division of the Azygos Vein

coaxial scissors below the azygos vein, which is then gently mobilized and its anterior edge grasped by an atraumatic grasper (Fig. 4.10 a). The vein is lifted from the underlying oesophagus and root of the right lung. Several small vessels require individual electrocoagulation (in the soft coagulation mode) before division by scissors during this separation. The azygos vein is then held down and the

The azygos vein may be ligated in continuity or stapled with the EndoGIA. We prefer ligature using 1/0 Dacron mounted on a push rod (Surgiwhip, USSC) and the Tayside external slip knot which is reinforced for added security by a half hitch. The first ligature is placed medially (Fig. 4.11 a) as near to the vena cava as possible and the second ligature laterally near the chest wall (Fig. 4.11 b). A large

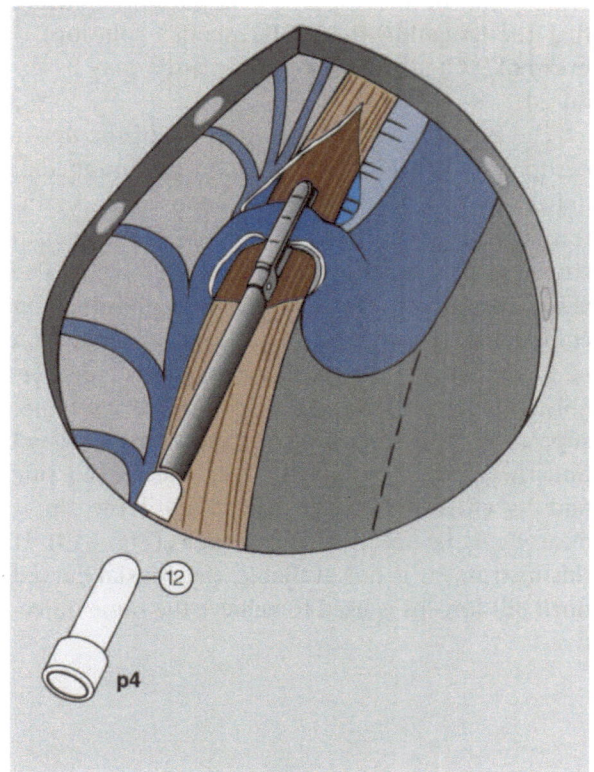

a

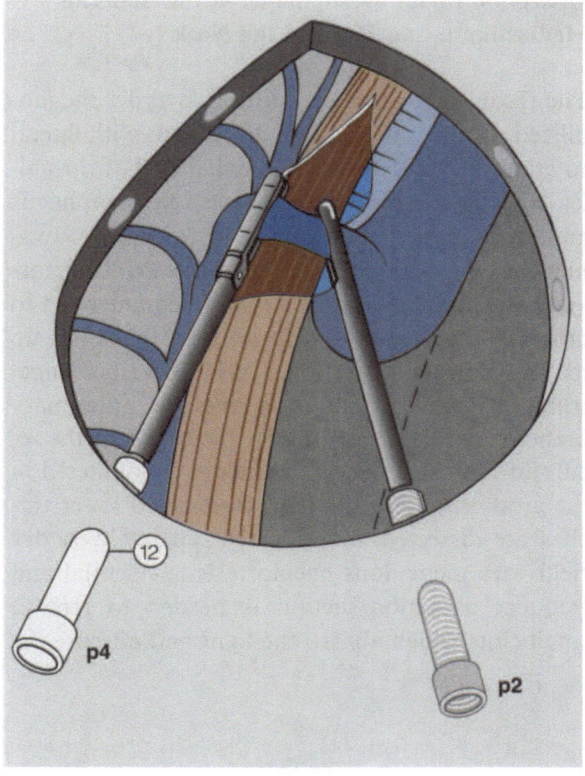

b

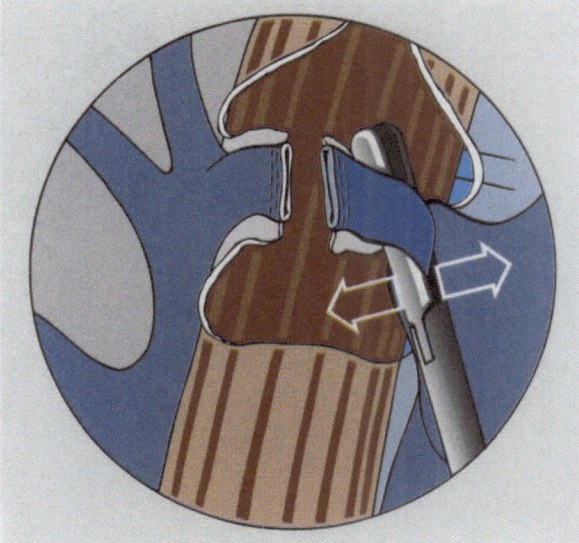

c

Fig. 4.12 a – c. Staple division of the azygos vein. **a** Positioning the limbs of the EndoGIA, **b** placing forceps before the instrument is fired, on the medial end of the vein, and **c** slowly releasing the atraumatic forceps after the vein has been cut and stapled

atraumatic forceps is placed on the medial end of the vein, before this is divided with scissors (Fig. 4.11 c). The grasper is then released slowly but reapplied immediately in the event of haemorrhage.

Alternatively, the azygos vein may be stapled. The opened limbs of the EndoGIA are positioned with the vein in the centre and then approximated (Fig. 4.12 a). Before the instrument is fired, an atraumatic forceps is placed on the medial end of the vein (Fig. 4.12 b). This is released slowly after the vein has been cut and stapled by the device (Fig. 4.12 c).

Dissection of the Oesophagus in the Superior Mediastinum and Root of the Neck

The flexible endoscope is withdrawn above the mobilized azygos vein and flexed forwards with lateral rotation to expose the anteromedial wall of the gullet. The dissection plane is between the oesophagus and the superior vena cava and trachea. A two-handed dissection with the curved coaxial scissors and insulated duck-bill forceps is recommended to mobilize the oesophagus from these structures up to the thoracic inlet (Fig. 4.13). The right·vagal trunk is identified before it gives the pulmonary branches and is divided below the origin of the recurrent laryngeal nerve. Any nodes encountered in the groove between the oesophagus and lower trachea are dissected and removed separately. A dry field with meticulous haemostasis is essential and frequent irrigation/suction is needed to remove small clots which absorb the light and obscure the visual field. In this respect it is important to ensure that the irrigating fluid (Hartmann's solution) is warm (37 °C) as otherwise bradycardia may be induced.

The exposure of the lateral aspect of the upper oesophagus is achieved by forward lift and medial deflection of the gullet by the endoscope. Again, this dissection is carried out with use of the coaxial curved scissors and duck-bill insulated forceps. The vessels are electrocoagulated before division. On completion of the lateral dissection, the separation of the remaining posterior attachment is considerably aided by the use of the variable curvature superelastic sling passer or dissector. This is passed underneath the oesophagus from the medial side and its curvature then extruded until the tip is clearly seen lateral to the oesophagus (Fig. 4.14). If this instrument is not available, the coaxial curved duck-bill forceps is used to achieve the same objective.

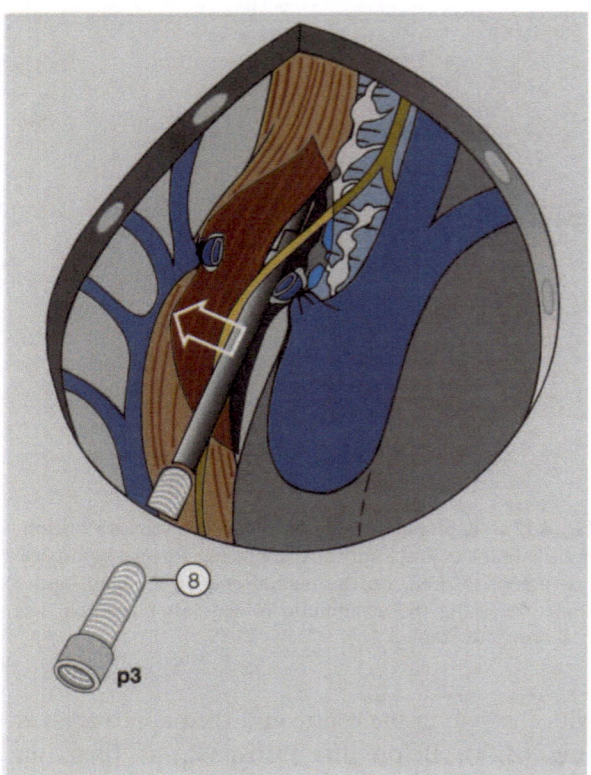

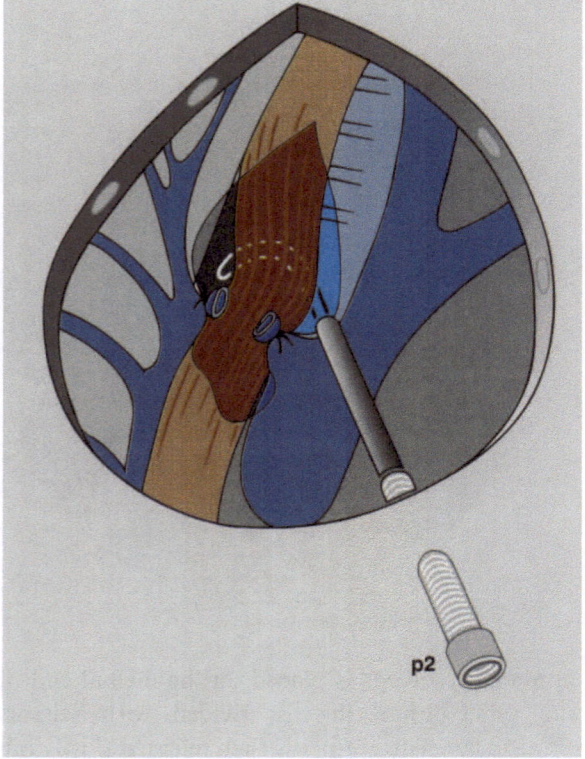

Fig. 4.13. Dissection of the plane between the oesophagus and the superior vena cava and trachea

Fig. 4.14. Insertion of variable curvature superelastic sling passer for the posterior dissection of the proximal oesophagus and passage of silicon sling

Insertion of Silicon Sling and Completion of Posterior Mobilization of the Upper Thoracic Oesophagus

A small stab wound is made in the midaxillary line at the fourth intercostal space with a pointed scalpel, and a vascular silicon sling loaded on the 3-mm needle holder is introduced into the right chest and passed around the mobilized upper oesophagus using the sling passer (Fig. 4.15). The internal end of the sling is then regrasped by the 3-mm needle holder and exteriorized through the same stab wound in the chest wall. Traction applied to the external limbs of the sling by means of an artery forceps lifts the posterior surface of the upper thoracic oesophagus from the superior mediastinum, completing the mobilization (Fig. 4.16).

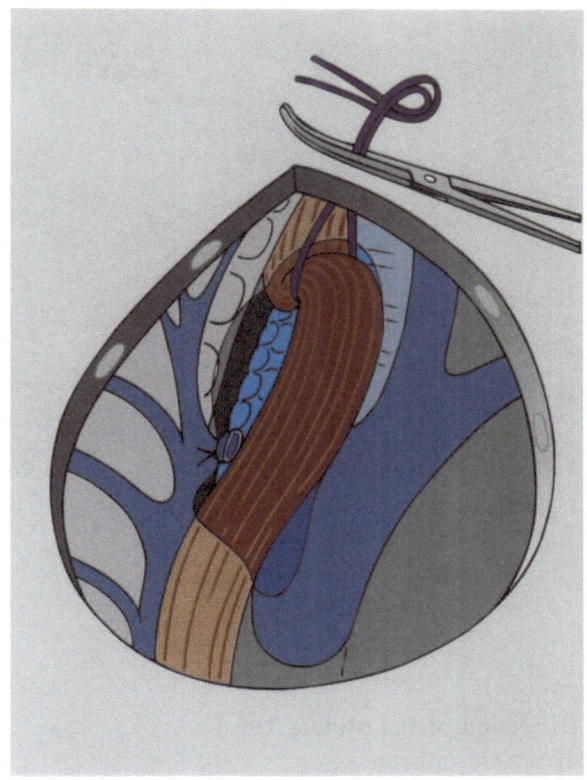

Fig. 4.16. Traction applied to the external limbs of the sling lifts the posterior surface of the upper thoracic oesophagus from the superior mediastinum and enables its complete mobilization

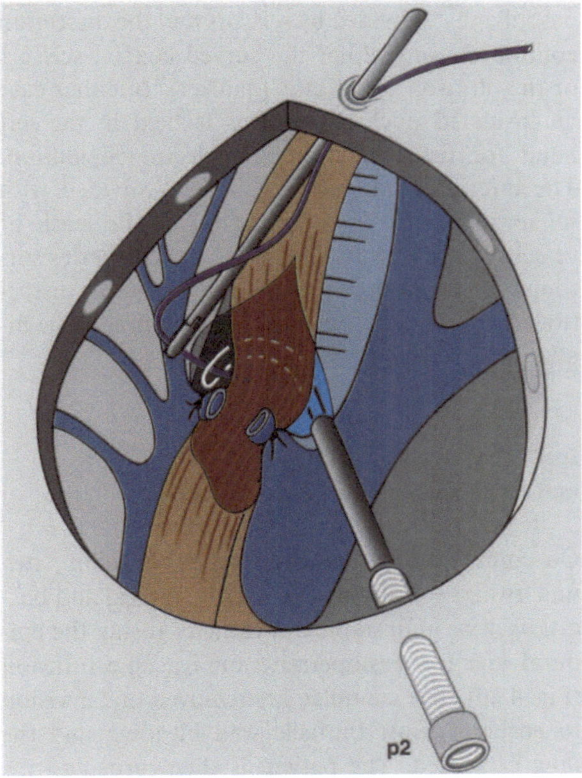

Fig. 4.15. Passage of silicon sling around the oesophagus by means of superelastic sling passer

Dissection of the Lower Cervical Oesophagus

The dissection of the cervical oesophagus is carried out in a manner which trails the flexible instrument (adjusted to the straight position). As blunt (suction probe, pledget or ultrasonic) dissection proceeds around the oesophagus beyond the thoracic inlet, the endoscope is withdrawn further up and the process continued inside the root of the neck up to the level of the thyroid lobes. The dissection plane is on the prevertebral fascia posteriorly, the trachea anteriorly and the recurrent laryngeal nerves and inferior thyroid arteries laterally (Fig. 4.17). Electrocoagulation must not be used during this stage of the operation because of the risk of damage to the recurrent laryngeal nerves. Bleeding is minimal if the correct planes are followed.

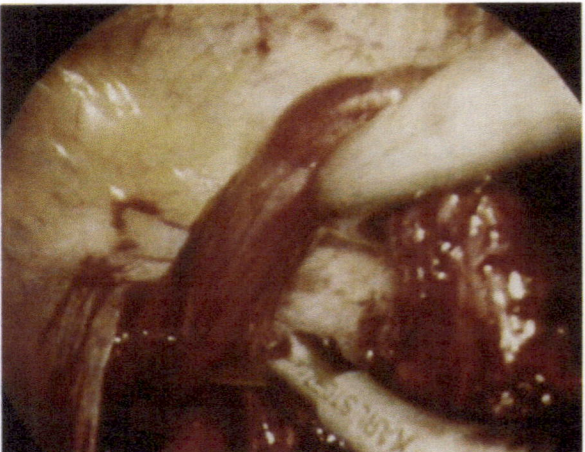

Fig. 4.17. Dissection of the lower cervical oesophagus

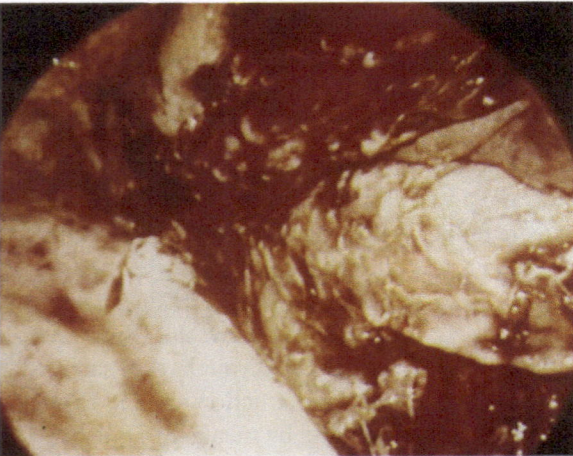

Fig. 4.18. Medial separation from the tracheal bifurcation and pericardium. The subcarinal lymph nodes and the middle oesophageal nodes are dissected and removed with the tumour or separately

Dissection of the Middle Third of the Oesophagus

On completion of the cervical dissection, the endoscope is advanced below the level of the azygos vein and the vascular sling slid down to the appropriate position for dissection of the middle oesophagus. During separation from the aorta, any sizeable, direct arterioles are clipped and divided. One such vessel is fairly consistently found at the junction of the upper with the middle third and runs in a straight posterolateral direction to the descending thoracic aorta. This vessel must be carefully dissected and doubly clipped on the aortic side before it is cut. On the medial side, for separation from the tracheal bifurcation and the pericardium a two-handed technique is preferred using the curved coaxial scissors and the duck-bill insulated grasper, with careful haemostasis throughout. The subcarinal lymph nodes and the oesophageal nodes are dissected and removed with the tumour or separately (Fig. 4.18). On the medial side as the pericardium is approached, electrocoagulation must be used sparingly because of the risk of cardiac arrhythmias. Posteriorly, the dissection is taken down to the left pleura. This is left intact unless it is involved or adherent, in which case the affected area is cut and removed with the tumour.

Dissection of the Lower Oesophagus

The mediastinal pleura on the right surface of the oesophagus is divided by scissors and the dissection continued using either the curved coaxial scissors or the ultrasonic dissector (quicker). In either case an insulated duck-bill forceps is held in the left hand for tissue traction and electrocoagulation. The inferior pulmonary ligament is divided with scissors after electroacoagulation of the leash of vessels within its fold (Fig. 4.19). Lymph nodes surrounding the oesophagus are included in the dissection, which is continued up to the diapragmatic hiatus.

Insertion of Chest Drains and Bupivacaine Intrapleural Catheter

On completion of the endoscopic dissection, two underwater seal drains are inserted (apical and basal), likewise an intrapleural catheter (using the epidural kit) for postoperative bupivacaine infusion (Fig. 4.20). The cannulae are removed under vision to ensure against thoracic wall bleeding and the lung expanded. The patient is then turned to the supine position for the second stage of the operation.

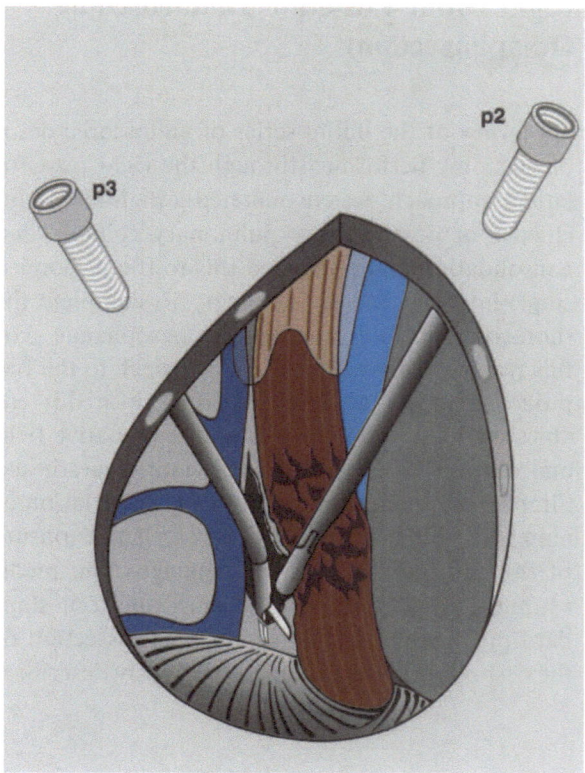

Fig. 4.19. Mobilization of the lower oesophagus and lymph nodes down to the diaphragmatic hiatus

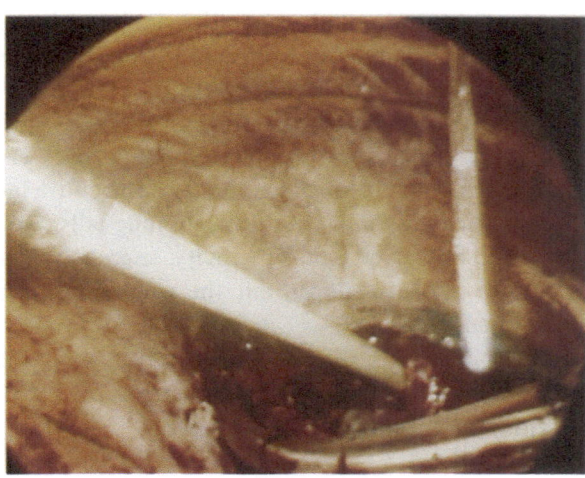

Fig. 4.20. Bupivacaine intrapleural catheter

Technique of Trial Dissection of Tumours Which Exhibit Fixation at Initial Thoracoscopic Assessment

The trial dissection starts in the vicinity of the tumour. Laterally, a plane is sought between the lesion and the vertebral column and descending thoracic aorta. If the tumour has not directly invaded these structures, gentle separation is achieved using the curved coaxial scissors and blunt dissection. If such a plane cannot be established because of infiltration, the lesion is inoperable. Medial separation is attempted only if the lateral aspect of the tumour has been mobilized. Often the tumour extends into the pericardium; this can be opened and the involved area removed with the lesion. Direct cardiac involvement indicates inoperability. The most difficult plane to separate in these large tumours is that between the lesion and the tracheal bifurcation and the left bronchus, as this space is frequently occupied by large nodal masses which bleed easily during dissection. If with care, separation of the tumour is achieved, the rest of the operation proceeds as previously described.

Second (Synchronous Combined) Stage

The cervical and abdominal procedures are carried out synchronously. After division of the skin, platysma, investing layer of the deep cervical fascia and omohyoid, the carotid sheath is retracted laterally. Following division of its middle vein, the thyroid lobe is lifted up and the oesophagus and, at least, one recurrent laryngeal nerve (usually left) identified. Very little, if any, further mobilization of the cervical oesophagus is usually needed.

The stomach and abdominal oesophagus are mobilized using the orthodox technique, preserving the right gastroepiploic arcade and ligature of the left gastric artery at its origin from the coeliac artery and removing the related lymph nodes. If the tumour encroaches the cardio-oesophageal junction, the upper lesser curve and adjacent cardio-oesophageal junction are removed, with closure of the gastric tube by hand suture or GIA 80 (Auto-Suture, UK). Pyloroplasty is not performed unless duodenal scarring is present. However, the right-crus of the diaphragmatic hiatus is cut antero-laterally between sutures unless there is a wide hiatus (due to a hiatal hernia).

On completion of the lower transection, the cervical oesophagus is pulled into the neck wound and stapled (TIA 50, AutoSuture, UK). Next, the end of a size 16 Ryle's tube is anchored by transfixation to the oesophagus distal to the staple line and the gullet transected above this level. The oesophagus and tumour are then delivered through the abdominal wound and the gastric fundus stitched to the end of the Ryle's tube. Following cervical gastric pull through, the anastomosis between the proximal oesophagus and the fundus is performed using a single-layer all-coats technique with polyamide sutures. A nasogastric tube is passed before the anterior wall of the anastomosis is completed and its tip placed in the intrathoracic stomach above the diaphragm. A Redivac drain leading to the anastomosis is inserted and the cervical and abdominal wounds are closed.

Postoperative Management

The patient is sent to the intensive care unit on recovery from anaesthesia and is ventilated overnight. In the absence of complications, the patients are extubated the following day and if stable are sent to the high dependency unit. Analgesia is met by intrapleural bupivacaine. Daily chest X-rays are performed during the first 4 days, and the apical chest drain is removed on the second day if the lung was expanded completely. At X-ray examination on the seventh day a Gastrografin is administered orally in order to check the integrity of the anastomosis. If there is no evidence of leakage, oral fluids are started and the neck and basal chest drains removed. Parenteral nutrition is maintained until oral feeding is commenced. Recently, we have opted for routine insertion of a feeding jejunostomy tube inserted at the time of surgery and have dispensed with parenteral nutrition.

Right Prone-Posterior Thoracoscopic Oesophagectomy

On review of the initial series of endoscopic oesophagectomy performed through the right posterolateral approach, we encountered a high (30%) incidence of postoperative pulmonary collapse and consolidation and attributed this to the prolonged single-lung anaesthesia necessary to complete the thoracoscopic dissection of the oesophagus. For this reason we have altered the approach to the full prone posterior jackknife position since this enables the lung to fall away from the operative field and obviates the need for single-lung anaesthesia. Simple lung compression with CO_2 insufflation at a pressure of 6.0 mmHg gives an excellent exposure of the entire intrathoracic oesophagus and mediastinum. This approach now constitutes our standard practice [12]. The technique of dissection of the oesophagus is the same as previously described.

Right Prone-Posterior Jack-knife

The patient is placed in the full prone jackknife position with supports beneath the epigastric and upper sternal regions to enable respiratory excursion of the chest walls. The upper arms are placed hanging on either side of the operating table, with the forearms and hands supported in a sling with the elbow flexed 90° or more. This results in lateral displacement of the scapula (Fig. 4.21). The right prone-posterior thoracoscopic approach gives excellent access to the mediastinum and the entire intrathoracic oesophagus. As the right lung falls away from the operative field by gravity, a good visual exposure is obtained without the need for single lung anaesthesia.

Position and Types of Access Ports

The same types and number of cannulae are used (Fig. 4.22). The optical cannula (10 mm) is placed through the intercostal space encountered below and lateral to the inferior angle of the scapula (usually the fifth). The flexible operating cannulae are inserted through the separate intercostal spaces

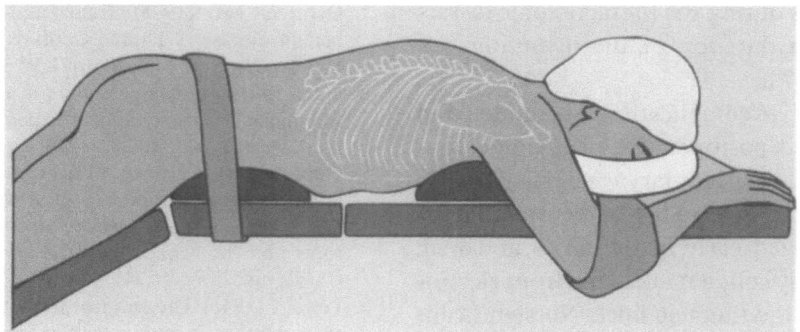

Fig. 4.21. Prone-posterior jackknife position

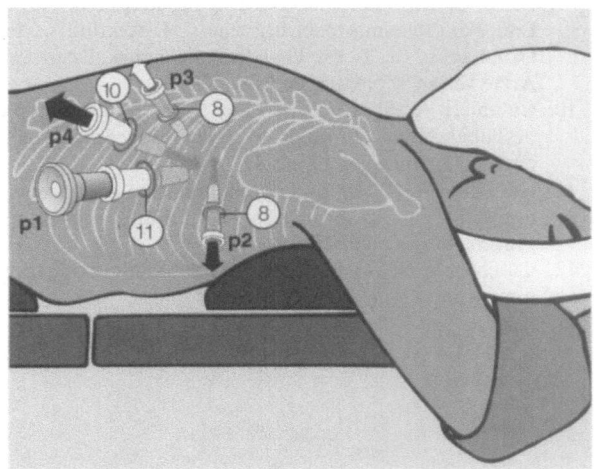

Fig. 4.22. Sites of access ports for right prone-posterior position

above and on either side of the telescope, some 5.0 cm from the spinous processes. A 10.5- or 12-mm cannula is placed laterally low down (seventh interspace). This is used by the assistant for retraction and for the introduction of the EndoGIA stapler when stapled division of the azygos vein is contemplated.

Clinical Results

Staging and Endoscopic Resectability

In a consecutive series of 34 patients with oesophageal cancer, two were found have hepatic deposits at laparoscopy and four were inoperable at thoracoscopic staging (pleural deposits $n = 2$, invasion of descending aorta $n = 1$, invasion of the myocardium $n = 1$). A further two patients had dense fibrous obliteration of the pleural cavity which precluded the endoscopic dissection. The first 20 were conducted through the posterolateral right thoracoscopic approach with one conversion due to aortic bleeding and the last six through the prone-posterior jackknife route. The distribution of the site of the tumours, the extent of mural involvement and lymph node staging is shown in Table 4.1.

In one patient with a large middle third neoplasm, massive aortic bleeding requiring immediate thoracotomy was encountered during its separation from the aorta. In all the others, there was no mea-

Table 4.1. Pathology of endoscopically resected tumours

	n
Site	
Middle third	19
Lower third	12
Pathological stage	
Mucosal tumour	1
Incomplete mural invasion	3
Complete mural invasion	27
Nodal disease	
N_0	12
N_{1-2}	19

surable blood loss during the thoracoscopic dissection. The median duration of the operation was 5.5 h, range 4.5–7 h.

The postoperative complications encountered in the series included postoperative pneumonic consolidation ($n = 3$), recurrent laryngeal palsy ($n = 2$) and anastomotic leak ($n = 1$). The recurrent laryngeal palsies occurred early in the series and were probably caused by collateral damage from electrocoagulation near the thoracic inlet. No significant pulmonary complications have been observed in the patients in whom the oesophagectomy was conducted by the prone-posterior jackknife approach. There were no postoperative deaths in the entire series. The median postoperative stay has been 12 days, range 9–30 days.

References

1. Turner GC (1933) Excision of the thoracic oesophagus for carcinoma with reconstruction of an extra-throacic gullet. Lancet ii:1315–1317
2. Orringer MB (1987) Transthoracic versus transhiatal esophagectomy: what difference does it make? Ann Thorac Surg 44:116–126
3. Orringer MB (1985) Transhiatal esophagectomy for benign disease. J Thorac Cardiovasc Surg 90:649–655
4. Stewart JR, Sarr MG, Sharp KW, Efron G et al. Transhiatal (blunt) esophagectomy for malignant and benign esophageal disease: clinical experience and technique. Ann Thorac Surg 40:343–348
5. Godfaden D, Orringer MB, Appelman HD, Kalish R (1986) Adenocarcinoma of the distal esophagus and gastric cardia. Comparison of transhiatal esophagectomy and thoracoabdominal esophagectomy. J Thorac Cardiovasc Surg 91:242–247
6. Lewis I (1946) The surgical treatment of carcinoma of the oesophagus with special reference to a new operation for growths of the middle third. Br J Surg 34:18–31
7. Tanner NC (1947) The present position of carcinoma of the oesophagus. Postgrad Med J 23:109–139
8. McKeown KC (1976) Total three stage oesophagectomy for cancer of the oesophagus. Br J Surg 63:259–262
9. Buess G, Kipfmüller K, Nahrun M, Melzer A (1990) Endoskopische-mikrochirurgische Dissektion des Ösophagus. In: Buess G (ed) Endoskopie. Deutscher Ärzte-Verlag, Cologne, pp 358–375
10. Cuschieri A, Shimi S, Banting S (1992) Endoscopic oesophagectomy through a right thoracoscopic approach. J Coll Surg Edinb 37:7–11
11. Cuschieri A (1993) Endoscopic subtotal oesophagectomy for cancer through a right thoracoscopic approach. Surg Oncol 2:3–11
12. Cuschieri A (1994) Thoracoscopic subtotal oesophagectomy. Endoscopic Surg 26:134–147

5 Thoracoscopic Pericardiectomy and Insertion of Epicardial Pacemaker Lead

A. CUSCHIERI

Introduction

Although it is difficult to predict the ultimate scope of thoracoscopic cardiac surgery with or without a small access thoracotomy (video-assisted thoracoscopic surgery), there is little doubt about its potential; single case reports of ligation of patent ductus are documented and experimental cannulation of the atrial chambers has been performed. In this chapter the technique of two simple cardiac procedures – pericardial fenestration for effusion and insertion of epicardial pacemaker lead – are outlined. Our limited experience with these two operations has been entirely favourable. Excellent results have also been reported from other centres [1].

Preoperative Work-up and Preparation

Anaesthesia

Both pericardial fenestration and insertion of epicardial pacemaker leads are conducted under general endotracheal anaesthesia. If the condition of the patient permits, single lung anaesthesia (trilumen tube) is ideal for exposure of the pericardial sac. These patients require expert anaesthesia with continuous cardiovascular monitoring and blood gas analysis during the procedure.

Instrumentation

Although thoracoscopic pericardial fenestration and insertion of epicardial pacemaker leads can be conducted with the use of standard straight laparoscopic instrumentation, the use of the coaxial curved instruments introduced through flexible metal cannulae greatly facilitates the execution of both operations. The endoscopic pericardial hook (Fig. 5.1) is very useful for tenting and stabilizing the pericardial sac prior to opening it. Especially when distended by serous effusion, the pericardium may be difficult to grasp with a dissecting forceps.

Positioning of the Patient and Skin Preparation

For both procedures, the patient is put in the left posterolateral position with the left arm well abducted on a rest and the operating table split (or the central bridge raised) to widen the intercostal spaces.

For pericardial fenestration, only the skin of the left chest wall is prepared with medicated soap and appropriate skin disinfectant and the area draped accordingly. In patients undergoing insertion of an

Fig. 5.1. Endoscopic pericardial hook (Storz, Tuttlingen, Germany)

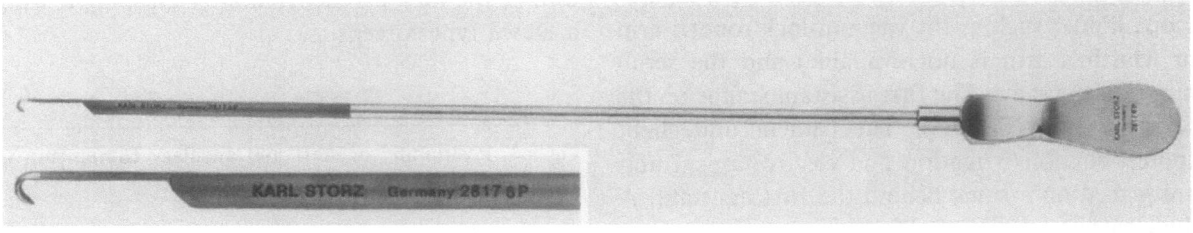

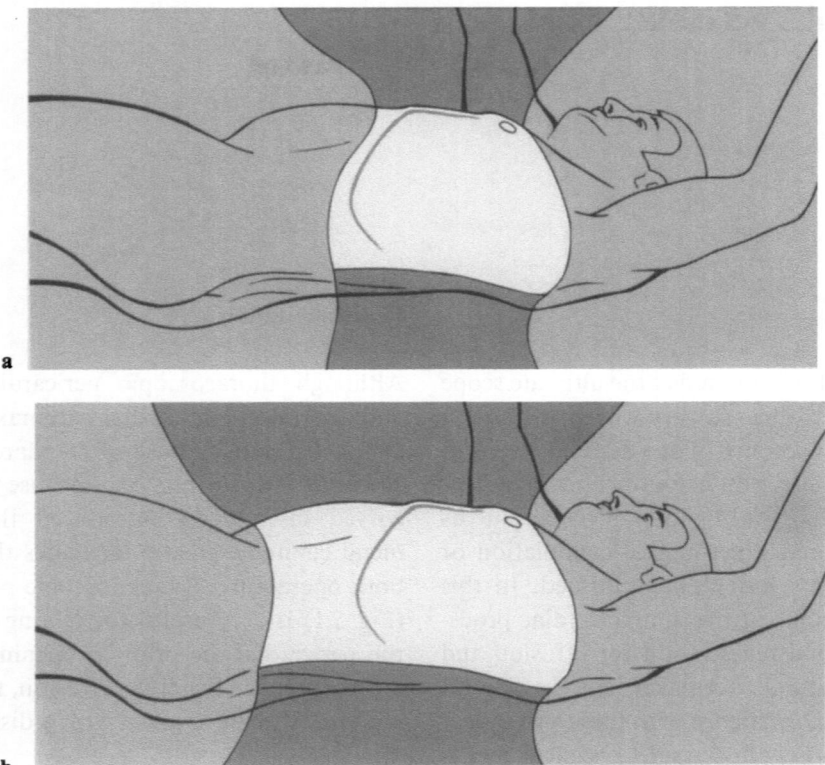

a

b

Fig. 5.2 a, b. Skin preparation and draping for pericardiectomy (**a**) and for thoracoscopic implantation of epicardial pacemaker lead (**b**) with the patient in the left posterolateral thoracic position

epicardial pacemaker lead, the skin preparation includes the left chest wall and the upper left quadrant of the abdomen (Fig. 5.2 a, b).

Layout of Ancillary Equipment and Postioning of Staff

The surgeon operates from the right side of the operating table with the camera person (if a laparoscope holder such as the vacuum-lock robotic arm or Martin's arm is not available) and the scrub nurse on the same. The first assistant stands on the opposite side (Fig. 5.3). The camera unit, light source, suction/irrigation and electrosurgical unit are placed on a stack behind the first assistant. A dual monitor display is ideal.

Sites of Trocar and Cannulae

Usually three trocar and cannulae are needed for either procedure. The telescope cannula (11-mm; p1) is inserted below and behind the angle of the scapula just in front of the angle of the left fourth rib. The two operating cannulae (metal flexible, 8-mm; p2, p3) are placed two intercostal spaces lower down anteriorly and posteriorly such that the tips of the instruments (introduced through them) meet at a right angle at the middle of the left pericardium. These two operating cannulae are inserted under vision (Fig. 5.4). Occasionally, a fourth cannula placed near the sternal edge above the anterior operating cannula is needed for retraction of the lung parenchyma after grasping it with a Duval type forceps.

Fig. 5.3. Positioning of staff and ancillary equipment; *S*, surgeon

Fig. 5.4. Sites of trocar and cannulae

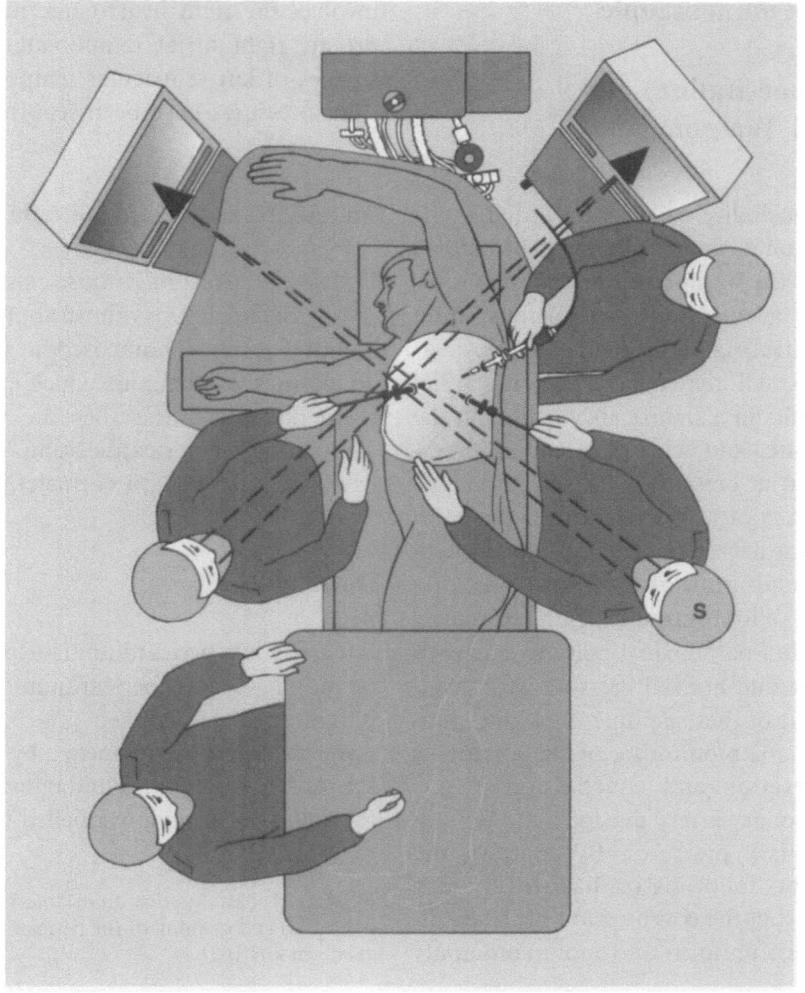

5.3

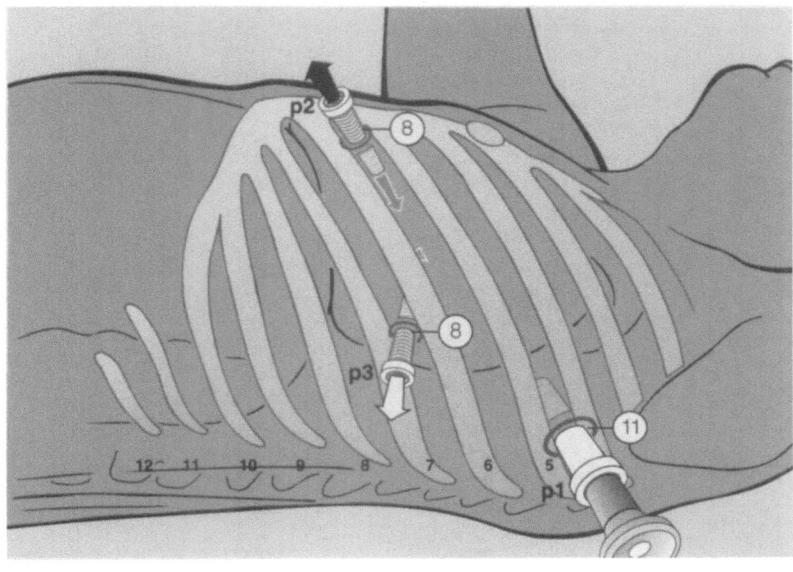

5.4

Technique of Thoracoscopic Pericardiectomy (Pericardial Fenestration) for Pericardial Tamponade

The limited distensibility of the pericardial sac is the principle factor in the development of cardiac tamponade when the intrapericardial volume is increased by the accumulation of serous fluid (uraemic, metastatic origin) or blood clots (postcardiac surgery). A small increment in the pericardial fluid volume results in a significant increase in the pericardial pressure, and when this equals or exceeds the right atrial pressure, cardiac tamponade ensures. In the case of serous effusions, the compression of the cardiac chambers is uniform, with elevation and equalization of the filling pressures of both ventricles, a low output state, raised central venous pressure and paradoxical pulse (decrease in the stroke volume and arterial pressure with inspiration and increase of these parameters with expiration) [2]. Swan-Ganz monitoring of these patients demonstrates elevation and equalization of the right atrial, pulmonary artery diastolic and pulmonary wedge capillary pressures. By contrast, the tamponade by clots following cardiac surgery may be localized such that the compression of the cardiac chambers is not uniform and more commonly involves the right heart (superior venal caval syndrome, right atrial tamponade) [3] although instances of left ventricular tamponade with normal right pressures have been reported.

Indications and Contraindications

Pericardial effusion is most commonly treated today by the open subxyphoid approach which avoids a thoracotomy. Thoracoscopic pericardiectomy is an alternative technique which can be employed in these patients unless they are very unstable [1]. Thoracoscopic pericardiectomy is also contraindicated in patients with constrictive pericarditis.

Operative Steps

After the left pericardium is exposed by retraction of the lingula, the pericardium anterior to the left phrenic nerve is hooked (Fig. 5.5; p2) and tented upwards before being opened by the curved coaxial scissors (Fig. 5.5; p3). Fluid immediately gushes out through the opening, propelled by the cardiac pul-

Fig. 5.5. Hooking pericardium anterior to the left phrenic nerve (p2) and opening of the pericardium by the curved coaxial scissors (p3)

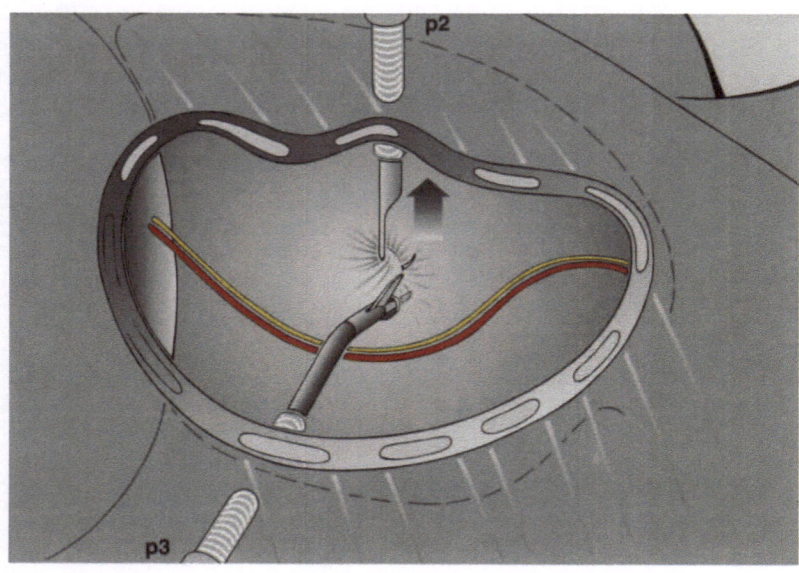

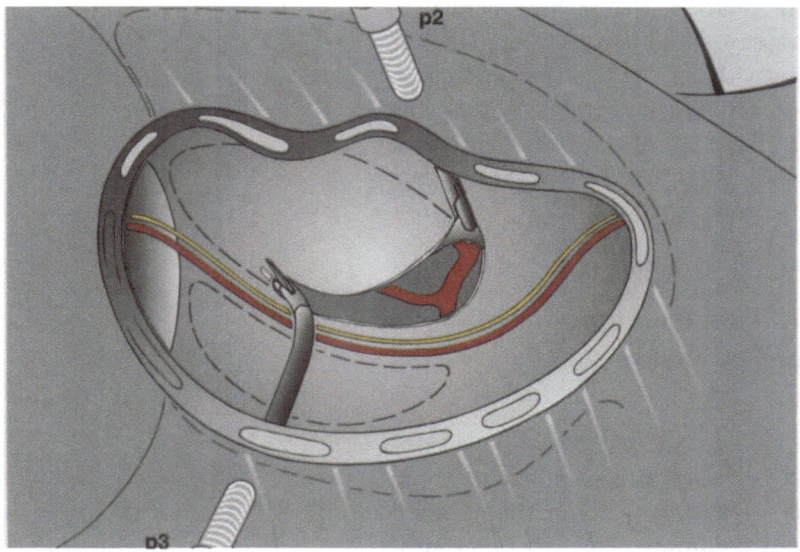

5.6

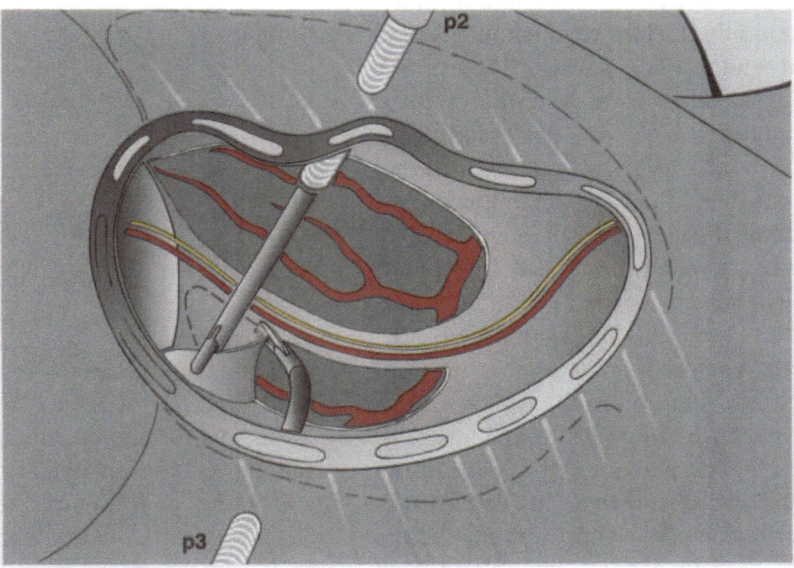

5.7

Fig. 5.6. Anterior pericardial fenestration. Start of the pericardial window

5.7. Extension of the completed pericardial fenestration behind the left phrenic nerve and accompanying vessels and to the tip of the ventricle

sations. It is sucked as it escapes into the pleural cavity. A specimen is obtained for culture and cytology. The cut pericardium is then picked with an atraumtic grasper and a sufficient window excised anterior to the left phrenic nerve and the pericardio-phrenic vessels (Fig. 5.6). Bleeding from the cut pericardial edges is controlled by soft electrocoagulation. Inspection of the pericardial sac and myocardium is best undertaken with a flexible choledochoscope introduced through the posterior operating cannula. The flexible endoscope is passed between the heart and the pericardium as this is tented upwards. Loculated fluid and especially clots can be identified in this fashion. Clots are best dislodged by irrigation with warm (37 °C)

Ringer's lactate solution. Severe bradycardia can occur if the irrigating fluid is cold (room temperature). If necessary, the pericardial resection can be extended behind the phrenic nerve and its accompanying vessels (Fig. 5.7). At the end of the procedure, a basal chest drain is inserted, the cannulae removed and the lung expanded.

Technique of Thoracoscopic Insertion of Epicardial Pacemaker

Permanent pacemaker implantation is needed in patients (usually elderly) with complete arteriovenous block, persistent and symptomatic bradycardia, the sick sinus syndrome, cerebrovascular insufficiency secondary to a low cardiac output, tachyarrhythmias and certain cases of myocardial infarction. Most commonly the intravenous route is used for permanent endocardial pacing, a procedure which is conducted under local anaesthesia under fluoroscopic control. However, epicardial leads (screw-in or fish-hook type) are more accurate and dependable, causing few late complications. Epicardial pacemaker leads are usually inserted via the subxiphoid approach and less commonly, transthoracically (left anterolateral, fourth space). An alternative, recently introduced, is the thoracoscopically guided approach to the left ventricle. Although implantation in the right ventricle can be performed (right thoracoscopic approach), we prefer the left approach because the walls of the left ventricle are thicker and there is consequently less risk of penetration of the endocardium and the electrode tip coming in contact with blood or a small haematoma forms, resulting in a poor threshold.

Our experience with thoracoscopic implantation is limited to the use of the "screw-in" type of sutureless epicardial lead. We have used the Medtronic (Minneapolis, USA) sutureless epicardial device, model 6917A-T, which has a corkscrew lead that is secured to the myocardium with two clockwise turns and a Dacron mesh diaphragm which allows fibrous ingrowth for additional fixation (Fig. 5.8). both unipolar (single) and bipolar (double) electrodes can be placed but they must be at least 1 cm apart.

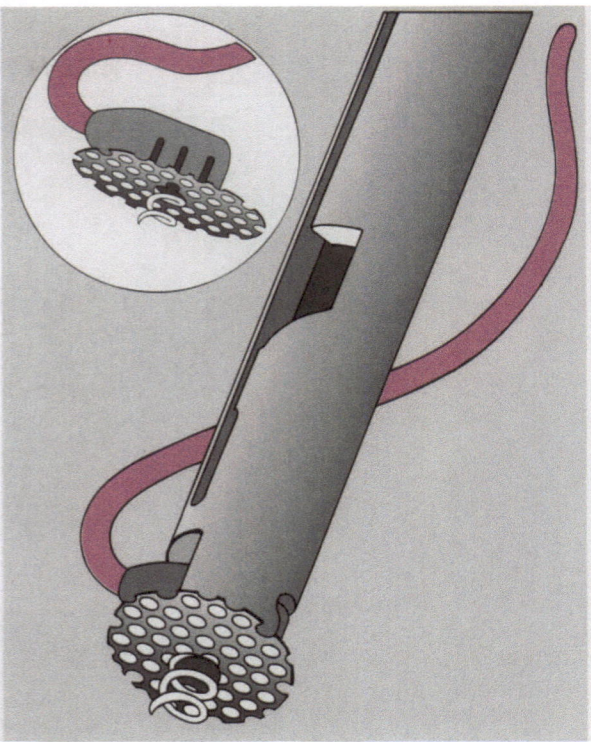

Fig. 5.8. Close-up of the Medtronic epicardial sutureless pacing lead (Model 6917A-T, Medtronic, Minneapolis, USA). The electrode head is slotted into the receiving space at the end of the handle

Indications and Contraindications

In our institution, epicardial leads are inserted when permanent ventricular or dual-chamber pacing is needed and attempts at permanent endocardial pacing by the cardiologists have been unsuccessful. Epicardial screw-in pacemaker implantation is contraindicated in patients with a thin-walled, heavily infarcted, or fibrotic myocardium or one which is extensively infiltrated by fat.

Preparation of the Lead

The lead is mounted before the operation is commenced. The Medtronic system consists of a handle and a tunneller. The electrode head is slotted into the receiving space at the end of the handle (Fig. 5.8). The pointed tip of the tunneller is then inserted inside the handle from the opposite end

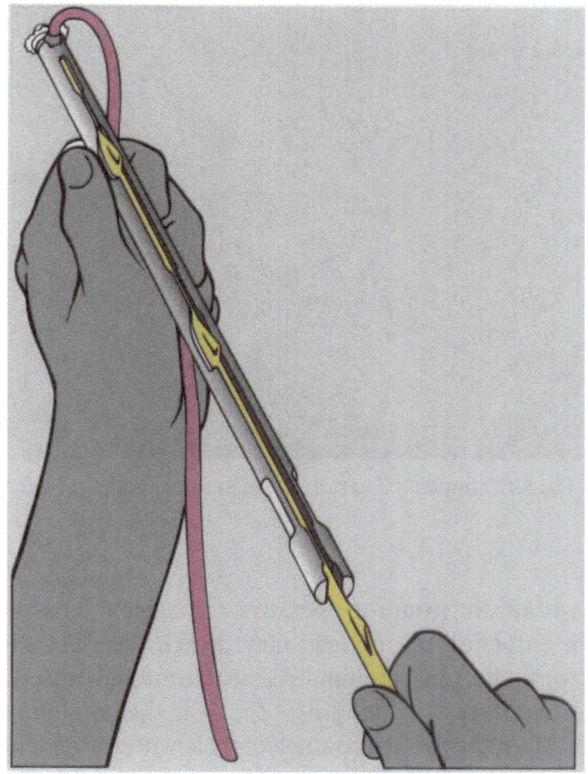

Fig. 5.9. Inserting the tunneller inside the handle from the opposite end such that the projections on the tunneller are in line with the notches on the handle

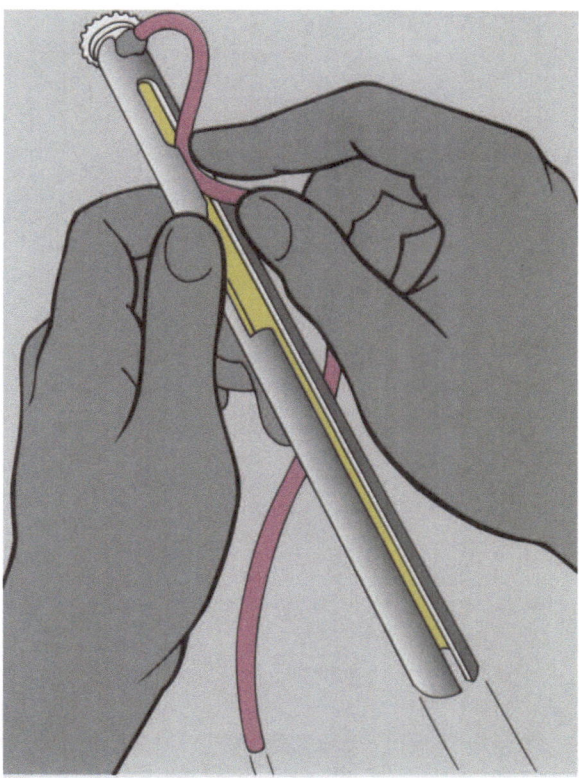

Fig. 5.10. Slotting lead from the electrode head inside the groove on the handle, leaving a small loop near the electrode head

such that the projections on the tunneller are in line with the notches on the handle (Fig. 5.9). The tunneller is then rotated anticlockwise and pulled back to engage the projections within the notches. The lead from the electrode head is then slotted inside the groove on the handle, leaving a small loop near the electrode head (Fig. 5.10). The mounted lead is then placed on the sterile trolley until required.

A cardiology technician should be present in theatre for testing of the lead once this has been implanted (satisfactory threshold, resistance and R wave potential).

Operative Steps

The exposure is the same as previously described for pericardial fenestration. After the pericardium is hooked, it is opened by curved coaxial scissors, starting in front of the phrenic nerve and extending

to the tip of the ventricle (see Fig. 5.7). Careful selection of the site of implantation is essential: the coronary arteries and veins must be avoided and an area of normal looking myocardium chosen (free from fibrosis and scarring). The previously mounted electrode (see above) is introduced into the left chest cavity through an appropriately sited intercostal incision. The tip of the electrode is approximated to the chosen site on the left ventricular myocardium as this is exposed by distraction of the cut pericardial edges. The surgeon then places the tip of the electrode on the myocardium, using only light pressure, and holds it in place with the right hand. The electrode is affixed to the myocardium with two clockwise turns on the handle (Fig. 5.11). Electrical measurements are taken before the lead is unloaded from the handle. If these prove unsatisfactory, they should be repeated after an interval of 10 min, when they often normalize as the acute cellular trauma subsides. Should the electrical mea-

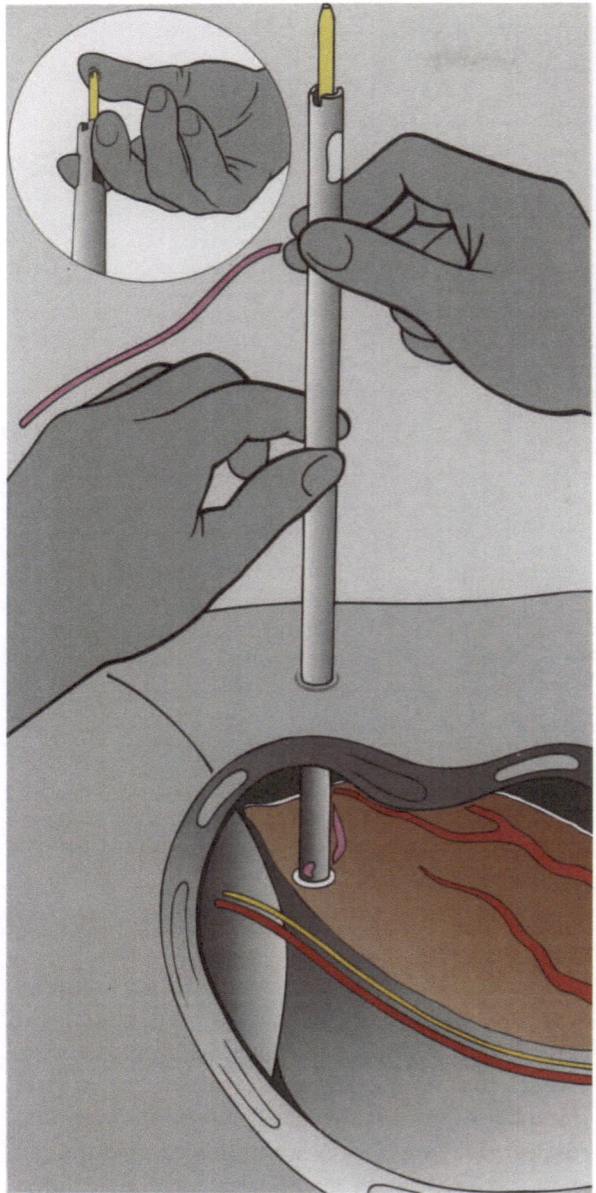

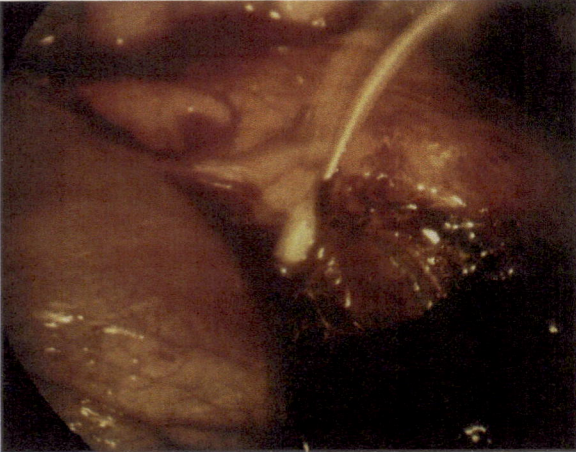

Fig. 5.12. Implanted detached Medtronic epicardial lead

Fig. 5.11. Affixing the electrode to the myocardium with two clockwise turns on the handle. The implanted electrode is released by gentle pressure on the tunneller against the butt of the handle

surements prove unsatisfactory after this interval, the electrode tip is released by two anticlockwise turns and another implantation site is selected. The implanted electrode is released by gentle pressure on the tunneller against the butt of the handle (Fig. 5.11). It is essential that the lead be totally disengaged from the handle before the latter is withdrawn from the operative site, since the resulting traction on the lead may detach the electrode from the myocardium. As an additional precaution, it is wise to grasp the lead gently by an atraumatic forceps as the handle is withdrawn. The implanted, detached lead is shown in Fig. 5.12. The pericardium is closed loosely by two interrupted sutures using Polysorb (USSC, Norwalk, USA) mounted on endoski needles.

The next step of the operation consists in the creation of a rectus sheath pocket for the pulse generator in the left subcostal region. It is important that this pocket not be fashioned too close to the costal margin as the implanted device will cause discomfort to the patient each time the chest is flexed when the pulse generator presses against the rib cage. A transverse incision is made in the skin, subcutaneous tissue and anterior rectus sheath. The rectus muscle is divided transversely by the electrosurgical knife. The exposed posterior rectus sheath is separated from the cut rectus muscle until a pocket of sufficient capacity to accommodate the pulse generator is created (Fig. 5.13). At this stage, the lead is passed subcutaneously from the intercostal wound to the rectus sheath pocket using the tunneller (Fig. 5.13). After the connector pin of the electrode lead has been detached from the tunneller, it is connected to the pulse generator, which is then placed in the rectus pocket such that the printed side (indifferent electrode) faces the rectus sheath; otherwise, painful contractions of the rec-

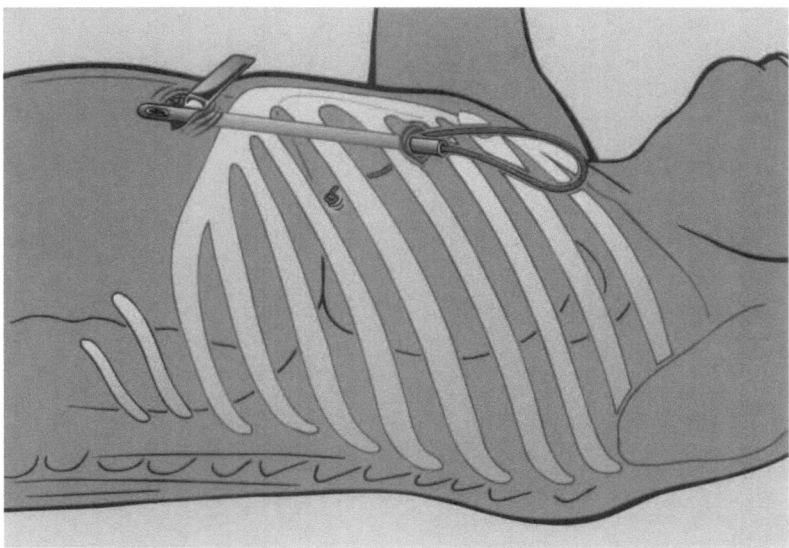

Fig. 5.13. Separating the exposed posterior rectus sheath from the cut rectus muscle until a pocket of sufficient capacity to accommodate the pulse generator is created. The lead is passed subcutaneously from the intercostal wound to the rectus sheath pocket using the tunneller

tus muscle are induced. Care is taken to ensure that there are no kinks or tension on the electrode lead before the wounds are closed. The anterior rectus sheath is closed over the pulse generator by continuous absorbable suture (polydioxanone or polyglycide) and the skin edges approximated by subcuticular suturing or skin clips. The lung is then expanded and the cannulae removed after the insertion of a chest drain.

Postoperative Care

Following implantation of an epicardial pacemaker, the patient's electrocardiogram should be monitored continuously for 1 week to ensure that the leads have not become dislodged, which is a well-recognized potential complication. The chest drain is removed in these patients as soon as full lung expansion is documented on the postoperative chest X-ray and there is no leakage of air from the intercostal underwater seal drain. In patients undergoing pericardiectomy, the chest drain is removed after full lung expansion and cessation of fluid drainage, usually within 24 h.

References

1. Hazelrigg SR, Mack M, Landreneau R (1992) Thoracoscopic pericardiectomy for pericardial effusion. Min Invas Ther [Suppl 1] 1:39
2. Reddy PS, Curtiss EL, O'Toole JD et al (1978) Cardiac tamponade: hemodynamic observations in man. Circulation 58:265–272
3. Bateman T, Gray R, Chaux A et al (1982) Right atrial tamponade caused by hematoma complicating coronary artery bypass graft surgery: clinical hemodynamic and scintigraphic correlates. J Thorac Cardiovasc Surg 84: 413–419

6 Endoscopic Procedures in the Mediastinum

K. MANNCKE, G. BUESS, and G. ROVIARO

Introduction

Besides the two different endoscopic techniques for oesophagectomy other diseases of the mediastinum can be treated or diagnosed thoracoscopically to diminish patient's pain and discomfort. There is a wide spectrum of procedures in mediastinal surgery with different technical difficulties, varying from simple removal of pedunculated neoplasms to more complex excisions of large masses or to extremely difficult resections of firmly adherent tumours infiltrating into the vicinity of important structures. This chapter describes procedures for the surgical treatment of benign tumours of the oesophagus and techniques of harvesting specimens for diagnostic purposes in patients with undiagnosed malignancies in the medastinum. Noninvasive, well encaspulated thymic neoplasms, nervous tumours at the costovertebral junction, dysontogenetic tumours (pleuropericardial cysts, bronchogenic cysts, enterogeneous cysts etc.) with a noninfiltrating tendency can be removed endoscopically.

Indications

Benign Tumours of the Oesophagus

Benign tumours of the oesophageal wall are rare and the clinical symptoms are caused by stenosis. Neoplasms can originate in all the different types of tissue in the layers of the oesophagus, so one can encounter lipomas, fibromas, and bronchogenic cysts, but most common are leiomyomas. Since malignancy has to be definitely excluded, these smooth muscle tumours always require excision. Biopsies taken via an oesophagoscope cannot reach the tumorous tissue, and snare excisions of these

and other mucosal lesions can lead to oesophageal perforation. Hence, none of these manipulations should be performed and the diagnosis confirmed instead by removal of the entire tumour. In open surgery this procedure entails thoracotomy, which seems inappropriate for such small tumours. In such cases the endoscopic approach is obviously far less traumatic.

Diagnostic Evaluation of Mediastinal Masses

Other tumors in the mediastinum can only be diagnosed by biopsy taken under endoscopic guidance. In contrast to traditional mediastinoscopy, thoracoscopic access permits much better orientation and overview and one side of the mediastinum can be inspected and dissected entirely. Specimens can be harvested from all parts, even those which are out of reach of mediastinoscopy. Dissection of lymph nodes and their removal in toto is feasible as is biopsy with a Tru-cut needle under endoscopic guidance. Control of bleeding is easier and safer. This technique is useful not only for the various types of lymphomas; the method has also been used to stage oesophageal and bronchial carcinomas.

Oesophageal Diverticulae

Diverticulae of the oesophagus are commonly located at the three physiological narrowings of the oseophagus, two of them in the mediastinum. In the presence of clinical symptoms such as regurgitation, resection is indicated. Again, conventional procedure requires a large and painful incision. In consequence the thoracoscopic technique has several advantages.

Preoperative Work-up

Benign Tumours of the Oesophagus

The preoperative work-up of benign tumours of the oesophagus includes radiological and endoscopic procedures. After first evaluating the clinical symptoms, a barium swallow is necessary in order to localize the tumour. This is followed by oesophagogastroscopy. It may be necessary to decide a biopsy should be taken or to leave the mucosa untouched. Computer tomography (CT) scan is essential to display the relationship to the surrounding tissues. If available, intraluminal ultrasound examination may be helpful. Intraluminal ultrasound is becoming increasingly important. The method is not very common yet, but as in examinations of the rectal wall, the anatomical relations to the different layers of the oseophageal wall can be displayed. A conventional X-ray of the thorax in antero posterior and lateral projection is necessary to obtain information about pleural adhesions and atelectases or other signs which may make thoracoscopy difficult. Since general anaesthesia is performed in most cases with double-lumen intubation and single-lung ventilation, extensive examination of pulmonary function completes the preoperative work-up.

Diagnostic Evaluation of Mediastinal Masses

For other conditions of the mediastinum and also when endoscopic biopsy is performed the site of the lesion must be known very precisely preoperatively. This requires, again, X-ray of the thorax and a CT scan. Intraluminal oesophageal ultrasound examination may also be helpful.

Oesophageal Diverticulae

The diagnosis of oesophageal diverticulae is usually confirmed by a barium swallow and oesophagoscopy. These two methods identify the location and the size of the diverticulum. In planning thoracoscopic procedures the choice of the side of approach is very important.

Preoperative Preparation

Patient Consent and General Preparation

As for other endoscopic procedures it is essential that patients are informed about the possibility of conversion to open access during surgery. In the two procedures involving the oesophageal wall, serious complications of lesions of the oesophageal mucosa and consequences such as mediastinitis must be known by the patient. In interventions in the upper mediastinum recurrent nerve palsies must be mentioned.

In contrast to other thoracoscopic procedures it is very important that oesophagoscopy can be performed intraoperatively. This is very helpful in identifying the site of the tumour or the diverticulum. Lesions and breaches of the mucosa can be detected intraoperatively. General anaesthesia has to be carried out with a double-lumen tube.

The best preparation of the patient for all kinds of thoracic procedures is by physiotherapy, if necessary bronchial dilators, mucolytics, administration of expectorants and abstinence from smoking.

Patient Positioning, Skin Preparation and Draping

As for other thoracoscopic procedures the patient has to be positioned on the contralateral side of the approach. Conversion to open access surgery must be possible at any time. Most patients require a three to four puncture procedure. The position of the trocars depends on the location of the tumour or diverticulum (Fig. 6.1). So the ipsilateral arm is elevated and abducted to displace the scapula. The table is split such that the ribs are splayed out (Fig. 6.2). Skin preparation is not different from other procedures in general surgery. Plastics drapes should not be used, however, so as to avoid any plastic material getting into the thoracic wall or the pleural cavity at the puncture site.

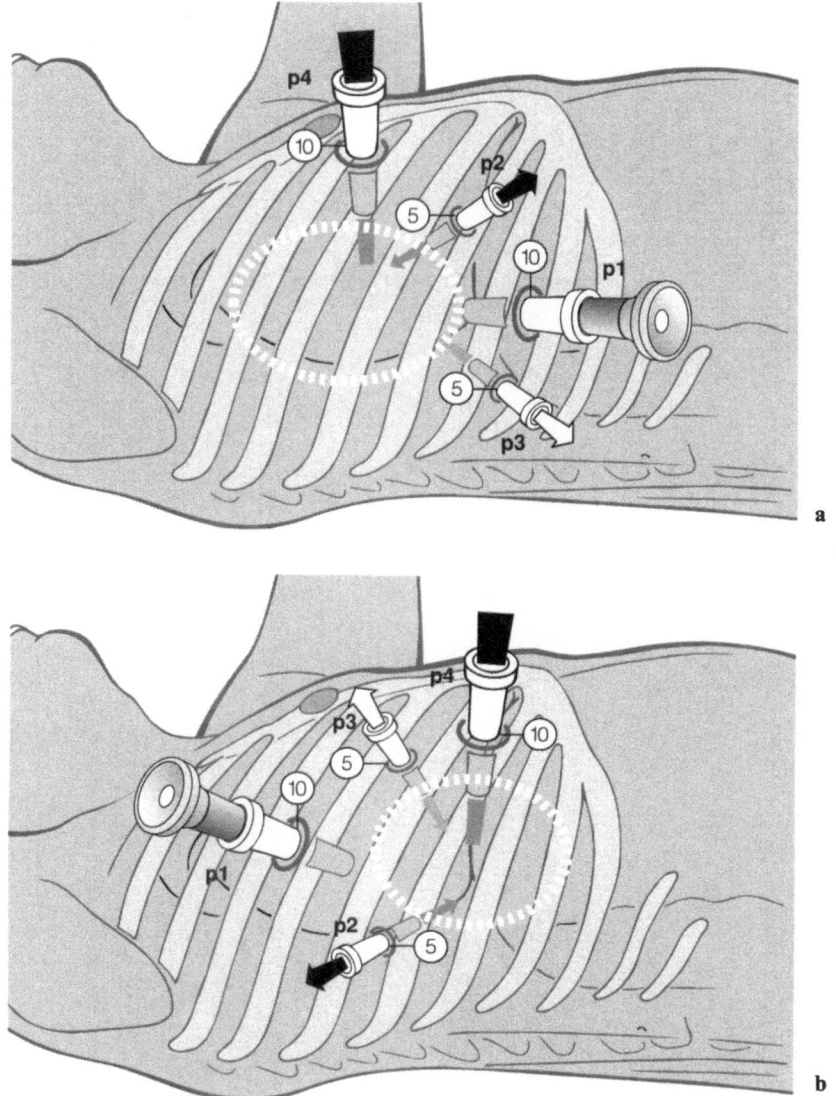

Fig. 6.1 a, b. Trocar placement in relation to the site of the tumour.
a Lesion of the proximal oesophagus; **b** lesion of the distal oesophagus

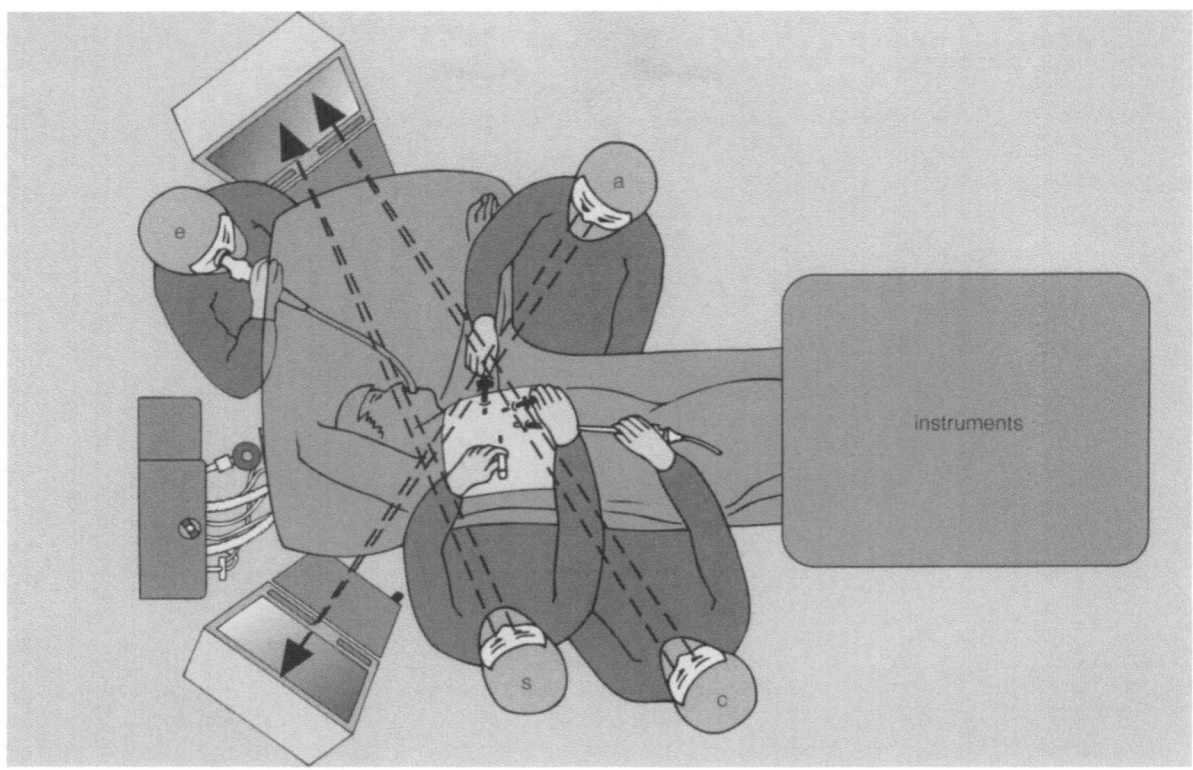

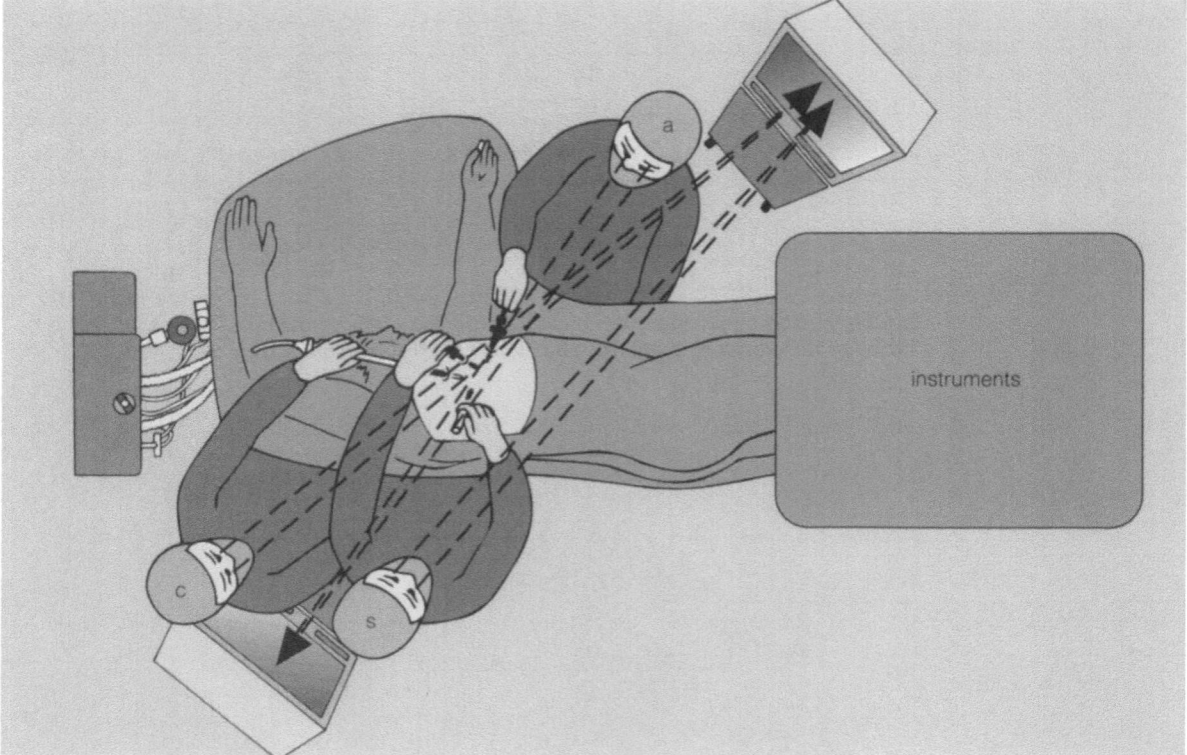

Fig. 6.2 a, b. Placement of the staff and positioning of patient. **a** Lesion of the proximal oesophagus; **b** lesion of the distal oesophagus

Layout of Ancillary Instruments and Positioning of Staff

For oesophagoscopy the endoscopic surgeon and equipment are positioned at the patient's head beside the anaesthetist. The procedures are usually performed by three surgeons. The second assistant stands on the opposite side and holds the lung-retracting instruments. The first assistant handling the endoscope and the camera and the surgeon are positioned at the dorsal side of the patient. In consequence, two monitors are located opposite the surgeons. Insufflation is, in principle, not necessary but initially helpful to accelerate the collapse of the lung. Besides this, a unit for rinsing and suction is required. This is also positioned opposite the surgeon. If the main monitor, the light source and the camera processor are installed in one unit they are positioned at the ventral side of the patient.

Specific Instrumentation

For thoracoscopic procedures several specific instruments have been designed, i.e. special trocars with blunt tips and flexible sleeves with a screw-like shape. In addition to the instruments developed by Cuschieri and produced by Storz (Tuttlingen, Germany) Inderbitzi of Berne, Switzerland, has designed a set of thoracoscopic instruments which is produced and distributed by Wolf (Knittlingen, Germany; Fig. 6.3). All the instruments are angled, so all parts of the thoracic cavity can be reached. Following similar principles Linder of Stuttgart, constructed another set in conjunction with the Duffner Company (Tuttlingen, Germany). Finally, Landreneau has designed in collaboration with PCI (Liptingen, Germany) his own thoracoscopic instruments. All of these have been developed specifically for thoracic and pulmonary surgery. In addition to these reusable instruments special disposable ones are also available (Fig. 6.4). For thoracoscopic surgical purposes the fan retractor and special grasping forceps are noteworthy. The force of these graspers is elastic via a spring, and the grip has been designed to avoid damage of lung tissue.

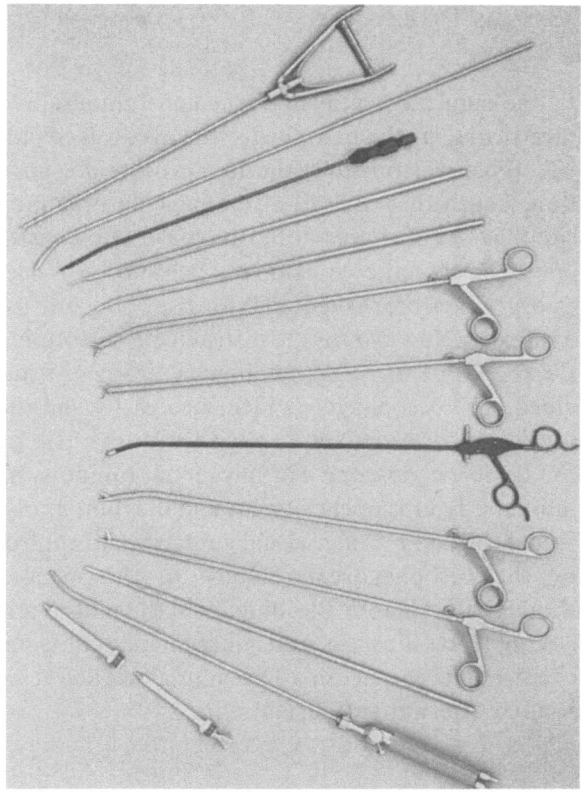

Fig. 6.3. A set of reusable thoracoscopic instruments (Wolf)

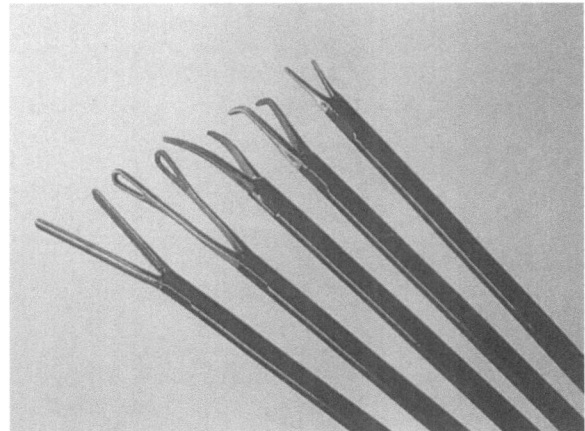

Fig. 6.4. Disposable instruments (Ethicon)

Various Procedures

In the surgical treatment of benign tumours and diverticulae of the oesophagus the access is identical. Whenever possible, the four trocars are positioned such that the site of drainage and the incision line of the thoracotomy are taken into consideration in case of conversion to open surgery is necessary. One trocar is required for the optic, one for a retractor, and two for the instruments performing the procedure. First the pulmonary ligament is divided. The oesophagus is identified easily and the tumour or diverticulum localized with the help of the flexible endoscope. For intramural tumours the muscular layer is opened (split) and the tumour dissected (Fig. 6.5). Under visual guidance and control by the oesophagoscope injury to the mucosa should be avoidable. Bleeding from the muscularis is stopped by clips, since coagulation may cause necrosis of the mucosa. The muscular defect is sutured afterwards (Fig. 6.6).

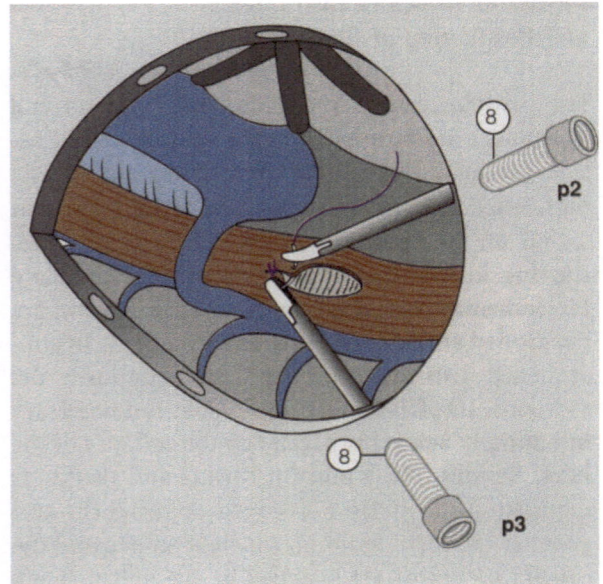

Fig. 6.6. Suturing of the muscular layer of the oseophagus

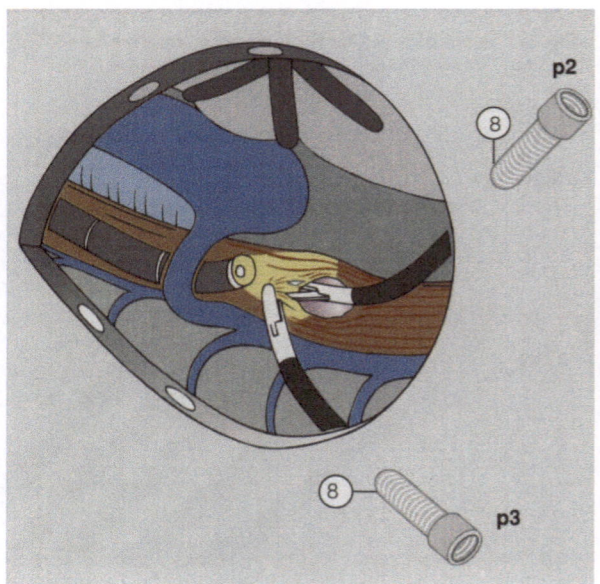
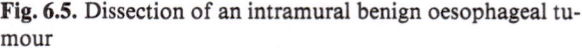

Fig. 6.5. Dissection of an intramural benign oesophageal tumour

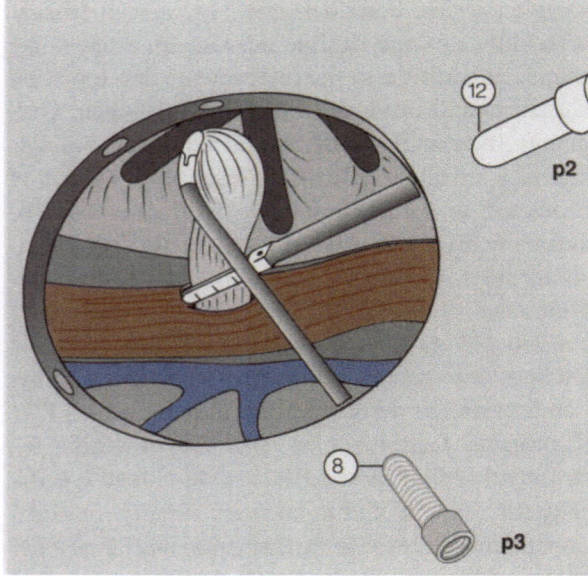

Fig. 6.7. Transection of an oesophageal diverticulum with a linear stapler

Diverticulae may be treated in different ways. One technique is resection with closure of the defect with a two-layer suture. Stapling (Endo GIA *) may be safer than suturing (Fig. 6.7), but is impeded by the rigid instrument having to be introduced at an inappropriate angle. With the advent of steerable linear staplers, for which prototypes already exist, this will be facilitated.

In infiltrating mediastinal masses, surgery often only involves diagnostic biopsy. So in most cases two or three puncture sites are suitable. Smaller lymph nodes at any location can be dissected and removed. They should be extracted incide the trocar sleeve or a bag to avoid contact with the tissues of the chest wall. Bleeding is controlled by coagulation or clips. If the mass is in the upper anterior mediastinum a core biopsy with a Tru-cut needle under thoracoscopic guidance may be the appropriate procedure. Larger masses of lymph nodes may cover the greater vessels. During the entire procedure the orientation of important structures of the mediastinum is essential.

Often mediastinal tumours are benign, well encapsulated and usually present distinct cleavage planes with adjacent structures which facilitates their isolation and can thus be easily removed, in contrast to infiltrating tumours. Typical examples are neurinomas, bronchogenic cysts and thymic neoplasms.

The most frequent site of neurinomas is the costovertebral junction but neurogenic tumours can develop elsewhere. They are usually subpleural and variable in size. Two operative trocars are generally sufficient to remove the mass with ease. The parietal pleura covering the tumour is incised around the mass with high-frequency electrocutting. It is then enucleated by dissecting the cleavage plane with a mounted swab. The procedure is usually dry, since the surrounding tissue has little blood supply. Smaller vessels can be easily electrocoagulated, while the intercostal artery, if injured, can be dissected and clipped. When preoperative examination or thoracoscopic exploration shows the tumour extending into the vertebral foramen, the extravertebral part of the tumour should be removed and the patient referred to a neurosurgeon to remove the rest of the tumour. The heterogeneous group of mediastinal cysts includes tumours which are simple to remove and others

which are very difficult to excise. Pleuropericardial cysts are the easiest to remove; they always have thin walls and originate at the cardiophrenic angle in close relationship with the pericardium. They are usually readily separable from the fatty aerial mediastinal tissue. Before dissecting the mass and particularly before using electrocoagulation or endograspers, it is very important to identify the phrenic nerve. Dissection of the cyst can be performed simply by using a mounted swab; rupturing the cyst sometimes facilitates the manoeuvre. When the cyst has been deflated following rupture or aspiration of the fluid, it can be extracted through the trocar.

Enterogeneous cysts usually have a more posterior or para-oesophageal location: some are only loosely attached to the oesophagus and are easy to dissect; others are more firmly adherent to the oesophagus and sometimes even to the mucosa. Accidental injury to the oesophageal mucosa must be repaired with an interrupted suture. If this is thoracoscopically impossible, conversion to open procedure is necessary.

Other mediastinal cysts (cystic teratomas, bronchogenic cysts) are removed by blunt dissection. In the presence of marked adhesions with pulmonary vessels, thoracotomy is advocated.

Thymic tumours represent 45% – 50% of all mediastinal tumours. They are often well encapsulated and readily cleavable, but some invade adjacent structures with variable degrees of adhesion. Their size varies, even becoming conspicuously large. Whether endoscopic removal is feasible depends more on the degree of infiltration rather than the size of the lesion, which, however, may impose further difficulties. Thymic tumours are almost always located in the anterior superior mediastinum, tending to extend downwards and to come in contact with the pericardium. Nevertheless they always remain connected to the innominate vein by thin vessels (veins of Keynes) which drain the thymus from its posterior surface into the anterior aspect of the innominate vein. These veins are variable in number and each must be isolated and clipped, avoiding excessive traction which might lead to accidental injury of the innominate vein.

In thymic surgery one trocar for the optic and two for instruments are sufficient. During inspection of the field, the lung must be displaced backwards so as to expose the mammary vessels anteriorly, the phrenic nerve posteriorly and the innominate trunk superiorly.

The procedure starts with an electrocoagulating incision of the mediastinal pleura around the tumour, usually beginning at the posterior aspect of the mass between the latter and the phrenic nerve, which must be identified and preserved. The incision then continues downwards to the pericardium and upwards parallel with the mammary vessels.

The loose and soft anterior mediastinal tissue presents a loose, avascular plane. The dissection of the tumour from the pericardium is sometimes facilitated by gentle traction on a thread transfixing the tumour when the endoscopic grasping forceps cannot hold the mass firmly enough without damaging the tissue. Adhesions are progressively divided, following an upward direction up to the superior thymic pole. Focusing the camera in maximum magnification, the superior thymic veins of Keynes are identified and then isolated one by one with the scissors. They are then divided after placement of two endoclips on the side of the innominate vein and a single clip on the thymic side. In large tumours it may be more advantageous to begin directly with the dissection of the superior peduncle, clipping and dividing the veins. This avoids torsion of the completely isolated tumour around its vascular pedicle and consequent twisting and stripping of delicate veins. The mass must be removed from the thorax by means of a small utility thoracotomy and prior insertion in a plastic bag to avoid tumour spread. Accurate haemostasis, positioning of chest drain and lung re-expansion conclude the operation.

Staging thoracoscopy in oesophageal cancer has been performed in a number of cases and can provide important information regarding the feasibility of radical surgery in future [1].

Postoperative Care

The postoperative care of patients undergoing such procedures is simple. Thorax drainage is common to all of them. Additionally, the oesophageal procedures require postoperative assessment by Gastrografin swallow. It may be necessary to insert a gastric tube, but this is not recommended routinely because of the many disadvantages.

Results and Discussion

Since benign tumours of the mediastinum and the oesophagus are rather rare only a few case reports have been published describing the individual thoracoscopic technique of the authors and the postoperative course of the patients [2, 3]. Bardini et al. [4] and Everitt et al. [5] reported the successful treatment of leiomyomas. The Tuebingen experience in the field of benign oesophageal lesions is limited to one case of a young man with a symptomatic stenosis of the oesophagus which was histologically diagnosed as a bronchogenic cyst. It was removed thoracoscopically under oesophagoscopic control. The postoperative course was uneventful.

In patients with mediastinal lymphomas we have harvested tissue for special histological examination. In one case of a suspected lymphoma we found a nodule of thyroid gland tissue after subtotal thyroidectomy. The Milan experiences have also been very positive. There is relatively little risk in cases of well encapsulated and noninfiltrating masses. Great caution is necessary to avoid damaging any of the major mediastinal vessels or the phrenic nerve. Patients are usually discharged on the third or fourth postoperative day.

References

1. Fiocco M, Krasna J (1992) Thoracoscopic lymph node dissection in the staging of oesophageal cancer. L Laparoendosc Surg 2:111–115
2. Landreneau RJ, Dowling RD, Castillo WM, Ferson PF (1992) Thoracoscopic resection of an anterior mediastinal tumor. Ann Thorac Surg 54:142–144
3. Lewis RJ, Caccavale RJ, Sisler GE (1992) Imaged thoracoscopic surgery: a new thoracic technique for resection of mediastinal cysts. Ann Thorac Surg 53:318–320
4. Bardini R, Segalin A, Ruol A, Pavanello M, Peracchia A (1992) Videothoracoscopic enucleation of oesophageal leiomyoma. Ann Thorac Surg 54:576–577
5. Everitt NJ, Glinatsis M, McMahon MJ (1992) Thoracoscopic enucleation of leiomyoma of the oseophagus. Br J Surg 79:643

7 Videoendoscopic Pulmonary Resections

G. ROVIARO, C. REBUFFAT, F. VAROLI, C. VERGANI, M. MACIOCCO, and S. M. SCALAMBRA

Introduction

The development of percutaneous automatic staplers has enabled the execution of anatomical and nonanatomical pulmonary resections by means of videothoracoscopic technique. In nonanatomical (wedge) resections, a "wedge" of pulmonary parenchyma containing the lesion is resected without isolation of any vascular or bronchial hilar structures. Videothoracoscopy has rapidly become the choice for this kind of intervention, which is, moreover, relatively simple to carry out.

Indications

The indications for thoracoscopically performed wedge resections are peripheral pulmonary lesions:

- Excisional lung biopsies in diffuse interstitial pulmonary disorders
- Inflammatory pulmonary nodules of uncertain diagnosis after fine needle aspiration
- Benign lung neoplasms (hamartomas, chondromas) or neoplasms of low-grade malignancy (carcinoid)
- Lung metastases of tumours not of pulmonary origin, if the primary lesion is resectable, or has already been excised and there is no recurrence
- Small primary lung carcinomas in patients with greatly compromised respiratory function.

Anatomical pulmonary resections (segmentectomies, lobectomies and pneumonectomies) may also be carried out with the assistance of videothoracoscopic techniques.

These interventions are technically much more difficult to perform due to the need for isolation, control and resection of important bronchial and vascular hilar structures. Thus they are still uncommonly performed thoracoscopically.

The indications for videothoracoscopically assisted lobectomy are:

- Inflammatory diseases (bronchiectasies)
- Congenital malformations (pulmonary arteriovenous fistula)
- Peripheral primary bronchogenic neoplasms staged $T_1N_0-T_2N_0$ when the lesion is limited to the segmental bronchi
- Benign peripheral lung neoplasms or metastatic lesions which are too deeply located to be removed by wedge resection.

The indications for videothoracoscopically assisted pneumonectomy are limited to small primary lung neoplasms staged T_2N_0 involving peribronchial structures near the bronchial division or the pulmonary artery within the fissure and would therefore necessitate a pneumonectomy in any case.

Involvement of the parietal pleura does not contraindicate thoracoscopy, as extrapleural cleavage is relatively easy to carry out. However, invasion of the costal segments requiring excision of the involved chest wall must be performed by the open approach.

Mediastinal lymphadenectomy is also feasible endoscopically.

Traditional thoracotomy incisions are carried out by section of important muscles and involve traction on the ribs which can result in fractures. This causes very intense postoperative pain, which is a problem, as reduction of respiratory excursions and consequent inefficacy of cough greatly impair the clearing mechanisms of the lungs. In its turn this favours stagnation of secretions and pulmonary collapse. Patients affected by bronchogenic neoplasms are usually elderly smokers with chronic bronchitis and thus have compromised respiratory function. In these cases reducing pain and a smoother postoperative course through a thoracoscopically assisted approach enhances the feasibility and safety of pulmonary resections.

Preoperative Work-up and Preparation

Preoperative investigations before pulmonary resections depend on the nature of the lesion (benign or malignant) and on the respiratory reserve. The degree of functional impairment will influence the nature of the intervention appropriate for the patient. Investigations for functional respiratory capacity are the same as for traditional surgery. In patients with malignant bronchial neoplasms, the disease is staged as for traditional surgery, and it is particularly important to exclude systemic metastatic disease.

Investigations more specifically concerned with videoendoscopic surgery are bronchoscopy and thoracic computed tomography (CT). In patients with bronchogenic neoplasms, bronchoscopy is necessary for accurate evaluation of the extent of bronchial involvement. This will determine the site of application of the automatic stapler, as manual assessment of the bronchus is impossible during thoracoscopy.

CT of the chest is considered indispensable in any patient harbouring pulmonary disease of surgical interest in view of the significant information it provides on the morphology, density and precise location of the mass. It can also give useful information on the state of the hilar and mediastinal lymph nodes.

Of particular interest for videothoracoscopically assisted surgery is high density CT with very thin sections. As well as providing more detailed morphologic information, it is the only method which allows scrutiny of the fissures and their relationship with the mass, this being of primary importance in videothoracoscopic surgery.

It is important to remember that conversion to thoracotomy may be necessary: the patient must therefore be prepared as for traditional open surgery. Respiratory physiotherapy, bronchial dilators, mucolytics, administration of expectorants and abstinence from smoking are therefore important.

Administration of anticoagulants and antibiotics for short-term prophylaxis begins 1 day before intervention.

In women, for an optimal cosmetic result, the site of a possible minimal thoracotomy (utility thoracotomy) is preoperatively drawn along the inframammary sulcus to avoid its displacement in the lateral decubitus position.

Anaesthesia

The patient is intubated before being positioned on his side. The use of a double-lumen Carlens tube allows single-lung ventilation and prevents the necessity of a CO_2-induced pneumothorax as the introduction of the first trocar results in collapse of the affected lung, while the contralateral continues to be ventilated. This greatly simplifies all endoscopic manoeuvres within the cavity.

Patient Positioning

The patient is placed in lateral decubitus as for a classic posterolateral thoracotomy (Fig. 7.1). The patient's arm on the side of access is raised upwards and anteriorly to shift the scapula, and a pillow is placed under the chest to further expose and spread the intercostal spaces. The operating table is slanted downwards from the centre on its distal end to lower the iliac crest as this can interfere with the movements of the camera.

The operating field is prepared by leaving the chest wall exposed between sternum and spinal cord, from the third to the ninth rib. This gives sufficient space for insertion of the operative trocars required for the intervention.

Layout of Ancillary Instruments and Positioning of Staff

Even though one monitor is enough, two videoscreens placed on either side of the patient's head ensure the best view for all members of the team. The position of the surgeon, assistants and scrub

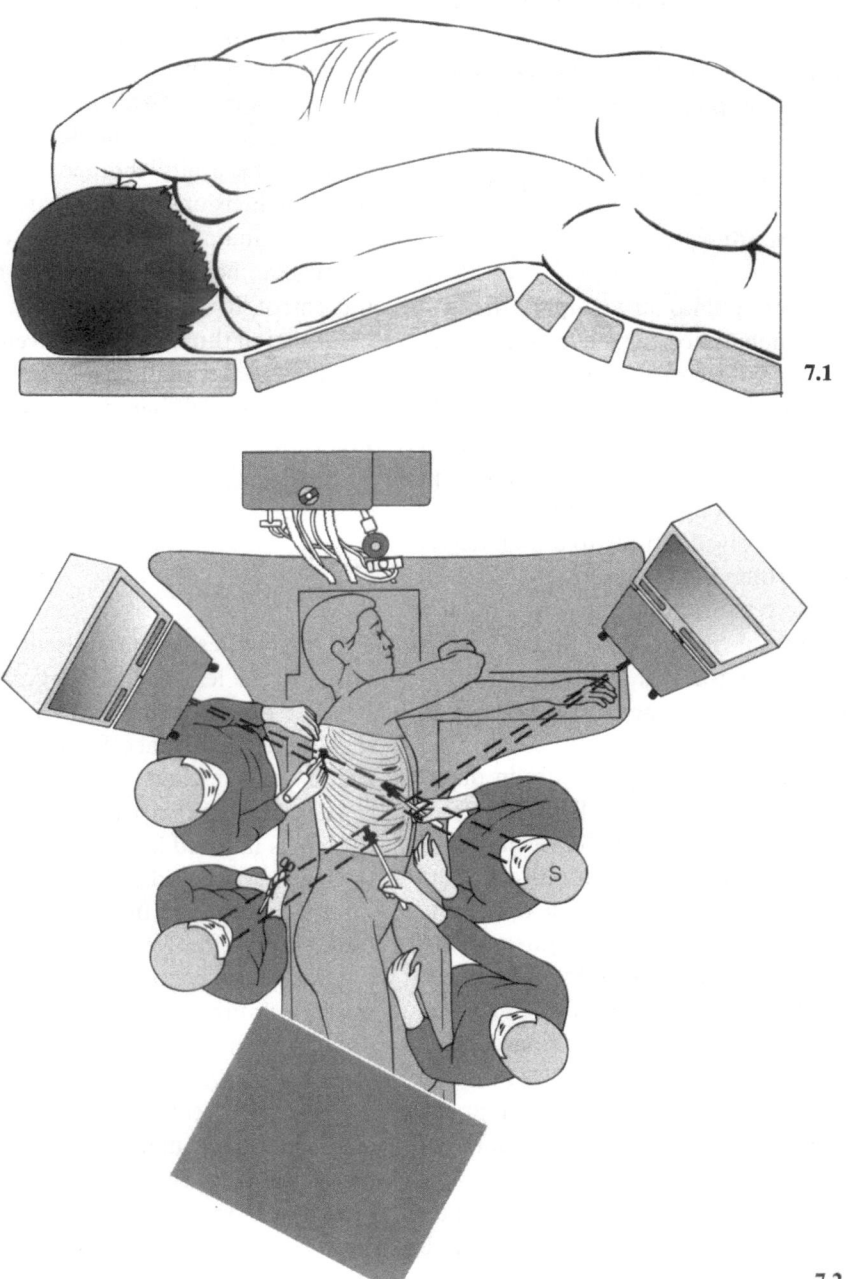

7.1

7.2

Fig. 7.1. Positioning of the patient on the operating table in lateral decubitus as for a classical posterolateral thoracotomy. The patient's arm on the side of access is raised upwards and anteriorly to displace the scapula, and a pillow is placed under the chest to further expose and spread the intercostal spaces. The operating table is slanted downwards from the centre on its distal end to lower the iliac crest, which can interfere with the movements of the camera

Fig. 7.2. Positioning of the operating team and apparatus; *S*, standard position of the surgeon

nurse is shown in Fig. 7.2, but the operator often needs to change position and sides during the intervention.

All the surgical instrumentation necessary for a thoracotomy must be prepared should conversion be necessary.

Specific Instrumentation

Videothoracoscopic pulmonary surgery depends on specific instrumentation which enable dissection, resection and suture of pulmonary parenchyma and great vessels both safely and with ease. This is now possible in thoracoscopic surgery with the introduction of endoscopic staplers and endoscopic clips appliers. Even though this sophisticated instrumentation has evolved rapidly to a high degree, it still requires further improvement.

An endoscopic version of instruments similar to those commonly employed in open surgery (such as atraumatic clamps, retractors dissecting forceps, and O'Shaugnessy ligature carriers) have been introduced only recently.

A forward viewing endoscope 10 mm in diameter is usually employed with excellent results. In special cases, optics with a 30° or 45° viewing angle can be helpful. However, we have no direct operative experience yet with the new flexible optics with distal charged couple device (CCD) camera, which should improve the visual quality by centring the field and enabling the best angle of vision.

The standard laparoscopic trocars have served well up to now, but the shorter atraumatic thoracic trocars recently introduced facilitate the manoeuvres and decrease the risk of injury to the intercostal vessels.

In addition to endoscopic shears and graspers, other useful instruments such as endoscopic Babcock grasping forceps and retractors are necessary to lift and retract the lung parenchyma.

A good washing-aspirating system is essential to keep the operative field clean. An endoscopic clip-applier is also necessary for haemostasis of small vessels. Endoscopic staplers with disposable vascular loading units permit closure/division of large vessels, and parenchymal loading units are required for stapling the lung. A suitable plastic bag in which to insert the resected lung avoids the need for morcellation and tumour implantation during extraction.

During these operations many conventional instruments are widely employed to overcome the present inadequacy of endoscopic instrumentation. Conventional instruments can be introduced through the utility thoracotomy but also through the skin incisions for the trocars. As there is no need to maintain positive pressure, the valved trocars can be removed to allow greater freedom of movement for the instruments. This can be very helpful even though these conventional instruments cannot be optimally employed (impossibility of opening the O'Shaugnessy ligature carrier etc.; Fig. 7.3).

Access

The patient lies in lateral decubitus on the side opposite to the lesion. The operation begins with collapse of the selectively intubated lung. This results in a large work space for manoeuvres despite the rigidity of the chest.

The first 10-mm trocar for introduction of the camera is inserted in the seventh or eighth intercostal space in the midaxillary line. A "low" insertion of the camera has many advantages: it allows an optimal position for immediate exploration of the pleural cavity; neither surgeon nor assistant have to watch a "mirror" image; it does not hinder introduction or manoeuvrability of instruments inserted at a later time.

Other operative trocars (5, 10, 12 or 15 mm in diameter) are usually positioned after trying out the chosen site with long, thin needles. As rigidity of the ribs and narrowness of intercostal spaces considerably limit the angulation which may be obtained, this can help to evaluate the angle which will be needed by the instruments to reach the operative field. Usually two operative trocars are inserted in the sixth intercostal space along the anterior axillary line, and in the fifth under the scapular tip (Fig. 7.4). Additional trocars may be placed in variable positions according to the site and characteristics of the lesion.

In pneumonectomy, lobectomy or removal of large specimens, a small thoracotomy incision is

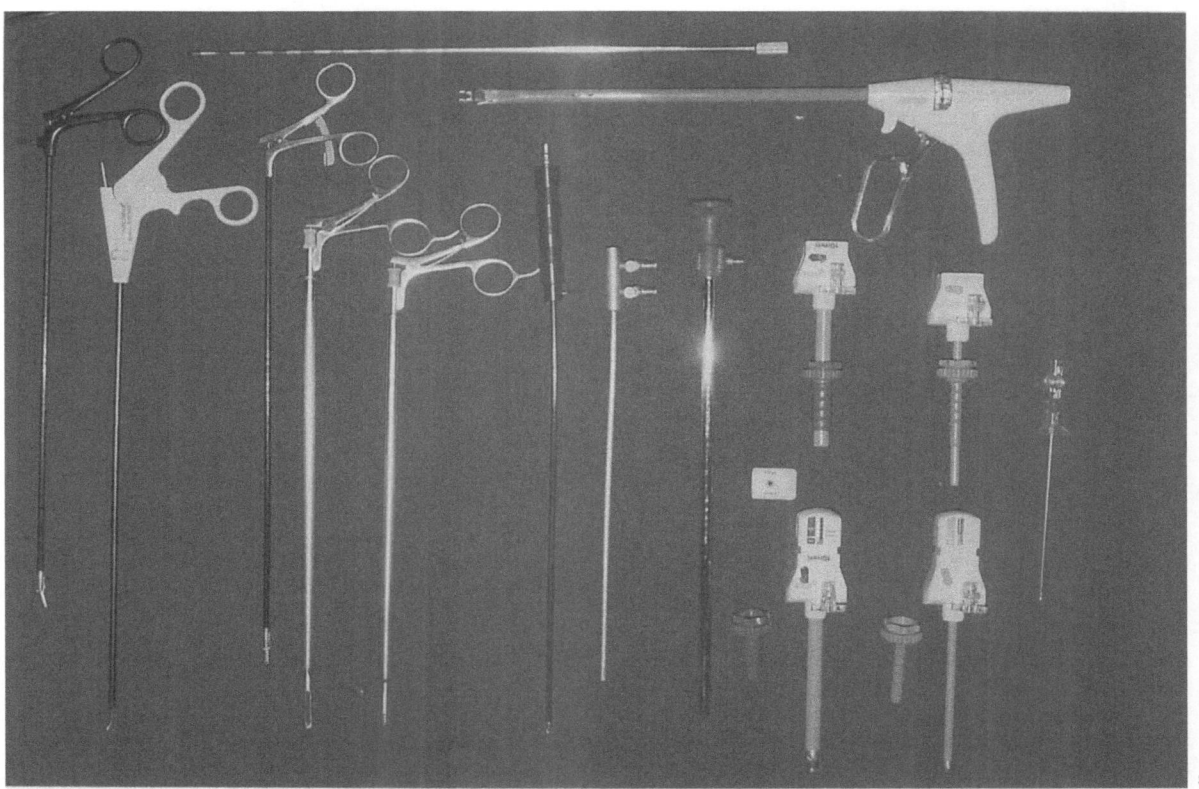

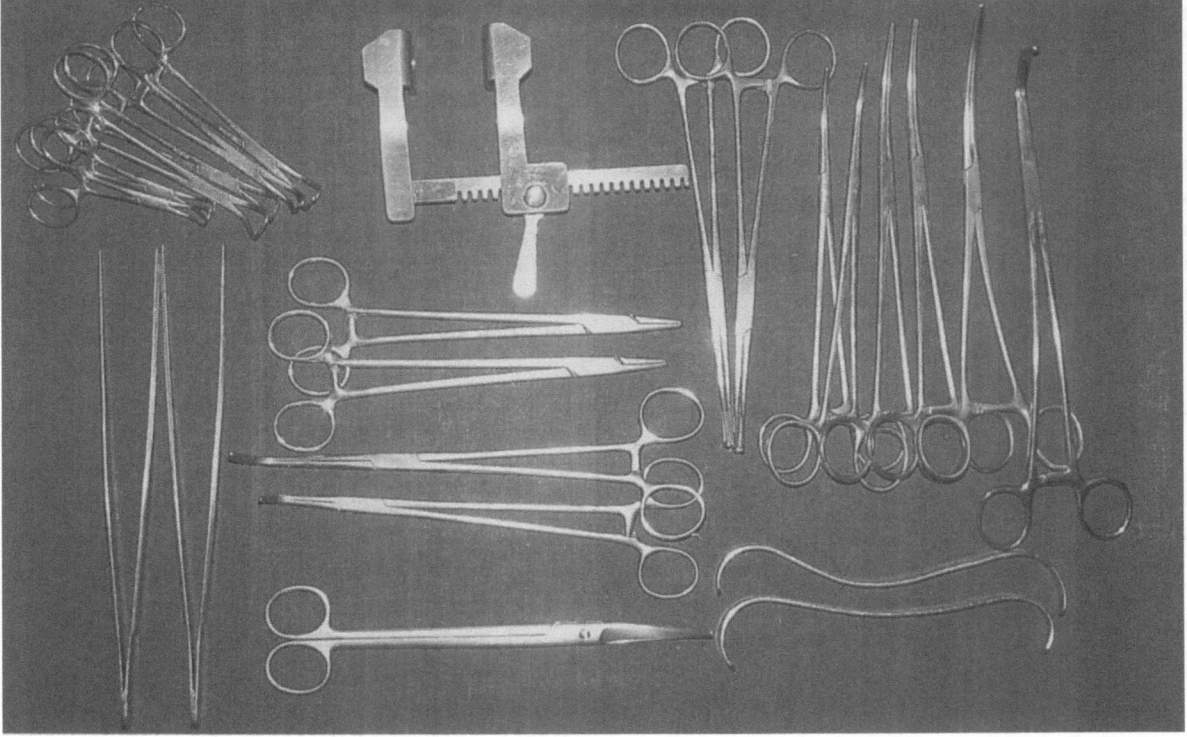

Fig. 7.3a, b. Endoscopic (**a**) and conventional (**b**) instrumentation necessary for major pulmonary resections

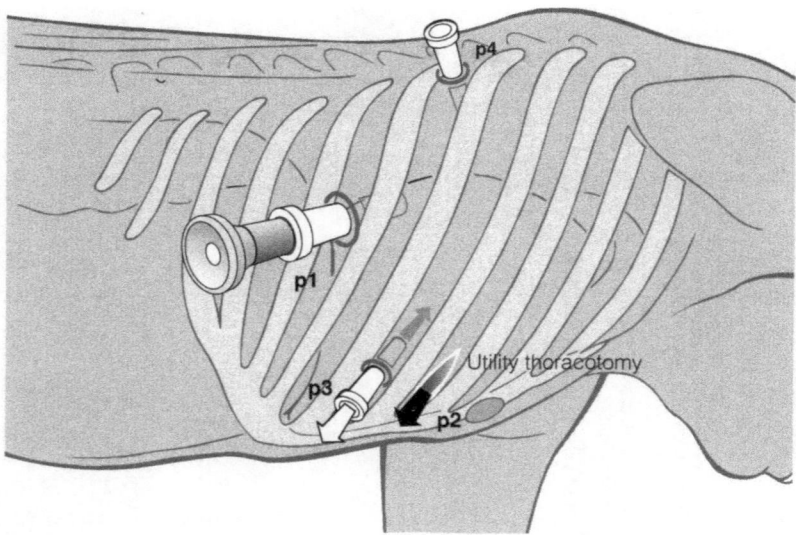

Utility thoracotomy

Fig. 7.4. Sites of insertion of the trocars and utility thoraco-tomy. A 10-mm trocar for the camera is inserted in the seventh or eigth intercostal space on the midaxillary line to provide the best exposure. Usually two other operative trocars are inserted in the sixth intercostal space anteriorly and posteriorly. Supplementary trocars can be positioned as required. A utility thoracotomy is usually performed along the inframammary sulcus

necessary for the extraction. This should be carried out right at the beginning of the operation so as to permit the use of nonendoscopic instruments if necessary, thus providing what we refer to as a "utility thoracotomy" (see p. 146).

Surgical Technique

Surgical technique for thoracoscopic nonanatomi-cal pulmonary resections (wedge resections) and anatomical videothoracoscopically assisted resec-tions (lobectomies, segmentectomies and pneumo-nectomies) follows the same steps and have the same indications as the equivalent thoracotomy procedures.

Nonanatomical Pulmonary Resections

Nonanatomical pulmonary resections (wedge resec-tions) are those in which the excision does not fol-low a definite anatomical plane. The most impor-tant points are control of bleeding and air leakage from the resection lines. Wedge resections are a rel-atively simple procedure when the lesion to be re-moved is small, peripheral and superficial, and thus at a good distance from any major bronchial or vascular structure. As size of the parenchyma in-volved increases, it becomes harder to obtain cor-rect haemostasis and aerostasis.

In traditional chest surgery the lesions are easily identified by manual palpation. By contrast, this can give rise to great difficulty during thoracosco-py, as instrumental palpation is considerably less sensitive, particularly if the lesion is soft and locat-ed deep in the parenchyma. Preoperative marking of the mass is extremely important so as to avoid prolonged thoracoscopic exploration. It is some-times necessary to introduce the fingers or even the hand for manual location of the lesion by means of a small thoracotomy. One of the simplest and safest methods is to preoperatively "hook" the lesion un-der CT scanning with a needle as for marking im-palpable tumours of the breast. Upon reaching the lesion, the needle is withdrawn, releasing its coaxial wire hook. Operation should follow this preopera-

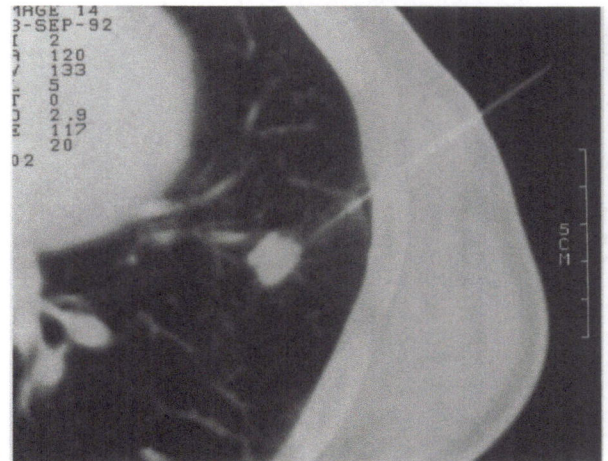

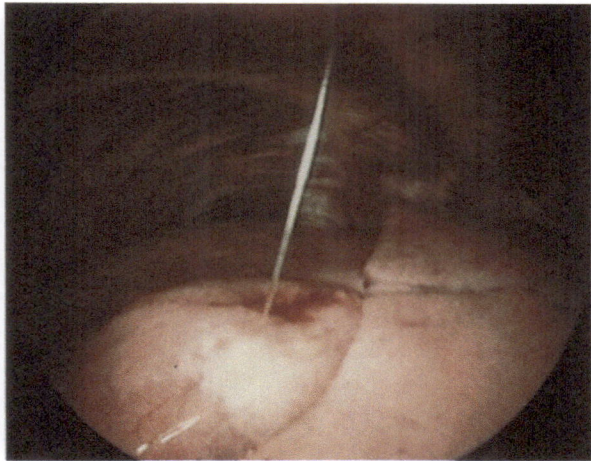

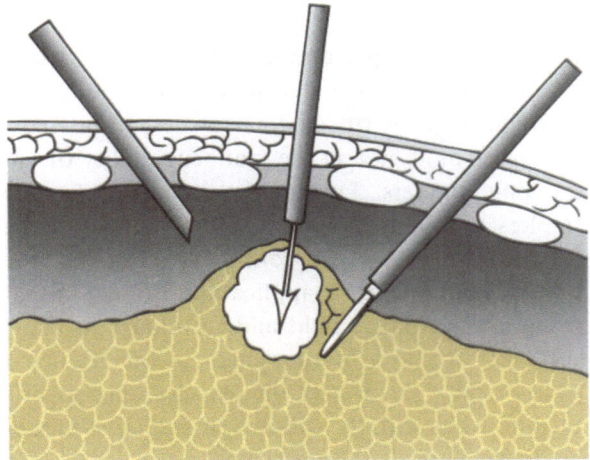

Fig. 7.5a–c. Identification of deep intraparenchymal lesions can be difficult in videothoracoscopic surgery due to the loss of manual palpation. Preoperative marking of the lesion is extremely useful. One of the simplest and safest methods is to preoperatively "hook" the lesion under CT scanning (**a**) with a needle as for marking impalpable tumours of the breast. Upon reaching the lesion, the needle is withdrawn, releasing its coaxial wired hook. Operation follows immediately to limit the risk of displacement of the hook and also to avoid a possible pneumothorax subsequent to the puncture. The "hooking manoeuvre" is illustrated in picture and drawing (**b, c**)

tive localization immediately to reduce the risk of displacement of the hook (Fig. 7.5).

The position of the trocars varies according to the site of the lesion. The first trocar is introduced with its valve open. This causes collapse of the lung excluded from ventilation by a double-lumen tube. The first trocar also serves to introduce the camera and is therefore placed in the seventh or eighth intercostal space where the thorax is wider and internal movements of the camera are facilitated.

Only two other trocars are needed for execution of the operation. The most frequently chosen site of insertion is the fifth intercostal space, anteriorly and posteriorly along the line which would serve for a classic posterolateral thoracotomy. The fourth intercostal space may be used for more apical lesions, or the sixth for lower ones.

Preliminary exploration is simple if the lesion is superficial, causes retraction of the pleura, or has been preoperatively hooked with a needle.

It is important to free the lung from any adhesions by section with scissors or by electrocutting. Diffuse adhesions, however, may cause considerable difficulty and require time and patience to separate. Complete adhesiolysis allows displacement of the lung with an endoscopic grasper or endoscopic Babcock grasping forceps, with care to avoid excessive traction which may damage or tear the delicate parenchyma. Lateral inclination of the operating table will facilitate exploration of more anterior or posterior segments.

Exploration of the inferior lobe can at times be hindered by the triangular ligament which can be sectioned with an endoscopic scissor right up to the

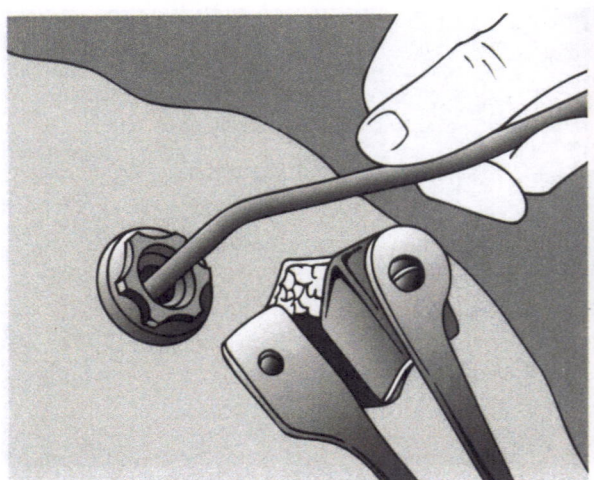
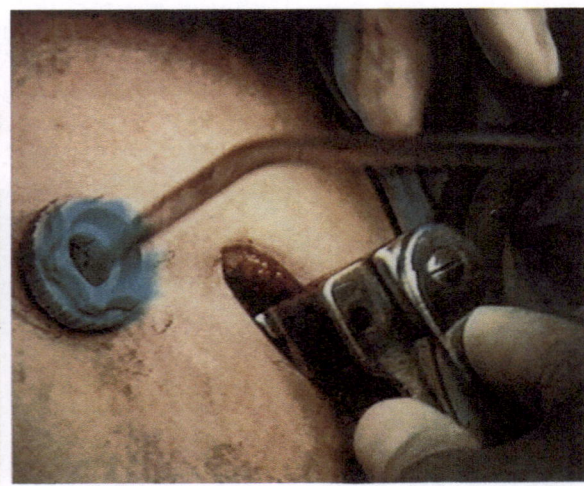

a   b

Fig. 7.6 a, b. Utility thoracotomy. The 3- to 4-cm incision is usually performed in the third or fourth intercostal space, lateral to the pectoralis major and medial to the serratus anterior along the inframammary sulcus, and is preoperatively marked with a dermographic pencil

inferior pulmonary vein, after electrocoagulation of the ligament's artery.

When the parenchyma which must be resected is abundant, a 3- to 4-cm utility thoracotomy must be performed anteriorly, between the midclavicular and the anterior axillary line (Fig. 7.6).

We have coined the term "utility thoracotomy" as we use this not only for removal of larger specimens, but also to introduce and employ those instruments not yet available for endoscopy. Moreover, in vascular lesions which may occur in major lung resections, a haemostatic clamp through this minimal incision can control the bleeding while conversion to thoracotomy is being effected. The utility thoracotomy is performed in the third or fourth intercostal space, lateral to the pectoralis major and medial to the serratus to avoid section of major muscles. Moreover, in this region the intercostal spaces are wider. The utility thoracotomy is performed under direct endoscopic vision so that it is made to face the fissure. For aesthetic purposes in women, the inframammary sulcus is preoperatively marked with the patient in an upright position.

Endoscopic staplers have permitted and greatly facilitated the performance of wedge resections.

However, certain precautions and technical details must be followed to render these interventions safe.

Rigidity of the ribs and narrowness of intercostal spaces limit greatly the manoeuvrability of endoscopic staplers. Further development of these staplers to enable rotation and angulation of the functional endpiece will considerably enhance the ease and safety of their application. Present instruments are too long, rigid and rectilinear to allow sufficient freedom of movement in the restricted pleural space. Whenever the affected lung is difficult to reach with the endoscopic stapler, it should be drawn towards the instrument.

It is also essential to check carefully that the thickness of the compressed parenchyma does not exceed the holding length of the clips as this would result in suboptimal closure, with leakage of air and blood when the lung is reinflated.

Wedge resection is very simple when there is just a small, superficial portion of lung to resect and may only need one application of the endoscopic stapler. As the parenchyma is held in gentle traction with an endoscopic grasper, the endoscopic stapler is applied across the base of the chosen segment, the jaws closed and the instrument then fired.

Sometimes the stapled segment remains attached at its distal end or even along the line of staples. Whenever this happens, division is completed with endoscopic scissors, taking care to cut the remaining fibres between the two rows of triple-staggered staples.

If the portion to be resected is large, several applications of the endostapler may be required. It is important in this case to check that the second application is not superimposed on the first line of staples. This may impair haemostasis and aerostasis, or even result in parenchymal lacerations on withdrawal of the stapler.

The parenchyma adjacent to larger or deeper lesions close to the vascular and bronchiolar branches is thicker when compressed by the stapler limbs and particular care is required to verify that closure of the jaws is complete, which indicates that the entrapped parenchyma comprised is not too thick or fibrous, for safe staple closure. By contrast if the approximation of the jaws is incomplete, the resulting closure will be unsafe.

For lesions 3–4 cm in size, the line of resection must include a wedge of parenchyma with the apex corresponding to the bronchovascular pedicle. This minimizes the risk of damage to the bronchial and vascular supply to surrounding segments.

When a wedge resection is not feasible because of an excessively large or central lesion, thoracoscopically assisted or thoracotomy-performed anatomical resection (lobectomy or segmentectomy) is necessary.

Thoracoscopically Assisted Lobectomies and Pneumonectomies: General Principles

Anatomical resective interventions (lobectomies and pneumonectomies) are the most difficult thoracoscopic operations and require long training in conventional thoracic surgery. The procedure and isolation of arteries, veins and bronchi follow the same steps as all open thoracic interventions and require the same technical support.

Endoscopic versions of automatic staplers, widely employed in conventional thoracic surgery, not only allow but greatly facilitate suture section of vessels and bronchi in thoracoscopically assisted interventions, too.

The operative procedure follows three main phases: (1) mediastinal, (2) fissural, and (3) bronchial.

Mediastinal Vascular Phase

Isolation, suture and section of mediastinal vessels usually follows a common procedure in the various kinds of resection and necessitates extensive knowledge of the anatomy of the main hilum. The difficulties are greater than those in conventional surgery and are mainly due to a small operative field, inadequate current endoscopic instrumentation such that traditional instruments have to be used through the trocars or through the "utility thoracotomy", and isolation of vascular elements must be more accurate and extensive to allow positioning of straight mechanical staplers which are, moreover, much thicker than a conventional O'Shaugnessy dissector. Excessive traction or rough, uncautious movements can result in vascular lesions which may be difficult to repair.

After introduction of the camera and cannulae, the pulmonary parenchyma is grasped and moved to stretch and divide any adhesions.

All preliminary manoeuvres are as described previously for atypical resections. The mediastinum must be accurately explored both visually and by palpation with forceps and swabs in search for lymph nodes.

The outer coat of pulmonary vessels consists of loose connective tissue extending from the pericardium. If this adventitia is thin, the vessels can be perceived through it and gentle swabbing towards the lung (never in the opposite direction) achieves isolation of their anterior and lateral aspects. If the adventitia is thicker and blunt dissection does not suffice, the adventitia is grasped and incised with scissors. Curved endoscopic scissors and dissecting forceps may then be used to obtain a plane of cleavage between the adventitia and the vascular wall which must be carefully and gently dissected (Fig. 7.7).

Once the vessel is isolated on its entire circumference, a thread is passed around it with a conventional O'Shaugnessy forceps or an endoscopic roticulator grasper (Fig. 7.8). Gentle traction on this sling will allow further exposure of the vessel and any posterior adhesions can then be cauterized and divided.

One of the most difficult and essential steps is the positioning of an endoscopic stapler. This often requires several attempts to find the correct angle,

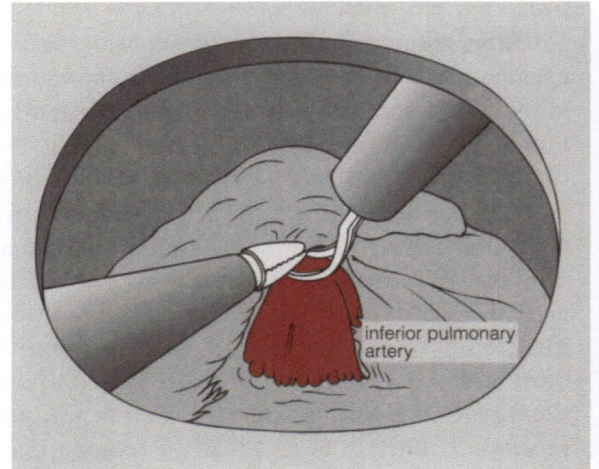

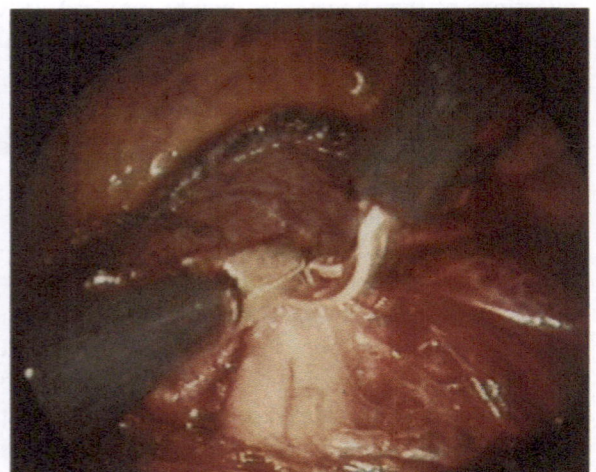

7.7a   **b**

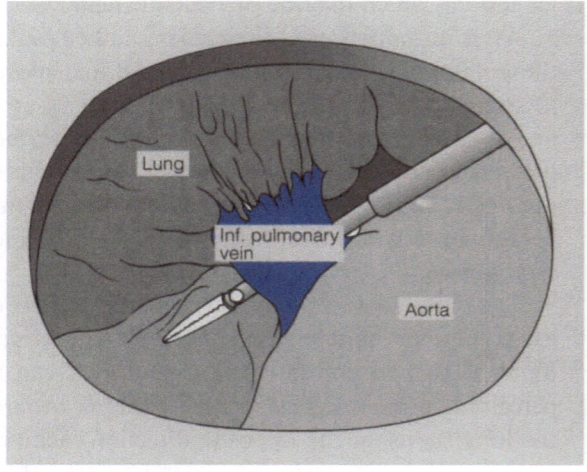

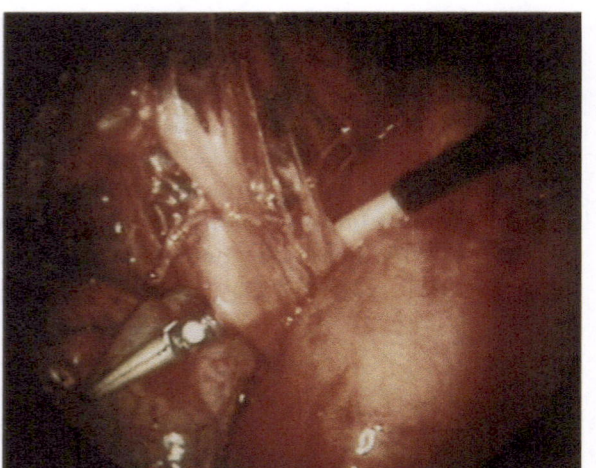

7.8a   **b**

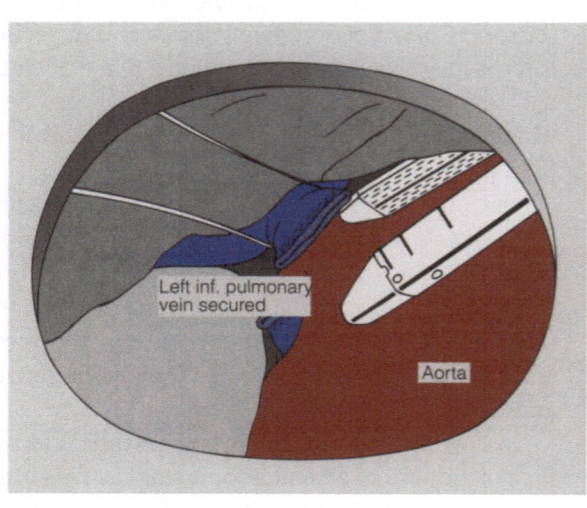

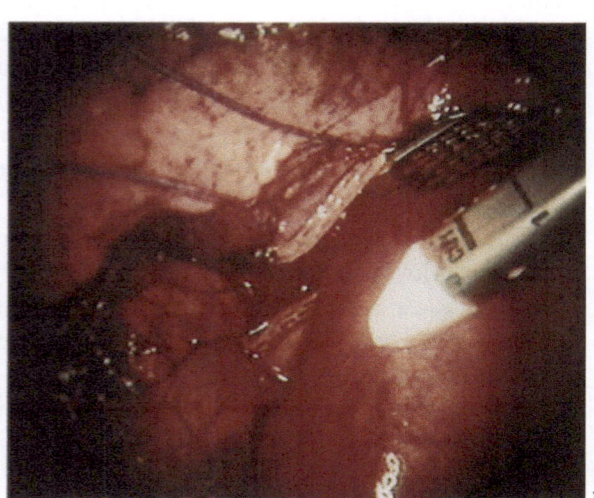

7.9a   **b**

as the tip of the instrument's jaws must go well beyond the vessel to ensure complete closure. To achieve this, the surgeon often has to change his position as well as the position of the endostapler through the trocars or through the utility thoracotomy. Optimal placement of the stapler is essential before firing.

If the correct technique has been followed and the vessel was adequately isolated, the section will be clean and the stumps will fall apart immediately after the endoscopic stapler is opened (Fig. 7.9). Residues of adventitial fibres can prevent the opening and extraction of the endostapler; they must therefore be sectioned with scissors between the two triple-staggered rows of staples. These are dangerous manoeuvres and extreme caution must be exercised to avoid damaging the vessel.

If isolation is sufficiently extensive, a vascular clamp can be introduced and applied proximally on the vessel. The clamp is removed only after checking that the staples are well placed and haemostasis on the distal stump (which can be seen) is perfect.

Pulmonary arteries and veins are isolated using a similar technique, but it is important to remember that the pulmonary arteries are more fragile than the pulmonary veins and thus require even greater caution.

Fissural Phase

Freeing the fissure to isolate the lobar artery is the most important phase when carrying out a lobec-

tomy. The lobar hilum is anatomically more complex than the primary hilum: it has more ramifications and it is located deeper and in closer connection with lymph nodes and bronchi. Inflammatory processes and subsequent peribronchial fibrosis may obscure the artery, making access and isolation very difficult.

In young patients the fissure is frequently well marked. The artery can be seen deep in the fissure or its pulsations may be perceived when covered by a thin layer of lung parenchyma. In older patients emphysema produces thickening of the fissure, thus making identification and isolation of the artery very difficult, even more so if large or calcified lymph nodes are present.

Loose or avascular adhesions present within the fissure are easily cauterized and sectioned. If the adhesions are thicker or diffuse, the dissection necessary to expose the artery can result in bleeding, which even though slight, is often very difficult to control. Whenever this occurs, continuation of the intervention by the thoracoscopic route is dangerous and conversion to thoracotomy is recommended.

Suture section of the artery, once it has been isolated, follows the same rules as described for the arteries during the mediastinal phase. Larger vessels must be stapled, while endoclips are sufficient for the lesser ones. Incomplete residual segments of fissure may be divided by stapling.

Bronchial Phase

After suture section of all vascular structures, the bronchus is the last element to be divided. As proposed by many authors, there are different techniques of bronchial suture. Automatic staplers have greatly simplified this choice, at the same time reducing the risk of fistulization.

Endoscopic staplers have the same characteristics as conventional automatic staplers, but at present endoscopic versions are limited to Endo GIA 30–60, 3.5–30 V staples, which are rather inadequate for suturing the bronchi, particularly the main stem ones.

As for conventional surgery, it is important not to devascularize the bronchial stump and not to leave an excessively long bronchial stump, which fa-

◄────────────────────

Fig. 7.7 a, b. Dissection of the lobar artery within the fissure. Isolation of the lobar artery is the most difficult step when performing a lobectomy. This can be done through a careful use of swabs, graspers and scissors to obtain a plane of cleavage between the adventitia and the vascular wall

Fig. 7.8 a, b. Once the vessel is isolated along its entire circumference, a thread is passed around it with a conventional O'Shaugnessy forceps or the Roticulator Endograsp. An endoscopic Roticulator grasper is inserted behind the left inferior pulmonary vein originating posterior to the descending aorta

Fig. 7.9 a, b. The left inferior pulmonary vein is surrounded with a thread to facilitate the insertion of the stapler and then secured. After the stapler has been fired, the vascular stumps fall apart. Here the lower stump is partially hidden by the aorta

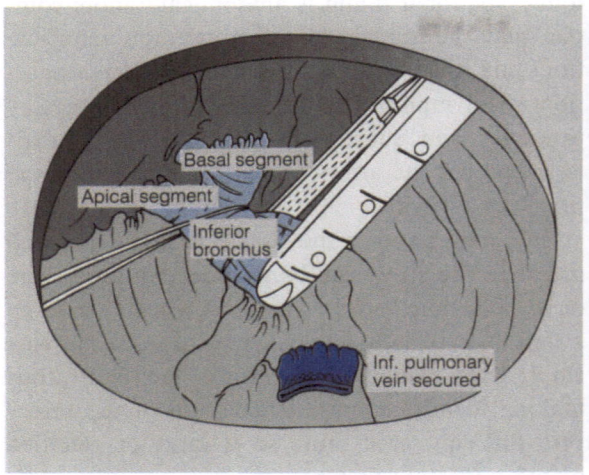
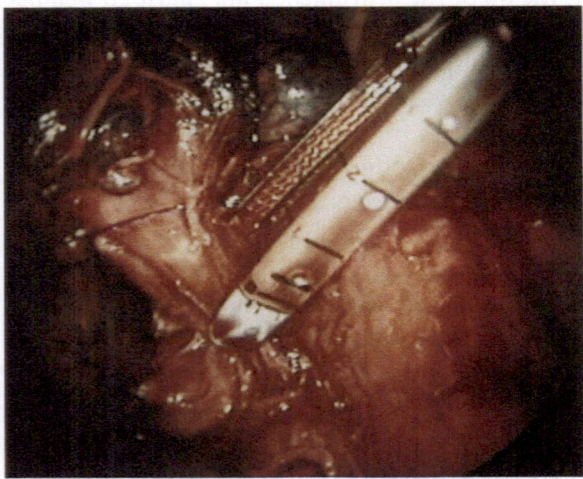

a   b

Fig. 7.10a, b. Once isolated, the bronchus is introduced in the endostapler's jaws and secured. Possible residual fibres can be sectioned with endoscopic scissors. The right inferior bronchus inserted in the stapler and the already secured inferior pulmonary vein are visible

vours stagnation of bronchial secretions and, consequently, the formation of a fistula.

The bronchus is isolated using a mounted swab with electrocoagulation of small vessels when these are encountered during dissection. Peribronchial lymph nodes are removed and the bronchial artery is isolated and clipped. The bronchus is introduced within the jaws of the endostapler and divided. Some residual connective fibres frequently remain between the two stapled bronchial edges and must be sectioned with endoscopic scissors.

Sometimes the bronchus for the apical lower originates higher, at the same level as the bronchus for the middle lobe. In right lower lobectomies, if the apical lower bronchus and the lower bronchus are sectioned off together with a single shot of endostapler (Fig. 7.10), there is considerable risk of stenosing the bronchus for the middle lobe. It is therefore more convenient to stable section with two separate applications: one for the apical lower bronchus, and one for the bronchus to the basal segments.

Suturing the main bronchus presents some peculiar problems. In our experience of videothoracoscopically assisted pneumonectomies (limited to few cases), endoscopic staples are too short for safe closure as the main bronchus is too thick and large.

Therefore after suture section of the vessels, the main bronchus is divided with scissors and the collapsed lung removed through the utility thoracotomy. The edges of the remaining stump are then grasped with two traditional clamps or two endoscopic grasp, drawn upwards and closed by a conventional 4.5 TA Roticulator inserted through the utility thoracotomy.

The angle of insertion of the TA Roticulator and traction on the grasper allow closure of the bronchus leaving only a short stump. Any residual tissue can be sectioned off with endoscissors a few millimetres from the suture line. Due to the limited space available for manoeuvres, closure of the bronchus with TA Roticulator is possible only after extraction of the lung (Fig. 7.11). After a careful check for haemostasis and re-expansion of the lung, a chest drain is placed after lobectomy. We do not usually place a drain after a pneumonectomy. Suture of the utility thoracotomy concludes the operation.

Types of Anatomical Pulmonary Resections: Particular Aspects

Right Upper Lobectomy

Right upper lobectomy is one of the most difficult lobectomies because the artery must be isolated both in the mediastinum and within the fissure.

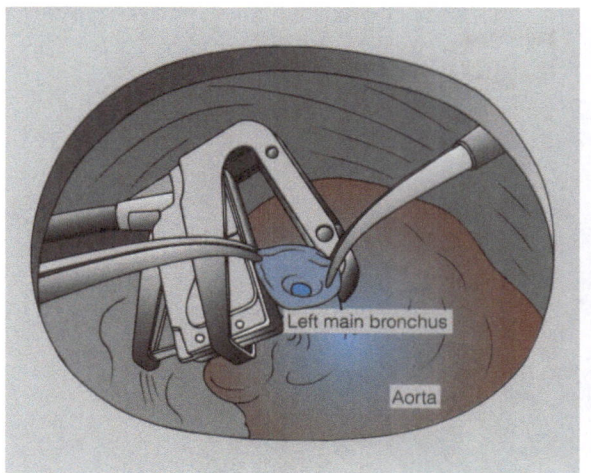
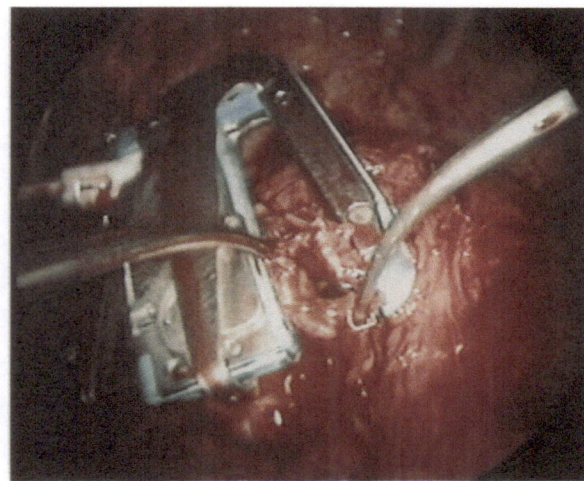

a   b

Fig. 7.11 a, b. Endoscopic staples are too short for a safe suture as the main bronchus is too thick and large. The latter is divided with scissors and the collapsed lung is removed. The bronchial stump is first drawn upwards with two graspers and then secured with a TA Roticulator inserted through the utility thoracotomy. Suture of the main bronchus is shown

The cannula for the optic is inserted in the sixth intercostal space and the two operative trocars in the fourth or fifth space, according to the level of the fissure. The utility thoracotomy is performed under direct vision in the third or fourth space so as to face the mediastinal vascular elements. The upper lobe is displaced posteriorly with endoscopic graspers or Babcock grasping forceps. The vena cava dominates the operative field and the vascular elements appear to originate beneath it. The mediastinal pleura is incised with graspers or endoscopic scissors. The vascular elements are identified. The superior pulmonary vein is the first element to be isolated as it is the easiest to free (Fig. 7.12). The vein must be dissected for as great a length as possible so that the trunk for the upper and middle lobes are freed as well. The truncus for the upper lobe is encircled with the Endograsp Roticulator after complete isolation of the venous trunk in order to avoid damage to the intermediate artery, which runs just behind the vein. The Endograsp Roticulator permits passage of a nylon thread around the vessel. This allows a gentle traction which facilitates the positioning of the endostapler and suture section of the superior pulmonary vein.

The anterior arterial trunk (of Boyden) is isolated with the endoscopic grasper, scissors and swabs. The dissection starts at the lower margin and proceeds to its terminal branches, using the same technique as for the superior pulmonary vein. The arterial trunk and the intermediate artery for fissure are now visible. The latter may then be followed within the fissure, which is carefully opened with electrocoagulating dissector and scissors. This manoeuvre can be very difficult and dangerous if the fissure is particularly thick and the posterior ascending artery is deeply located. The posterior ascending artery usually has a small calibre and can be severed between clips. The superior lobe is then grasped and displaced anteriorly to expose the posterior mediastinum thus exposing the azygos vein and the main bronchus. The mediastinal pleura is incised with scissors and the upper bronchus is isolated over an adequate distance. Possible bronchial arteries are clipped and severed. The bronchus is surrounded with the Endograsp Roticulator. This facilitates placement of the endoscopic stapler. The division of fissure between the upper and the middle lobe anteriorly, and the lower lobe posteriorly, can be completed with the endostapler.

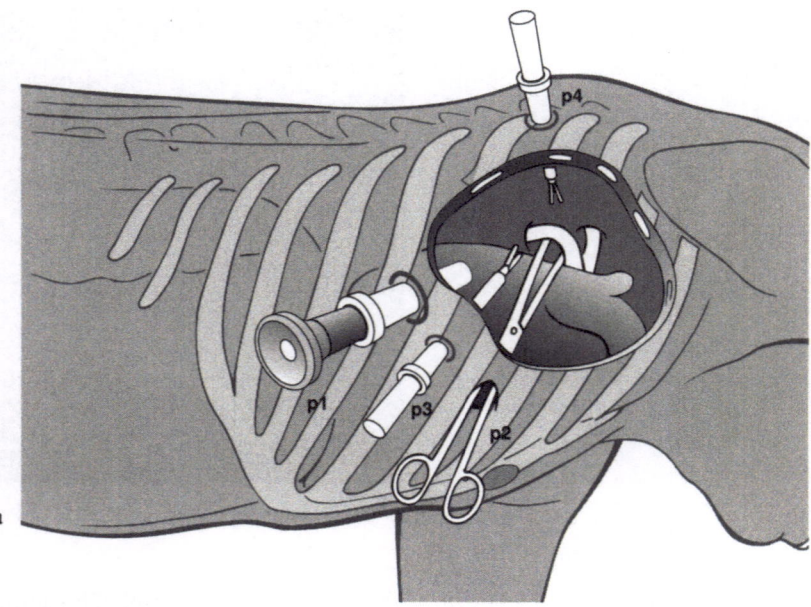

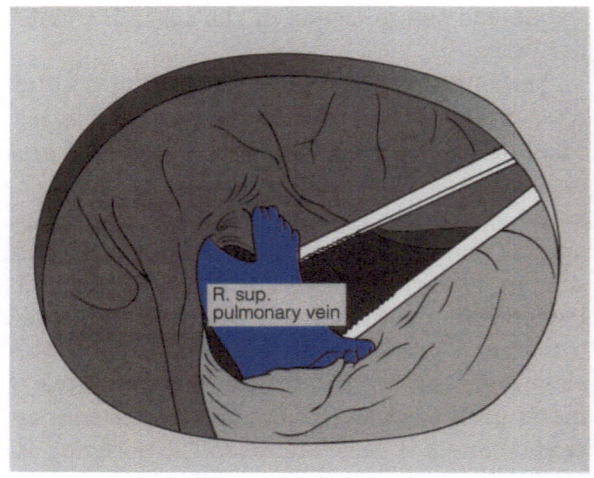

R. sup.
pulmonary vein

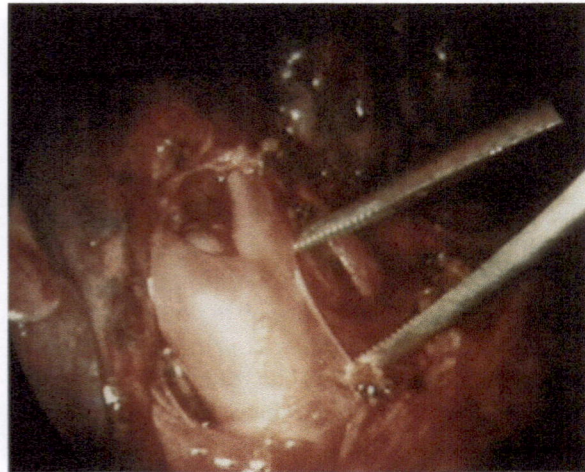

Middle Lobectomy

In the middle lobectomy the first 10-mm trocar for the optic is inserted in the sixth intercostal space along the midaxillary line. Two other trocars for the instruments are positioned in the fifth space. The utility thoracotomy is carried out under direct vision so that it is made to face the lower lobe fissure.

The middle lobe is grasped with the endoscopic grasper or Babcock grasping forceps and displaced posteriorly. The mediastinal pleura is then incised with endoscopic swabs or scissors, thus uncovering

Fig. 7.12. a Isolation of the right superior pulmonary vein. The superior pulmonary vein is the first element to be isolated during a right upper lobectomy as it is the easiest to free. Endoscopic scissors or dissectors can be used to obtain a cleavage plane between the adventitia and the vascular wall which must be gently dissected. **b, c** Intraoperative magnified picture and relative drawing

the superior pulmonary vein. The venous branch for the middle lobe is isolated with the same instruments and encircled with an Endograsp Roticulator carrying a nylon thread. This sling is used to exert gentle traction. As the calibre of this venous branch is usually small, it can easily be sectioned with endoscopic scissors after placement of two endoclips. If the branch is larger, it is secured with an endoscopic stapler.

The fissure between the middle and the lower lobe is opened with electrosurgical dissection to isolate the artery for the lower lobe and the middle lobe. The latter is isolated over an adequate distance and is sectioned using the same technique as for the vein. The possible presence of a second and more anterior artery for the middle lobe must always be considered. The middle lobar bronchus is now identifiable by instrumental palpation and can be dissected with an endoscopic swab inserted through the trocar port or the utility thoracotomy. A thread is passed around the bronchus to facilitate the positioning of the endoscopic stapler, which is used to effect it closure. The main fissure can be completed with the endostapler.

Right Lower Lobectomy and Left Lower Lobectomy

Right and left lower lobectomy are described together as they present many common anatomical and technical aspects.

The first cannula for the optic is inserted in the seventh intercostal space and the two operative cannulae anteriorly and posteriorly in fifth space, right on the line of the classical posterolateral thoracotomy. The utility thoracotomy is performed under video control usually in the fourth or fifth space, so as to face the fissure.

The operation starts by isolating the inferior pulmonary vein. Pointing the camera downwards, the diaphragm and the base of the lung are exposed. The lung is then grasped with an endoscopic grasper and drawn upwards to achieve mild tension on the inferior pulmonary ligament. This is divided up to the inferior pulmonary vein. The camera is again pointed upwards and the inferior pulmonary vein is isolated using the same procedures as for the pulmonary ligament. The vein can be surrounded with an Endograsp Roticulator to pass a thread which will facilitate the insertion of the endostapler and subsequent transection of the vein. Division of the inferior pulmonary vein increases the mobility of the lower lobe.

The dissection of the artery within the fissure is a difficult step and follows the same procedures previously described in the general section.

During a *right lobectomy* the artery must be isolated until the branches for the middle lobe and the apical lower segment have been identified. The right arterial trunk to the basal segments runs without divisions for a longer distance than the equivalent branch on the left.

The artery is isolated with endoscopic graspers or scissors for a sufficient distance to be encircled by a thread passed with an Endograsp Roticulator. By traction on the sling section of posterior adventitial fibres is facilitated, as is the positioning of the endostapler. The branch or branches to the apical lower segment are severed between clips.

During a *left lobectomy*, isolation must be more accurate due to the necessity for isolation of all the arteries to the lingula, and the artery must be followed in the fissure for a long distance. All the branches to the basal segments and to the apical lower segment must then be clipped and severed.

After securing the arteries, the lung is displaced anteriorly to free the lower bronchus with endoscopic scissors and swabs with electrocoagulation of the small vessels. The endostapler is positioned with the same precautions already described for the other procedures and the bronchus is closed and transected. The anterior part of the fissure can be completed with applications of endostapler.

Left Pneumonectomy

The first trocar for the camera is inserted in the seventh intercostal space along the midaxillary line, and the pleural cavity is explored to evaluate the site of the tumour and its anatomical relationship with the mediastinal structures. The utility thoracotomy is performed under direct endoscopic vision, usually in the second or third intercostal space so as to face the main pulmonary artery. Once the operability is ascertained, the surgical steps are similar to those of a classical pneumonectomy. Complete mobilization of the lung and division of the inferior pulmonary ligament is achieved by using either electrocoagulation with endoscopic scissors or blunt dissection with endoswabs. Major vascular structures are dissected with Endograsp

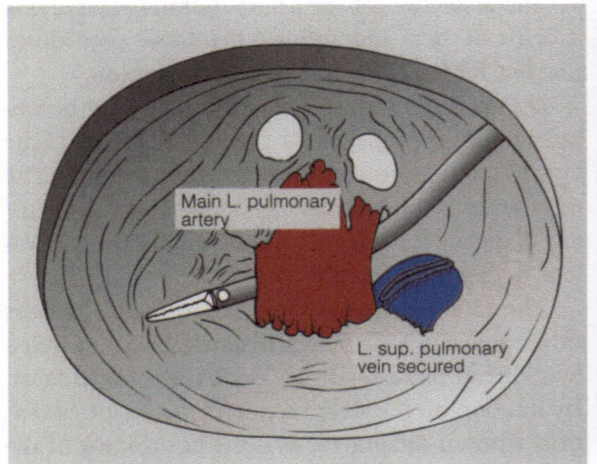

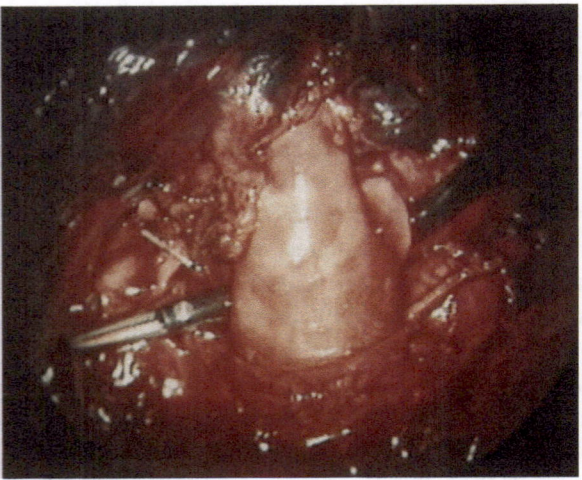

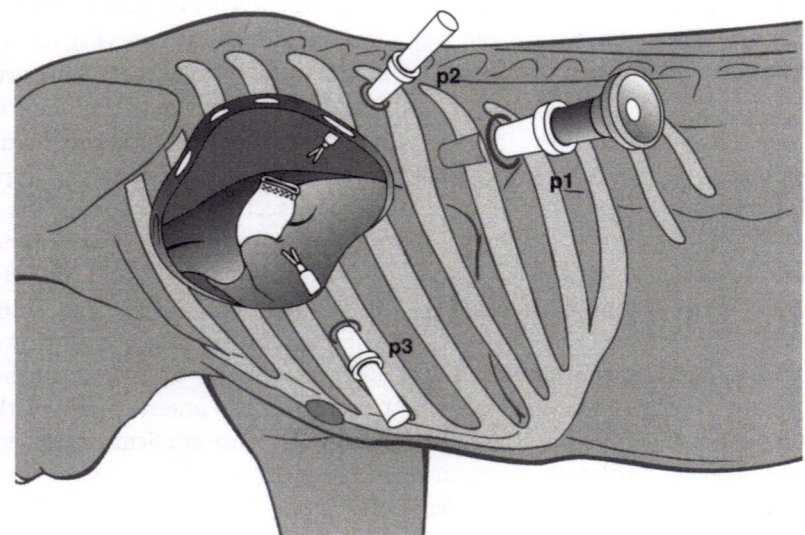

Roticulator forceps or O'Shaugnessy ligature carrier and encircled with a thread, which allows a gentle traction so as to facilitate the positioning of the stapler. We always place a vascular clamp underneath the endostapler before staple section to prevent severe haemorrhagic complications in case of stapler dysfunction. The lower pulmonary vein is transected with the endostapler bearing 2.8- or 3-mm vascular staples, and the vascular clamp is removed.

The upper pulmonary vein is then dissected on its anterior aspect while the lung is retracted downwards and posteriorly. Using a Roticular Endograsp the vein is completely isolated, encircled with a thread and secured with an endostapler.

Fig. 7.13 a – c. Dissection of the main pulmonary arteries is the most difficult step in videothoracoscopic left pneumonectomy. As shown in **a** and **b**, the left main pulmonary artery has been isolated and encircled with a Roticulator Endograsp to enable passage of a thread which will facilitate positioning of the stapler

Dissection of the main pulmonary artery is the most difficult step in videothoracoscopic left pneumonectomy (Fig. 7.13). Absence of adequate endoscopic instrumentation makes it difficult to find the plane of dissection. Once completely free, the artery is transected with an endoscopic stapler. It may be difficult to find the correct angle of positioning the stapler. When this is achieved, dissec-

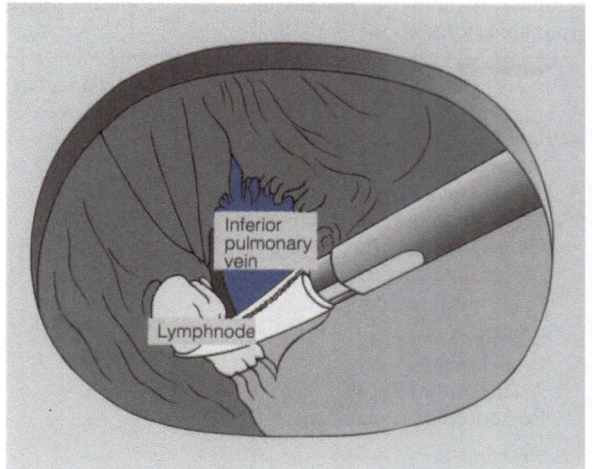

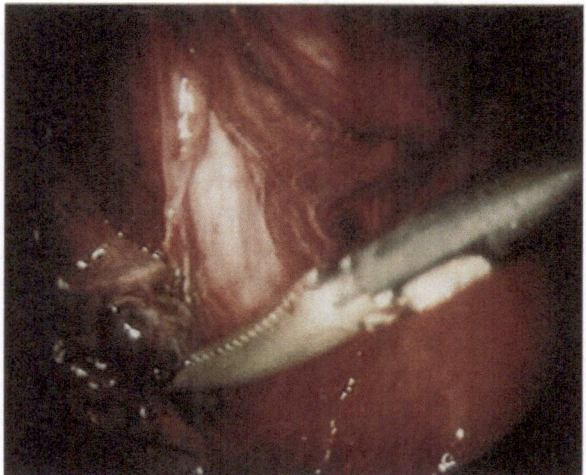

a   b

Fig. 7.14a, b. Lymphadenectomy. Lymph nodes can be removed by combined sharp and blunt dissection. The partially isolated inferior pulmonary vein is visible behind the
grasper holding a lymph node

tion is clean and the arterial stump immediately
falls after opening the stapler. Eventually the main
bronchus is dissected for a sufficient length while
the bronchial arteries are electrocoagulated or
clipped. The bronchus is severed using one or two
triple rows of staples and endoscissors. Due to
thickness of the main bronchus, endostaplers at
present do not guarantee a safe suture. For this reason the collapsed lung is grasped with two Duval
clamps and gently coaxed through the utility
thoracotomy. The edges of the residual bronchial
stump are grasped with two conventional clamps or
two endoscopic graspers, drawn upwards and closed with a conventional 4.5 TA Roticulator inserted
through the utility thoracotomy (Fig. 7.11).

In the course of all the above-described procedures, lymph nodes encountered are removed with
a technique similar to that for open surgery. In
videoendoscopic operations they are magnified and
even the smallest ones can be easily excised
(Fig. 7.14).

Postoperative Care

The postoperative course of thoracoscopically assisted pulmonary resections differs from open thoracic interventions in that trauma is minimal, pain
is drastically reduced and recovery is accelerated.
At the end of the operation a control X-ray is done
to rule out any endothoracic collections, to check
the re-expansion of the lung and in pneumonectomy cases to establish the position of the mediastinum. In partial resections, the drain is placed under water seal and connected to suction. It is usually removed 24 h later if there is no air leakage. After
pneumonectomy the pleural cavity must be kept at
a slight negative pressure of 1–12 cm of water so
as to favour displacement of the mediastinum and
compensatory overexpansion of the remaining
lung.

As previously mentioned, the great reduction of
pain compared to traditional "open" resections ensures a smooth postoperative course by improving
effective coughing and expectoration of bronchial
secretions which otherwise tend to stagnate, leading
to secretional airway obstruction and postoperative
bronchopneumonia.

Complications and Results

Complications of videothoracoscopic pulmonary resections are the same as in conventional surgery.

From October 1991 to March 1994, 78 patients underwent thoracoscopically assisted surgery with the intent of performing major pulmonary resection in our department. Out of these, 71 major pulmonary resections proved to be possible: one right apical lower segmentectomy, 65 lobectomies (14 right lower lobectomies, nine middle lobectomies, 16 right upper lobectomies and 18 left lower lobectomies) and three left pneumonectomies and two right pneumonectomies. These operations were carried out in patients with an average age of 52.9 years (range 11–74 years).

Eleven patients (15%) had benign pulmonary disease, four (6%) had pulmonary metastases non-resectable by a wedge resection and 56 (79%) were suffering from primary lung neoplasms at TNM clinical stage 1. In all these patients lymphadenectomy was performed, and in 16 (28.5%) cases pathological findings revealed N1 disease (Table 1).

In our experience, diffuse pleural adhesions rarely represent an insuperable problem, since they can usually be divided. Fissural isolation of the artery is the most difficult step and often determines whether a major videoendoscopically assisted resection is feasible. In our series, five patients required conversion to open procedure. In one of them, after having isolated and secured the superior pulmonary vein and the anterior arterial trunk, displacement of the double-lumen orotracheal Carlens tube caused a sudden and irreversible re-expansion of the lung, thus preventing fissural isolation and completion of the procedure. In three other patients inflammatory changes had obliterated the fissure, thereby precluding a safe dissection of the artery. In three cases moderate bleeding from a lobar artery was controlled by positioning a vascular clamp, but the fibrotic fissure did not permit isolation and transection of the artery.

In our series there was no peri- nor postoperative mortality, and no reinterventions were necessary. Out of 71 patients submitted to videothoracoscopic resections, 62 (87%) had an uneventful postoperative course and the chest drain was removed on the fifth postoperative day (range 2–10). One

Table 1. Pathology of major videothoracoscopically assisted pulmonary resection

Disease	Patients (n)
Primary lung tumors	*56*
Squamous cell carcinomas	7
Adenocarcinomas	16
Bronchiolo-alveolar carcinomas	4
Undifferentiated large cell carcinoma	3
Atypical carcinoid	2
Plasma cell granuloma	1
Benign lung diseases	*11*
Bronchiectasis	9
Arteriovenous fistula	1
Pseudotumor (sarcoidosis)	1
Lung metastasis	*4*
Endobronchial metastasis from renal clear-cell carcinoma	1
Colonic adenocarcinoma	2
Skin melanom	1

patient with bronchiectasis and diffuse inflammatory changes needed a postoperative blood transfusion but otherwise the postoperative course was uneventful. In nine (13%) cases prolonged air leakage was observed (mean: 21 days; range: 12–45 days) and a pleural infection occurred in one patient. Protracted air leakage should not be considered as a specific postoperative complication as the candidates for this kind of surgery are often afflicted by impairment of respiratory function and emphysema, and therefore prone to this kind of event.

Two patients had haemorrhagic pleural effusion after chest drain withdrawal (on third and fourth postoperative day). One of these required insertion of a new drain under CT control; the other did not require any active measures and his postoperative course was not prolonged.

The postoperative course of these patients is enormously improved mainly because of the near absence of pain, which allows good respiratory function and therefore efficacy of cough is maintained. Rapid recovery and resumption of normal activity are the norm in patients with good preoperative respiratory reserve. Patients with contraindications to conventional open surgery derive particular advantage from the minimal functional impairment and smooth postoperative course.

References

1. Roviaro GC, Rebuffat C, Varoli F, Vergani C, Mariani C, Maciocco M (1992) Videoendoscopic pulmonary lobectomy for cancer. Surg Laparosc Endos 2 N 3:244–247
2. Roviaro GC, Rebuffat C, Varoli F, Vergani C, Maciocco M, Grignani F, Scalambra SM, Mariani C (1993) Video-endoscopic thoracic surgery. Int Surg 78:4–9
3. Roviaro GC, Rebuffat C, Varoli F, Vergani C, Maciocco M, Grignani F, Scalambra SM, Mariani C (1993) Video-thoracoscopic pulmonary lobectomies for cancer. In: Steichen FM, Welter R (eds) Minimally invasive surgery and new technology. Quality Medical Publishing 1994, pp 700–703
4. Roviaro GC, Varoli F, Rebuffat C, Maciocco M, Vergani C, Scalambra SM, D'Hoore A (1993) Videoendoscopic major pulmonary resections: pneumonectomies and lobectomies. Ann Thorac Surg 56:779–783
5. Landreneau R, Hazelrigg S, Ferson P et al (1992) Thoracoscopic resection of 85 pulmonary lesions. Ann Thorac Surg 54:415–420
6. Mack M, Aronoff R, Acuff T, Douthit M, Bowman R, Ryan W (1992) Present role of thoracoscopy in the diagnosis and treatment of dieseases of the chest. Ann Thorac Surg 54:403–409
7. Miller D, Allen M, Trastek VF, Deschamps C, Pairolero PC (1992) Videothoracoscopic wedge excision of the lung. Ann Thorac Surg 54:410–414

8 Laparoscopic Liver Surgery

A. CUSCHIERI

Introduction

Currently, laparoscopic liver surgery is in its infancy and is confined to limited, nonanatomical resections for small tumours, deroofing of large simple cysts and pericystectomy for accessible hydatid disease. There is, however, little doubt that with the use of the emerging, advanced ancillary technologies, the scope of laparoscopic liver surgery will be extended such that major resections, which are currently experimental, will be performed clinically in the near future.

The important ancillary technological advances which will play a significant role in the development of laparoscopic liver surgery are: contact ultrasound scanning, ultrasonic dissection, water jet dissection, argon and helium ion plasma coagulation, cryotherapy and laser dissection with photocoagulation.

Ancillary Technology

Laparoscopic Contact Hepatic Ultrasound Scanning

Contact laparoscopic ultrasound scanning is discussed in Chapter 14 of this volume. As in open liver surgery, contact laparoscopic ultrasound scanning of the liver parenchyma using high definition (7.5-MHz) linear array probes is necessary not only for the diagnosis of hepatic lesions but also to map out the resection margins during segmental and lobar resections for tumours [1]. Contact ultrasonography is also essential during the application of cryotherapy for the destruction of hepatic tumours whether this is performed by the open or the laparoscopic route [2].

Ultrasonic Dissection and Ion Plasma Coagulation

The advantage of ultrasonic dissection for division of the hepatic parenchyma during open liver surgery has been well established [3, 4]. The ultrasonic probe divides parenchymal cells (because of their high water content) by the cavitational effect without injury to structures with a high content of fibrous tissue, e.g. bile ducts and blood vessels. Once skeletonized by the probe, these are then clipped if large or coagulated if small. The combined use of the argon or helium ion plasma coagulation (Chap. 4, Vol. 1) and the ultrasonic probe results in virtually bloodless division of the hepatic parenchyma. Laparoscopic hand-pieces for ultrasonic dissection are now available and the Selector probe (Surgical Technology Group; Andover, UK) has been evaluated by us in a number of clinical situations [5]. This endoscopic probe employs a light-weight, high-efficiency piezoelectric ceramic transducer to provide energy for motion at a resonant frequency of 24000 Hz. A full-wavelength titanium alloy extension is inserted between the step amplifier and the tip section to provide the reach required for endoscopic use. A black delrin shroud with a 10 mm outer diameter and 278 mm overall length ensures adequate reach for endoscopic use following its insertion through a standard 10.5-mm cannula (Fig. 8.1a). The hand-piece delivers ultrasonic vibration at operating amplitudes up to 240 µm together with simultaneous aspiration and irrigation. The grip of the hand-piece has a control valve which is operated by the thumb and is used to occlude the aspiration tube. The Selector probe is introduced with the aspiration control valve closed until the tip of the hand-piece is in the operating field and ready for activation of the ultrasonic en-

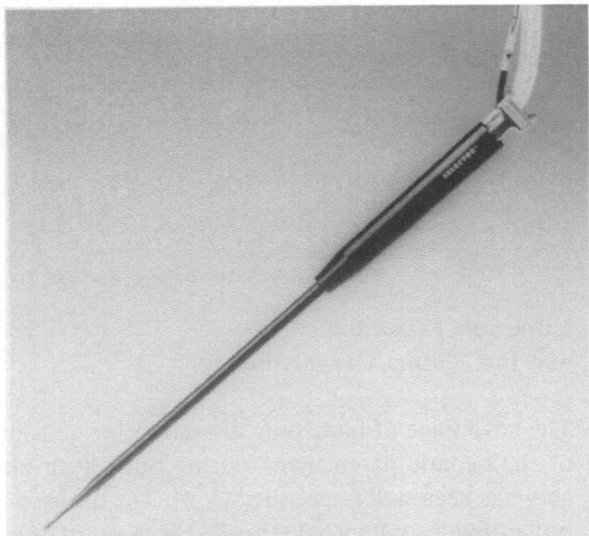

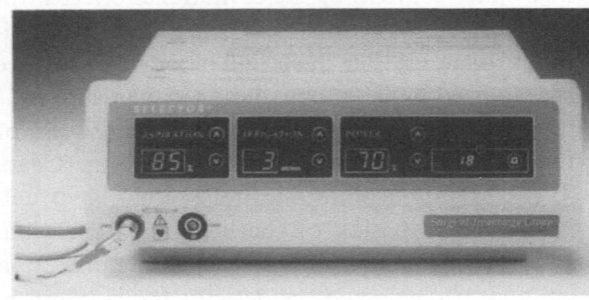

Fig. 8.1. a Selector ultrasonic hand piece for endoscopic surgery. **b** Ultrasonic console (Surgical Technology Group, Andover, UK)

ergy. The probe is used with the standard Selector ultrasonic surgical aspirator console (Fig. 8.1 b).

As the ultrasonic probe does not cut peritoneal membranes and fascial layers (low water content), the Glisson's capsule of the liver has to be incised by the electrosurgical knife before ultrasonic division of the hepatic parenchyma is commenced.

Hydro (Water-Jet) Dissection

Hydrodissection has been in use for a while in pelvic endoscopic surgery to open tissue planes and is useful in lymph node dissections. High-pressure water-jet dissection was first reported by Papachristu and Barters [6] as a quick and efficient technique for disruption of the liver parenchyma during open hepatic resections. A purpose-designed hydrodynamic device has been developed by Baer et al. [7, 8] for high-pressure, high-velocity water-jet hepatic parenchymal dissection which facilitates major hepatic resections and enables the exposure of intraparenchymal bile ducts for segmental bilioenteric anastomosis. The device is now on the market (ME Medical Exports AG, Unter Altstadt 3, Zug, Switzerland). Three operating nozzles (20–70 µm) are available, including one for laparoscopic use. The device delivers water at a high pressure (6×10 Pa). This results in an outflow stream from the nozzle which has an initial velocity of 300 m/s. The water jet is only coherent for a short distance from the tip of the nozzle (30 mm). Thereafter, it fans out to an intermediate zone of microdroplets and at a variable distance (40–80 cm) from the nozzle, the jet becomes a spray. Thus when the instrument is applied close to the tissue (3–4 cm), deep, sharp cutting of all structures (including blood vessels) is achieved, but as the nozzle is withdrawn, this effect is replaced by washing and gentle separation.

A laparoscopic dedicated water-jet dissector developed by Storz (Tuttlingen, Germany) is currently under evaluation. It operates at a lower pressure than the Baer system, which was designed for open surgery. Consequently, the jet is coherent (i.e. cutting) for only a short distance beyond the nozzle (<1 cm). The Storz system also includes important safety features of the applicator to eliminate the risk of inadvertant deep cutting.

It is not possible to arrive at any conclusion on the value of hydro-jet dissection as there has not been any report of experience with it in endoscopic surgery and even the experience in open hepatic resections is very limited. The most important consideration with the current Baer system is its safety margin during laparoscopic surgery as distances between the tip of the operating nozzle and the tissue can be difficult to assess with the current two-dimensional TV image of the operating field. This problem may be reduced, though not abolished, when three-dimensional imaging becomes established routinely and by the incorporation of a back stop. Only systems which incorporate a backstop as an intrinsic feature of the applicator will be safe for use in endoscopic surgery. Another problem with water-jet dissection is the storm effect, whereby the reflected spray, aside from fouling the optic, disseminates droplets containing parenchymatous debris and cell clumps all over the operating field. The risk of tumour dissemination and implantation during resections for tumours are obvious. As the volume of water delivered is small even during long procedures, the problem of excessive hydration does not arise. Obviously comparisons between water-jet and ultrasonic dissection in open and laparoscopic liver surgery are required.

Laser Dissection

Laser dissection with photocoagulation using contact and free beam modes is undoubtedly an elegant method of resecting hepatic parenchyma. The new linear array diode lasers which are small, portable and require very little maintenance, have largely overcome all the major disadvantages of the gas vapour lasers. The current device delivers laser light at a fixed wavelength of 750 nm and has a maximal power output of 25 W (Fig. 8.2). Advances in non-linear crystal technology will soon make it possible to produce tunable diode lasers.

Cryotherapy

Hepatic cryotherapy with liquid nitrogen probes has been used in a limited fashion in a number of pioneering centres as an alternative to resection for secondary metastatic disease [2, 9, 10] and less frequently in the management of primary liver cancer [11]. The cell-destructive effect of cryotherapy is primarily due to the formation of intracellular and extracellular ice crystals, the relative ratio of which within a cryolesion depends on the rate of freezing. A slow rate of freezing results in ice crystal formation in the extracellular space, whereas a rapid freeze induces intracellular ice crystal formation. The latter causes immediate mechanical disruption of cell membranes and organelles. By contrast, extracellular ice crystal formation leads to cell damage by creating osmotic gradients with resulting cell shrinkage and high ionic intracellular concentrations. Within a cryolesion, a high intracellular to extracellular ice crystal ratio results in maximum tissue necrosis and underlies the confirmed observation that a rapid freeze is more effective than a slow one. The rewarming (thaw component) is also important as during a slow thaw, the growth of intracellular ice crystals continues during the early phases of the rewarming process [12, 13].

In addition to a rapid freeze-slow thaw cycle, repeated freezing of the same area increases the size of the iceball and thus the extent of tissue necrosis produced. Animal studies have demonstrated that this effect is caused by increased thermal conductivity and rapid enlargement of residual intracellular ice crystals [12, 13].

The secondary effects of cryotherapy include denaturation of lipid-protein complexes and changes in the microcirculation of the frozen tissue. Although after rewarming, blood flow through the damaged tissue is maintained initially, extensive intravascular thrombosis with platelet and fibrin deposition occurs within 1 h such that the cryolesion behaves like a sterile infarct. In the early stages, the necrosed tissue is separated from viable hepatic parenchyma by a zone of granulation tissue. The granulation tissue zone subsequently matures to a fibrous capsule that contracts to a fibrous scar within 6−8 weeks as the soft liquefied cellular debris is absorbed [14, 15].

Rapid freezing (temperature fall by 30 °C/min) of liver parenchyma and hepatic tumours can only be obtained by liquid nitrogen probes. The maximum size of the hepatic iceball achieved depends on the probe size and type (surface or implantable trocar). Experimental work in primates by Neel [16] has shown that the iceball diameter can also be increased by inflow occlusion (portal vein and hepatic artery) during freezing.

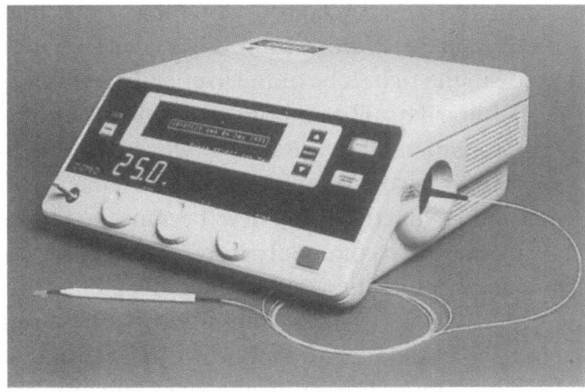

Fig. 8.2. Diode array laser (Diomed, UK)

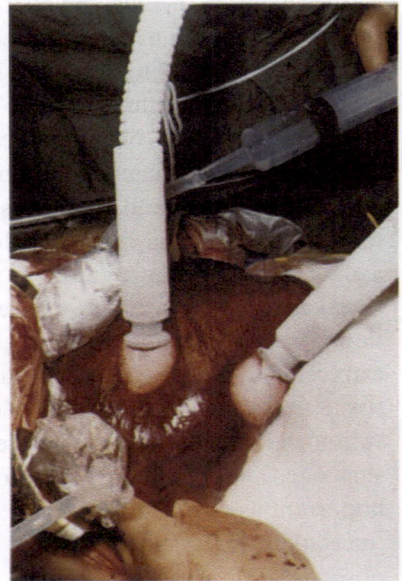
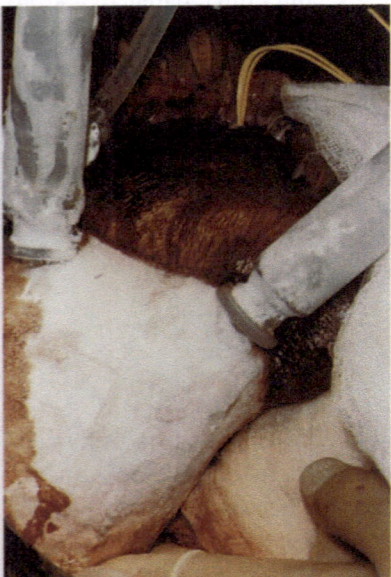

a

b

Fig. 8.3a, b. Extensive freezing of hepatic tumour in the human using multiprobe cryotherapy (Surgical Technology Group, Andover, UK). **a** Commencement of cryotherapy; **b** completed iceball

During therapy, the size of the iceball is monitored by contact ultrasonography using high resolution (7.5 MHz) linear array probes. The interface between the frozen and unfrozen tissue is highly reflecting of ultrasound waves and appears as a well-defined hyperechoic margin. The collective experience to date suggests that hepatic cryotherapy is safe and is well tolerated with few complications.

The limitation of the available cryosystems and probes is the size of the iceball achieved which rarely exceeds 5 cm. In conjunction with the Surgical Technology Group (Andover, UK), we have developed a closed nitrogen cryogenic system which has the following attributes: use of multiple, high-efficiency implantable probes (2−3 mm) to freeze large volumes of liver tissue, pressurized high-flow nitrogen delivery and probe rewarming for safe dislodgement from the hepatic parenchyma. Experimental evaluation of the prototype device has enabled volumes of hepatic parenchyma equivalent to 30% of the hepatic parenchyma to be frozen inside 1 h. The system has now been used in six human patients. In the human we have obtained iceballs measuring 12×15 cm (Fig. 8.3).

Laparoscopic probes which are introduced through 11-mm ports and which effectively avoid freezing of the abdominal wall have been developed and are currently being evaluated in patients with hepatic metastases. The potential for laparoscopic cryotherapy of patients with secondary deposits in the liver is now being realized and will carry considerable advantages over open cryodestruction or resection, as the procedure can be repeated.

Deroofing of Simple Liver Cysts

Simple hepatic cysts are generally considered to be congenital malformations. By definition, they do not communicate with the biliary tree, are lined by a single layer of cuboidal or columnar epithelium and contain clear serous fluid. They occur predominantly in the right lobe of the liver and may be uni- or multilocular. The majority of these cysts are asymptomatic and are usually discovered accidentally during imaging of the liver for some other condition. Nonetheless, a few become large and cause symptoms commonly in elderly females, although symptomatic cysts are well documented in younger patients. The manifestations include dull ache, upper abdominal discomfort, dyspepsia and a palpable mass usually in the right subcostal region. Less frequently, acute pain and jaundice may

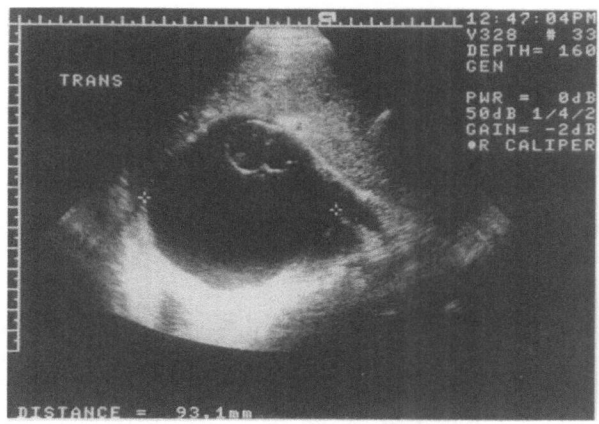

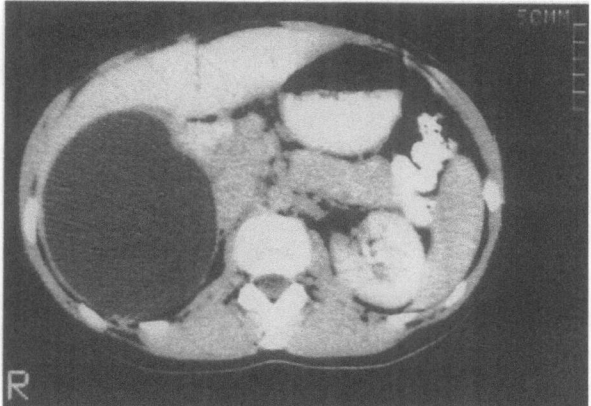

a   b

Fig. 8.4a, b. Large simple hepatic cyst with daughter cysts. **a** Ultrasound appearance; **b** CT scan

be encountered. The investigation of patients with such symptoms must include ultrasonography, CT scanning of the liver and determination of α-fetoprotein levels to exclude malignancy, particularly, cystic adenocarcinoma of the liver. The typical findings on ultrasound and CT examination reveal a uniform unilocular or multilocular uniform cystic lesion usually to the right of the gallbladder which is often displaced anteromedially (Fig. 8.4). The features which increase the likelihood of malignancy are septation and calcification.

Percutaneous ultrasound-guided drainage is invariably followed by recurrence and is not recommended. The standard surgical management of these symptomatic cysts is suction drainage and partial excision of the dome of the cyst (deroofing). This is preferred to total excision, which can be difficult because the interface between the intrahepatic portion of the cyst and the liver parenchyma is usually ill defined and dissection of this plane is attended by bleeding and the risk of bile ductal damage with subsequent biliary fistula [17, 18]. Furthermore, large cysts which extend throughout the right lobe are unresectable.

The deroofing of simple nonparasitic hepatic cysts can be undertaken laparoscopically with complete safety and excellent results [19, 20].

Sites of Trocar and Cannulae

The exact position of the trocar cannulae depend on the location and size of the cyst. For the typical right lobe lesion, the desired positioning is shown in Fig. 8.5: umbilical, 11 mm for the telescope; 5.5 mm midclavicular below the lower margin of the cyst; 5.5 mm left paramedian. Occasionally another cannula (right subxiphoid) may be necessary for retraction.

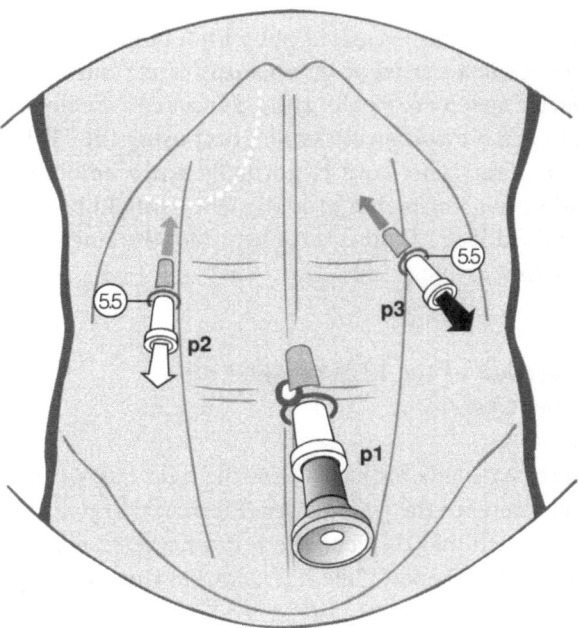

Fig. 8.5. Sites of trocar and cannulae for deroofing of simple hepatic cyst

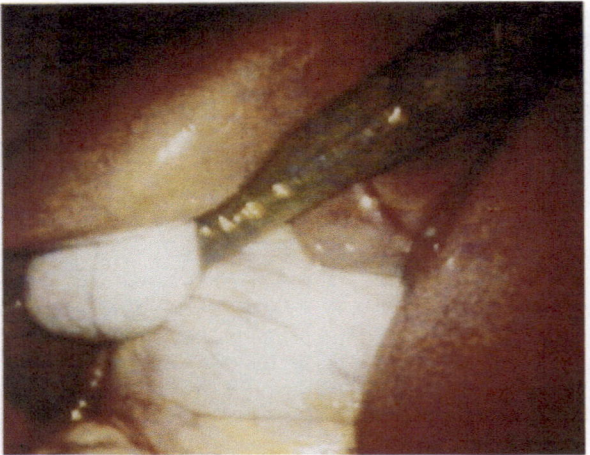

Fig. 8.6. Cyst projecting below the right lobe of the liver lateral to the gallbladder

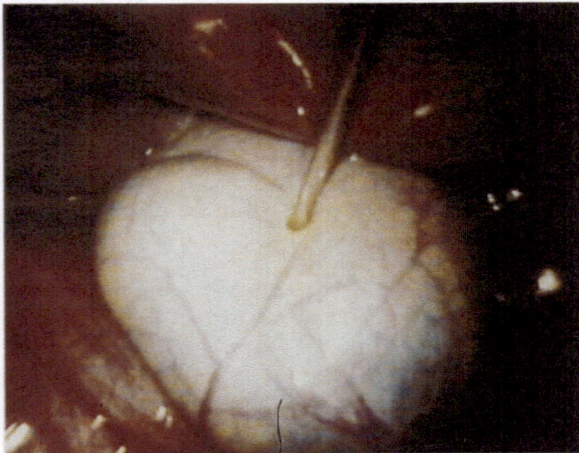

Confirmation of the Diagnosis

After the creation of the pneumoperitoneum and insertion of the laparoscope, the cyst is identified as a dark yellowish brown swelling underneath the liver with fine vessels traversing its fascial coverings. The remainder of the liver is inspected for other cysts. The first step consists of sampling the cystic fluid. This can be carried out with a lumbar puncture needle inserted percutaneously. The fluid is inspected macroscopically and a specimen is sent for immediate cytological examination using the Diff-Quik stain. The fluid is normally straw coloured and serous. Suspicion of malignancy should be entertained if the fluid is turbulent, blood stained, or contains atypical cells.

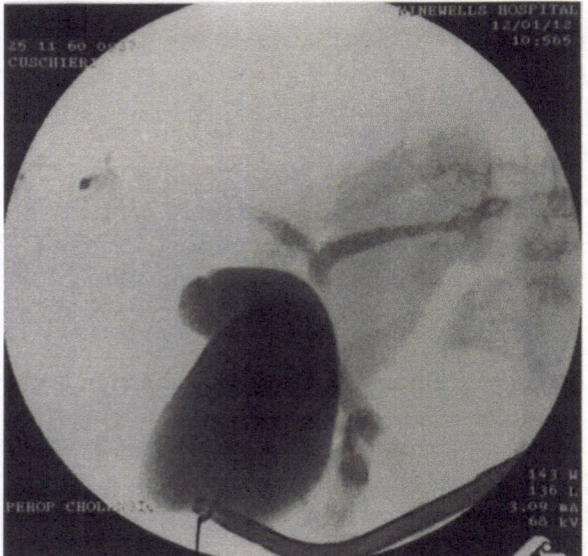

Dissection of the Extrahepatic Portion of the Cyst

The cyst usually projects below the right lobe of the liver lateral to the gallbladder (Fig. 8.6). Large cysts can stretch and displace the porta hepatis, including the extrahepatic bile duct, so that the anatomy becomes considerably disturbed. In this situation

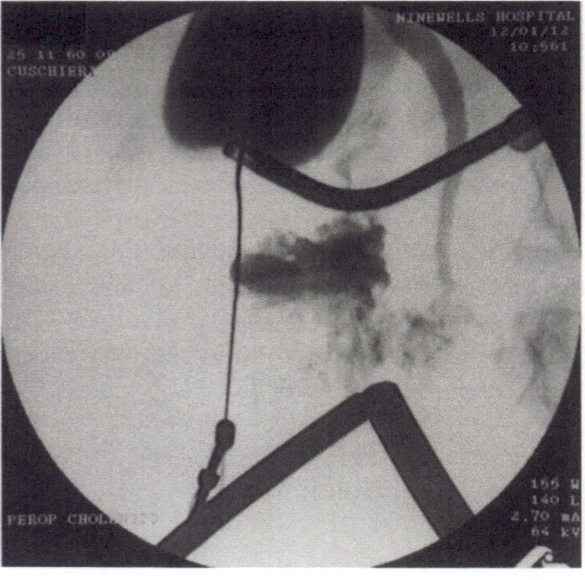

Fig. 8.7. **a** Gallbladder puncture for cholecystocholangiogram. **b, c** Contrast study excluding communication with the biliary tract

and whenever there is any doubt concerning communication of the cyst with the ductal system (fluid aspirated from cyst is bile stained), a cholecystocholangiogram should be performed (Fig. 8.7 a, b). In one of our patients, the common bile duct and the hepatic artery required mobilization from the anterior cyst wall. The extrahepatic portion of the cyst is covered by peritoneum and several layers of fascial coverings. The division of these layers exposes the cyst wall. A large enough area (5.0 × 5.0 cm) must be exposed to effect an adequate deroofing. Once this has been achieved, the sucker is placed close to the cyst wall for the next stage of the operation.

Aspiration and Inspection of the Cyst

A small incision is made with scissors or an electrosurgical hook knife, the sucker tip introduced into the cyst cavity and the fluid aspirated as completely as possible. The opening is then enlarged to admit the 30° oblique 10-mm viewing telescope for visual inspection of the interior of the cyst, which should have a smooth shining appearance. Sometimes multiple grape-like bunches of "daughter cysts" are encountered projecting into the main cyst lumen (Fig. 8.8). These require decompression, and whenever possible, they should be partially excised. The excision of daughter cysts is considerably facilitated by the use of the curved coaxial scissors.

Deroofing of the Cyst

The exposed anterior wall of the extrahepatic portion of the cyst in then grasped by an insulated atraumatic forceps and excised either by scissors with electrocoagulation of the vessels within the cyst wall or by means of the electrosurgical hook knife using a cutting blended current (Fig. 8.9). The excised cyst wall and any daughter cysts are sent for histological examination.

After the deroofing is completed, a portion of the greater omentum is transposed inside the cyst and held in place with a suture to the anterior cyst wall (Fig. 8.10). Some surgeons insert a drain routinely. This is unnecessary unless there has been considerable oozing during the operation.

Laparoscopic Treatment of Infected Simpled Cysts and Abscesses

Infected Simple Cysts

Infected simple cysts become adherent to surrounding organs, especially the hepatic flexure and duodenum. When located in the posterior segments of the right lobe, they stick to the diaphragm. Laparoscopic treatment begins by freeing enough superficial wall of the cyst or abscess wall from the

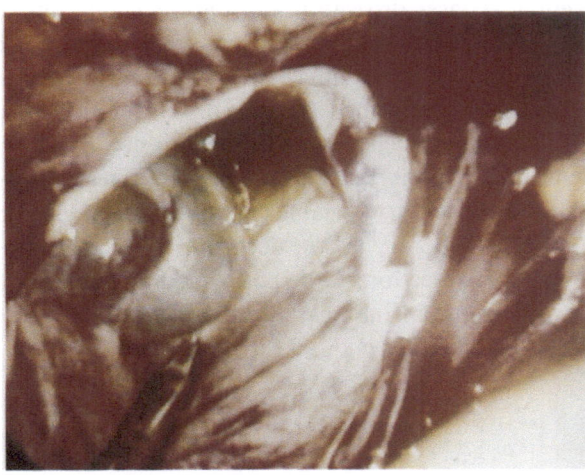

Fig. 8.8. Daughter cysts projecting into the main cyst lumen

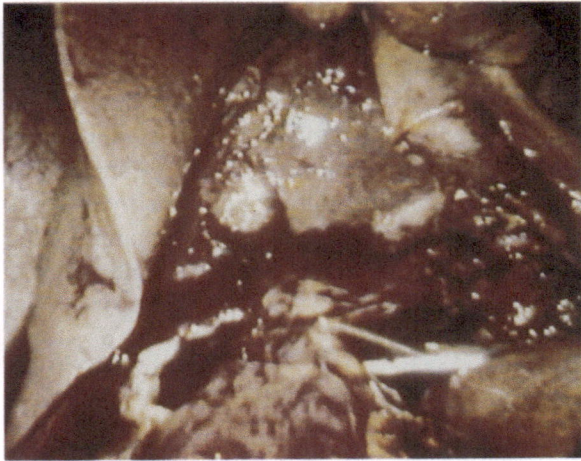

Fig. 8.9. Deroofing of the cyst

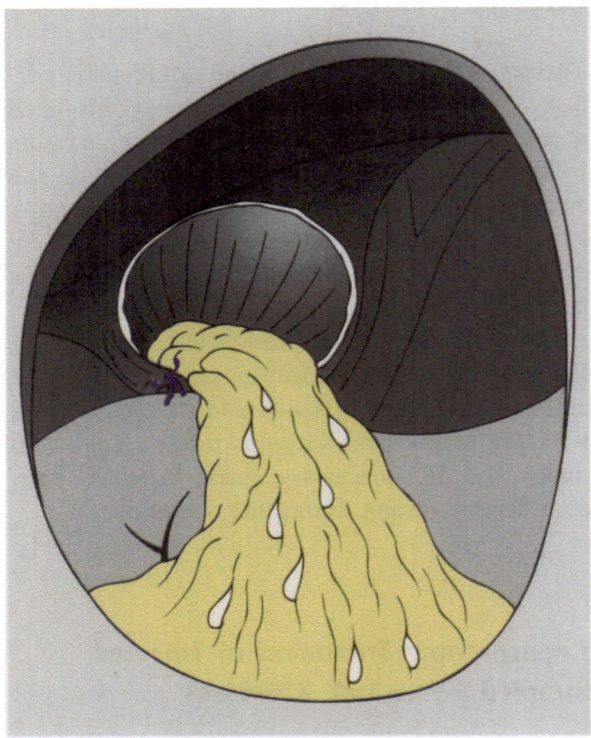

Fig. 8.10. Omentum transposed inside the cyst and held in place with a suture to the anterior cyst wall

adherent structures. This is followed by aspiration, preferably with the Veress needle with an intervening trap attached to the suction line. When the cyst or abscess is emptied, the suction line is disconnected from the Veress needle and saline injected slowly by syringe into the cyst cavity and then aspirated. This is repeated until the returning fluid is clear. A small portion of the cyst wall is then excised and sent for histological examination. After inspection of the interior of the cyst, a silicon drain is placed inside its cavity. The purulent fluid is examined immediately by microscopy after Gram's staining and a specimen sent for culture and sensitivity tests. Thorough lavage with saline or Hartmann's solution is performed before desufflation and removal of the cannulae.

Hepatic and Subphrenic Collections and Abscess

Provided access can be obtained, which is the case in the majority of these patients, pathological purulent collections can be dealt with laparoscopically. As in many instances, the pus is under tension, a sucker placed near the summit of the abscess must be ready for activation as soon as the needle is applied to the swollen portion. As the walls of these collections are soft, gentle pressure by the sucker tip over the perforation caused by the sampling needle often results in entry of the sucker into the abscess cavity when the contents are aspirated. Following evacuation, irrigation and aspiration of the cavity is undertaken until all necrotic debris has been removed. A drain is then placed into the abscess cavity and the peritoneal gutters lavaged with a clean irrigating/suction cannula.

Technique of Laparoscopic Liver Resections

Currently laparoscopic resections of the liver parenchyma are limited to small nonanatomical resections (cysts and small tumours) and to segmental resections on the left side (segments 2 and 3). The technique used by the author relies on the use of the ultrasonic dissector probe (Selector; British Technology Group; Andover, UK), the Argon Beamer (Beacon Labs) and the Endoclip applier (USSC; Norwalk, USA). An alternative technique employs laser dissection and photocoagulation.

More major resections using specially designed laparoscopic liver sling-type haemostatic clamps have been performed successfully in the dog [21]. Techniques which permit the laparoscopic mobilization of the portal vein and hepatic artery by use of shape-memory variable curvature instruments to enable temporary inflow occlusion will enable major lobar resections to be performed by the laparoscopic route in the near future.

References

1. Solomon MJ, Stephen MS, White JH, Eyers AA (1991) A new classification of hepatic territories using intraoperative ultrasound. Am J Surg 163:336–338
2. Ravikumar TS, Kane R, Cady B et al. (1987) Hepatic cryosurgery with intraoperative ultrasound monitoring for metastatic colon carcinoma. Arch Surg 122:403–409
3. Puttnam CHW (1983) Techniques of ultrasonic dissection in resection of the liver. Surg Gynecol Obstet 157:475–478
4. Hodgson WJB, DelGuercio LRM (1984) Preliminary experience in liver surgery using the ultrasonic scalpel. Surgery 95:230–234
5. Cuschieri A, Shimi S, Banting S, Van der Velpen G (1993) Endoscopic ultrasonic dissection for thoracoscopic and laparoscopic surgery. Surg Endosc (in press)
6. Papachristu DN, Barters R (1982) Resection of the liver with a water jet. Br J Surg 69:93–94
7. Baer HU, Maddern GJ, Blumgart LH (1991) Hepatic surgery facilitated by a new jet dissector. HPB Surg 1991; 4:137–144
8. Baer HU, Maddern GJ, Dennison AR, Blumgart LH (1992) Water-jet dissection in hepatic surgery. Min Invas Ther 1:169–172
9. Ravikumar TS, Steel GD (1989) Hepatic cryosurgery. Surg Clin North Am 69:433–436
10. Charnley RM, Doran J, Morris DL (1989) Cryotherapy for liver metastases: a new approach. Br J Surg 76:1040–1041
11. Zhou XD, Tang ZY, Yu YQ, Ma ZC (1988) Clinical evaluation of cryosurgery in the treatment of primary liver cancer. Cancer 61:1889–1892
12. Farrant J, Walter CA (1977) The cryobiological basis for cryosurgery. J Dermatol Surg Oncol 3:403–407
13. Whittaker DK (1984) Mechanisms of tissue destruction following cryosurgery. Ann Coll Surg Engl 66:313–318
14. Healey WV, Priebe CJ, Farrer SM, Phillips LL (1971) Hepatic cryosurgery, acute and long term effects. Arch Surg 103:384–392
15. Gilbert JC, Onik GM, Hoddick WK et al (1986) Ultrasound monitored hepatic cryosurgery. Longevity study on animal model. Cryobiology 23:277–285
16. Neel HB, Ketcham AS, Hammond WG (1971) Ischaemia potentiating cryosurgery of primate liver. Ann Surg 174:308–318
17. Doty JE, Tompkins RK (1989) Management of cystic disease of the liver. Surg Clin North Am 69:285–295
18. Lai ECS, Wong J (1990) Symptomatic non-parasitic cysts of the liver. World J Surg 14:452–465
19. Z'graggen K, Metzger A, Klaiber C (1991) Symptomatic simple cysts of the liver: treatment by laparoscopic surgery. J Surg Endosc 5:224–225
20. Cuschieri A, Berci G (1992) Laparoscopic biliary surgery, 2nd edn. Blackwell, London, pp 190–194
21. Zamora A, Mucio M (1992) Partial hepatectomy by laparoscopy: experimental phase. Min Invas Ther 1:389–391

9 Laparoscopic Bilioenteric Bypass

A. Cuschieri

Introduction

The incidence of pancreatic adenocarcinoma is increasing. The vast majority of cases are incurable and 90% of patients are dead within 1 year of the diagnosis [1]. Although small tumours are resectable in a small cohort of patients and 5-year survival rates of up to 30% have been reported in this small selected subgroup following radical resection [2], for the vast majority of patients, treatment entails palliation of jaundice and itching, pain and, less often, vomiting due to duodenal obstruction. Pain is an important feature of inoperable pancreatic cancer and is best managed by percutaneous paravertebral coeliac plexus block together with oral long-acting opiates or bilateral thoracoscopic splanchnicectomy.

Currently, the options for the relief of jaundice and itching include radiological/endoscopic stenting or open surgical bypass. Although one previous randomized study had indicated advantages for endoscopic stenting over surgical biliary bypass in terms of reduced morbidity and hospital stay, a recent study has failed to demonstrate any difference [3]. Nonetheless, endoscopic stenting is currently the most widely practised treatment in these unfortunate patients. Technical progress in endoscopic stenting, such as the introduction of the expanding wire wall stents [4] as distinct from the traditional plastic types, have further increased the scope of endoscopic stenting. However, growth of the tumour through the interstices of the wire wall stents can lead to occlusion and recurrence of symptoms [5]. The use of covered wire wall stents, which should prevent this complication, is being evaluated.

Irrespective of the nature of stents employed, there are problems related with this form of management. These stem from the inevitable formation of a bacterial biofilm [6, 7], which leads to infection with episodes of cholangitis and stent encrustation and blockage with calcium bilirubinate, necessitating stent replacement. Despite intense studies involving various prophylactic measures, including impregnation of stents with chemicals and antibiotics, use of oral bile salt therapy, etc., the problem remains unresolved. Thus, case selection in the palliation of these patients with inoperable pancreatic cancer is important. Most would agree that fit patients in whom life expectancy is considered to extend over several months are better managed by open surgical bypass as their quality of life is undoubtedly better by this treatment [8]. Furthermore, in those patients with coincident symptoms due to duodenal obstruction, the case for open surgical bilioenteric bypass and gastrojejunostomy is beyond argument. A minority surgeons limit endoscopic stenting to patients with metastatic disease [9]. Laparoscopic bilioenteric bypass [10–13] has to be seen against this background, since although technically demanding, it carries all the benefits of open surgery without the morbidity associated with laparotomy and, in addition, it avoids the complications of stent insertion.

Indications

Laparoscopic bilioenteric bypass is indicated in all patients with proven inoperable pancreatic cancer. It may be conducted during the same session as the laparoscopic staging (see p. 172) if the disease is demonstrated to be incurable (presence of hepatic or peritoneal metastases, invasion of portal vein) and the diagnosis is confirmed histologically by frozen section. If the latter is equivocal, it is wise to postpone the procedure until confirmation of the histology of the primary or the secondary lesions from fixed paraffin sections has been obtained.

Preoperative Work-up and Preparation

The preoperative work-up includes liver function tests, ultrasonography, CT scanning and ERCP. At this stage, the patient is prepared for laparoscopic assessment of operability with biopsy confirmation and, preferably, bilioenteric bypass in the one session. The clotting disorder manifested by a prolonged prothrombin time caused by malabsorption of vitamin K due to the cholestasis is corrected by the intramuscular injection of vitamin K analogues. Prophylaxis is also needed for the prevention of renal failure, which is common after surgery in these patients. This consists of adequate hydration with intravenous crystalloids, catheterization of the urinary bladder to measure hourly urine output and the administration of an osmotic (mannitol) or loop diuretic (frusemide) with induction of anaesthesia. As jaundiced patients are particularly susceptible to infection, antibiotic prophylaxis, usually with a third-generation cephalosporin, is also administered at the time of induction of anaesthesia, with a second dose 12–24 h later.

Anaesthesia

Laparoscopic staging and bilioenteric bypass are performed under general anaesthesia with endotracheal intubation. The exact details and premedication vary with the practice of the anaesthetist. A size 16 F Salem sump nasogastric tube is inserted and positioned in the distal antrum of the stomach. It is kept under continuous low suction to ensure deflation of the duodenal bulb and stomach during the procedure. An accurate check of the urinary output is kept throughout the operation and the urinary catheter left in situ after the procedure has been completed. Further doses of mannitol or frusemide may be needed postoperatively to maintain the urinary output above 30 ml/h.

Patient Positioning and Skin Preparation

The patient is operated upon in the supine position with a slight (15°) head-up tilt. The skin of the abdomen is prepared with medicated soap and then disinfected with antiseptic. The area prepared in this fashion extends from the nipple line to the suprapubic region. Draping is such as to leave exposed the upper three quarters of the abdomen.

Layout of Ancillary Instruments and Positioning of Staff

The layout of the ancillary instruments, the positioning of staff are outlined in Fig. 9.1. The surgeon operates from the left side. If an adjusting camera holder is used (Martin's arm or vacuum lock device), this is mounted on the left side of the operating table. Otherwise, the camera person stands on the same side as the surgeon. The first assistant and the scrub nurse stand on the opposite site facing the surgeon. The instrument trolley is situated beyond and behind the scrub nurse. The insufflator, light and camera unit, electrosurgical generator and suction irrigation system are arranged in a stack behind the surgeon. A dual monitor display is essential.

Details of Specific Instruments and Consumables for the Procedure

In addition to the basic set of laparoscopic instruments, the following are required:

1. 10 mm 30° forward oblique telescope
2. Pair of needle holders
3. Rubber shod suture holder
4. Abdominal wall/round ligament lift device
5. Dipping endoretractor (for choledochojejunostomy)
6. Reducing tube

The following consumables are needed:

1. Atraumatic endoski laparoscopic sutures
2. EndoGIA (USSC, Norwalk, USA).

The selection of good quality ergonomic needle drivers is essential. The author's preference is for spring-loaded tapered instruments which have flat rough diamond surfaces on their jaws without any serrations (Fig. 9.2). Needle drivers of any description which have serrated jaws cause damage and fraying of the suture. The rubber-shod suture holder (Fig. 9.3) is used by the first assistant to keep uni-

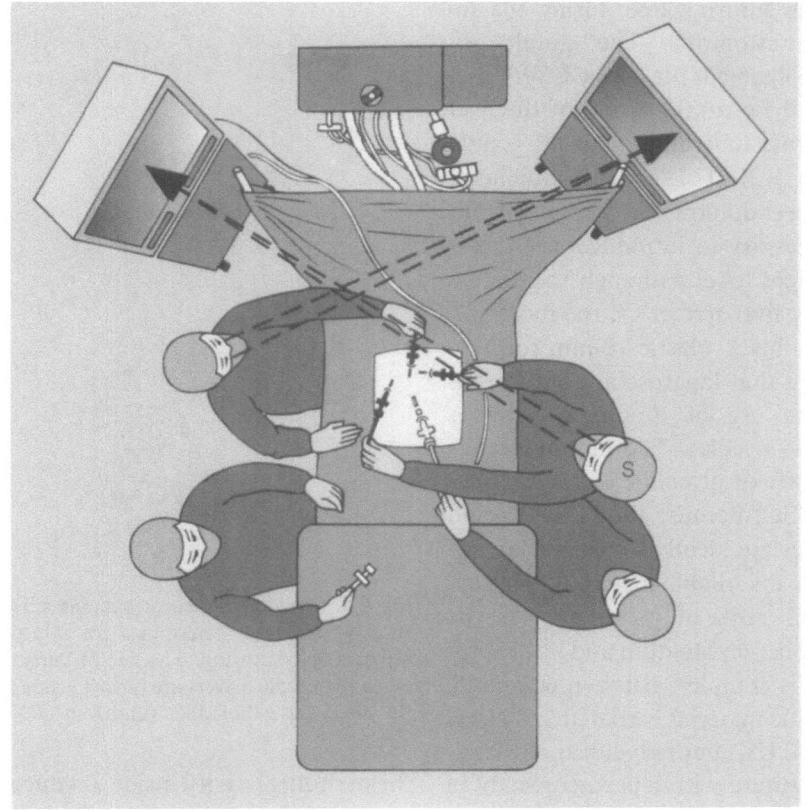

9.1

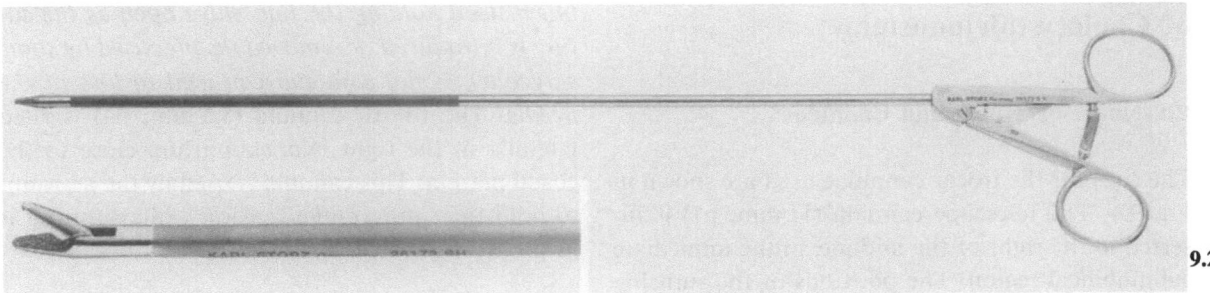

9.2

Fig. 9.1. Layout of ancillary instruments and positioning of staff

Fig. 9.2. Tapered spring-loaded needle holders (drivers) with flat (nonserrated) diamond surfaces on their jaws (Storz, Tuttlingen, Germany)

Fig. 9.3. Rubber shod suture holder (Storz)

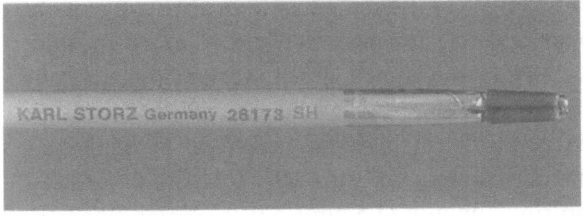

9.3

form tension on the suturing line during the fashioning of the anastomosis. The simple abdominal wall/round ligament lift device is very useful for elevation of the central portion of the liver including the quadrate lobe and enhances greatly the operative field [12]. For choledochojejunostomy, if the dipping endoretractor is not available, an extra port is necessary to introduce a retractor needed to lift the right lobe. Although there are a variety of expanding liver retractors, the most useful and safest is the black plastic 10-mm rod.

There is no doubt that laparoscopic suturing is made easier by the use of atraumatic sutures mounted on endoski needles. The author prefers 3/0 synthetic polyester of glycolide and lactide sutures (Polysorb; USSC) because the handling and knotting charactistics are ideally suited for laparoscopic suturing with absorbable materials. This suture material retains 50% of its original tensile strength at 2 weeks postimplanation and its absorption (by hydrolysis) is complete between 60 and 90 days. Another suitable material is coated 3/0 vicryl (Ethicon, Edinburgh, UK) but polydioxanone is extremely difficult to suture with laparoscopically in view of its high memory and spring-like qualities.

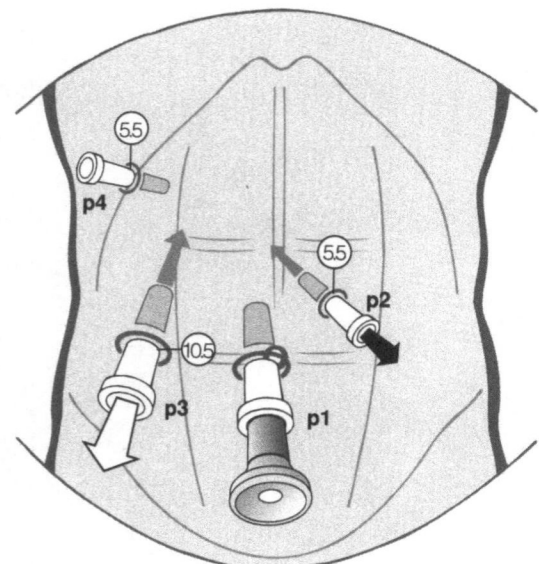

Fig. 9.4. Sites for the trocar/cannulae. The positions of the suturing cannulae determines the ease or difficulty of the laparoscopic suturing. The site of entry must be such that when the needle drivers are placed inside the abdomen, their tips meet the gallbladder fundus at 60°–90° (p2, p3)

Operative Steps of Cholecystojejunostomy

Placement of Trocar and Cannulae

The sites for the trocar cannulae used are shown in Fig. 9.4. The telescope cannula (11 mm; p1) is inserted to the right of the midline, in the immediate subumbilical region. The positions of the suturing cannulae are crucial as this is the most important factor in determining the ease or difficulty of the laparoscopic suturing. The site of entry must be away from the right hypochondrium (p2, p3) and the position is such that when the needle drivers are placed inside the abdomen, their tips meet the gall bladder fundus at 60°–90° (Fig. 9.4). The left suturing cannula (5.5 mm; p2) is placed along the linea semilunaris well down at umbilical level, the right (11 mm; p3) in the equivalent ipsilateral position. A large suturing cannula on the right side ensures safe insertion and removal of the suture from

the peritoneal cavity inside a reducer tube. A reducer tube should be used for this purpose with both disposable and nondisposable cannulae as it prevents entanglement of the suture or needle by the valve of the cannula. *Not using the reducer tube, but instead holding the flap valve open as the suture is introduced or removed (as practised by some surgeons), is not safe and can lead to loss of the needle.* The fourth cannula (5.5 mm; p4) is sited laterally in the right hypochondrium close to the costal margin. This cannula is used by the assistant to hold the suture under tension while suturing is in progress.

Laparoscopic Staging and Cholangiography

The laparoscopic staging of pancreatic cancer has three components: detection of hepatic and peritoneal spread, inspection of the tumour and biopsy for histological confirmation (Chap. 13). Any free fluid is aspirated in a suction trap and subjected to cytological examination. The local assessment of the tumour and visualization of the pancreas is carried out in an orderly fashion. Particular attention is paid to duodenal involvement as this necessitates

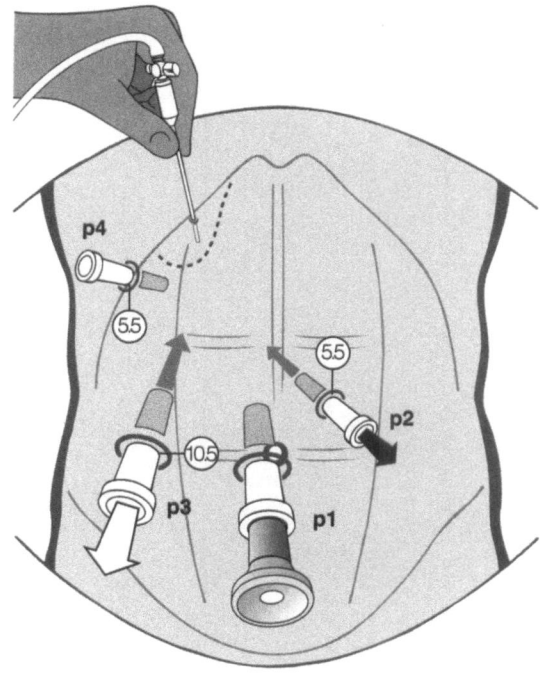

Fig. 9.5. Percutaneous introduction of Verres needle attached to a suction line into the fundus of the gallbladder

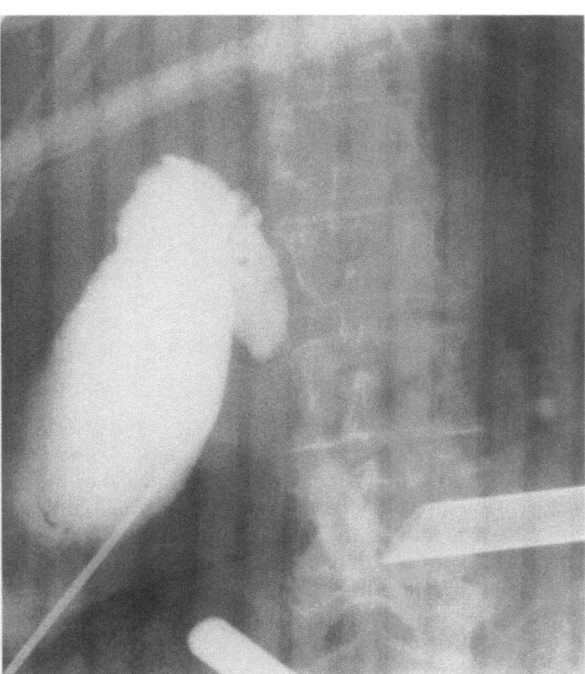

Fig. 9.6. Cholecystocholangiogram showing that the cystic duct insertion into the common bile duct is clear of the upper limit of the tumour

a gastrojejunostomy in addition ot the bilioenteric bypass. Duodenal involvement is assessed by lifting the anterior wall with an atraumatic forceps.

Having established inoperability, the next step consists in performing a cholecystocholangiogram to determine whether the cystic duct is patent and that its insertion has not been invaded by the tumour. A Veress needle attached to a suction line is introduced percutaneously into the fundus of the gallbladder (Fig. 9.5). After aspiration of bile, some of which is sent for culture, 50−70 ml 20% sodium diatrizoate is injected to obtain a cholecystocholangiogram. Cholecystojejunostomy is indicated only if the cystic duct is patent and its termination into the common bile duct is clear of the upper limit of the tumour by at least 1.5 cm (Fig. 9.6). Otherwise a choledochojejunostomy is performed. On completion of the cholangiogram, the gallbladder contents are aspirated completely before the Veress needle is removed.

Insertion of Abdominal Wall/Round Ligament Lift

The external frame consists of two horizontal struts which are attached by chucks to the rail on either side of the operating table. These support a transverse bar with a sliding hook attachment (Fig. 9.7). When mounted, the frame is covered by sterile drapes. The instrument itself consists of a curved 4-mm metal trocar-point introducer attached to a length of tubing (Fig. 9.8). A small stab wound is made with a pointed scalpel 2.5 cm from the midline, high up near the left costal margin. The exact spot is determined by finger point depression while viewing the anterior abdominal wall and the falciform ligament with the optic. The correct site should be about 2 cm above the lower margin of the liver and just lateral to the falciform fat. Once the curved introducer has penetrated the peritoneal cavity, it is manoeuvred around and below the falciform ligament to reach the anterior abdominal wall on the opposite side. The sharp point of the introducer is then impaled in the anterior abdominal wall at a point equivalent to the entry site and the curved introducer exteriorized through the parieties. As it is withdrawn completely, the curved introducer trails behind it the tubing which now

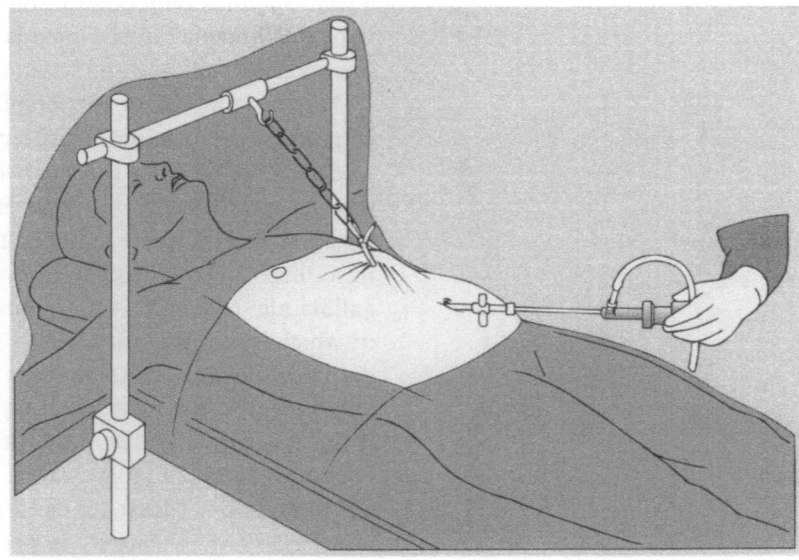

9.7

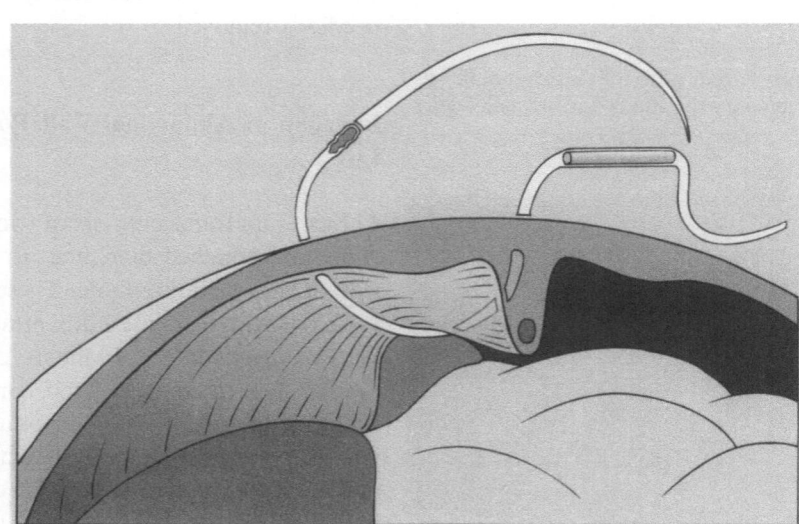

9.8

forms a sling around the central part of the abdominal wall and the falciform-round ligament complex (Fig. 9.9). Following detachment from the introducer, the two ends of the tube are tied and the loop thus formed engaged in the hook and chain assembly. The abdominal wall is then lifted and the appropriate loop of the chain affixed to the hook on the horizontal bar of the frame (Fig. 9.7). The resulting lift by pulling the abdominal wall and round ligament together elevates the central portion of the liver and the quadrate lobe (Fig. 9.10).

Fig. 9.7. External frame mounted at the head end of the operating table used for the abdominal wall/round ligament lift. The two ends of the tube are tied and the loop thus formed engaged in the hook and chain assembly. The abdominal wall is then lifted and the appropriate loop of the chain affixed to the hook on the horizontal bar of the frame

Fig. 9.8. Abdominal wall lift device. This consists of a curved 4 mm metal trocar point introducer attached to a length of tubing

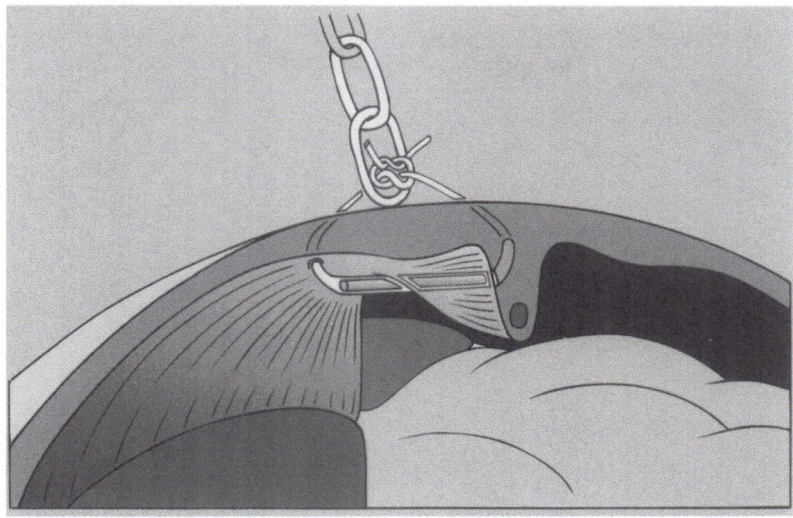

9.9

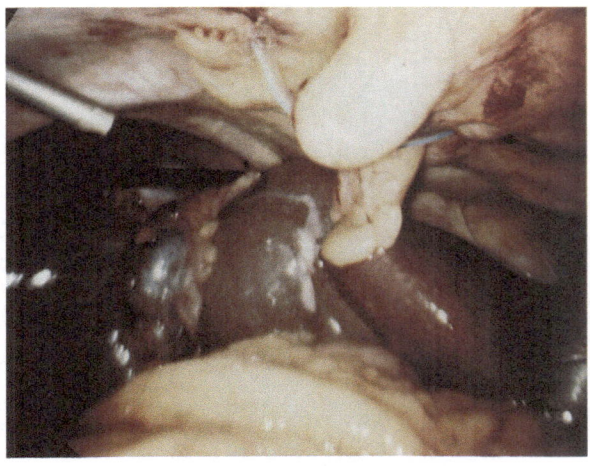

Fig. 9.10. The resulting lift by pulling the abdominal wall and round ligament together elevating the central portion of the liver and the quadrate lobe

Fig. 9.9. The tubing now forms a sling around the central part of the abdominal wall and the falciform-round ligament complex

bladder to ensure sufficient reach such that a tension-free anastomosis can be formed between the two organs (Fig. 9.11). If the patient also requires a gastroenterostomy because of duodenal involvement, the selected loop should be at least 15 cm longer.

Selection of Jejunal Loop

A loop of jejunum some 50 cm from the ligament of Treitz is selected for anastomosis to the gallbladder. To achieve this, the left part of the transverse colon and mesocolon are elevated to reveal the upper jejunum, which is then traced upwards by two graspers until the ligament of Treitz and the duodenojejunal junction are identified. A floppy loop some 40 cm in length is selected and its apex grasped and brought up antecolically to the gall-

Hand-Sutured Anastomosis

The method used for hand-sutured anastomosis consists of a single-layer, deep seromuscular, continuous suturing technique using two sutures — one each for the posterior and anterior walls of the anastomosis. This technique, which was first evaluated in an animal model [10], is safe and is now routinely employed at our institution [11]. The principles governing endoscopic suturing are outlined in Vol. 1. A starter loop knot (Dundee jamming loop knot, see Vol. 1, Chap. 7) can be fashioned externally or a standard microsurgical surgeon's knot formed and tied internally to start the anastomosis. If a preformed jamming loop knot is intended, the length of the suture must be 30 cm as the knot requires 10 cm of length from the tail in order to fashion and draw easily. If an internal sur-

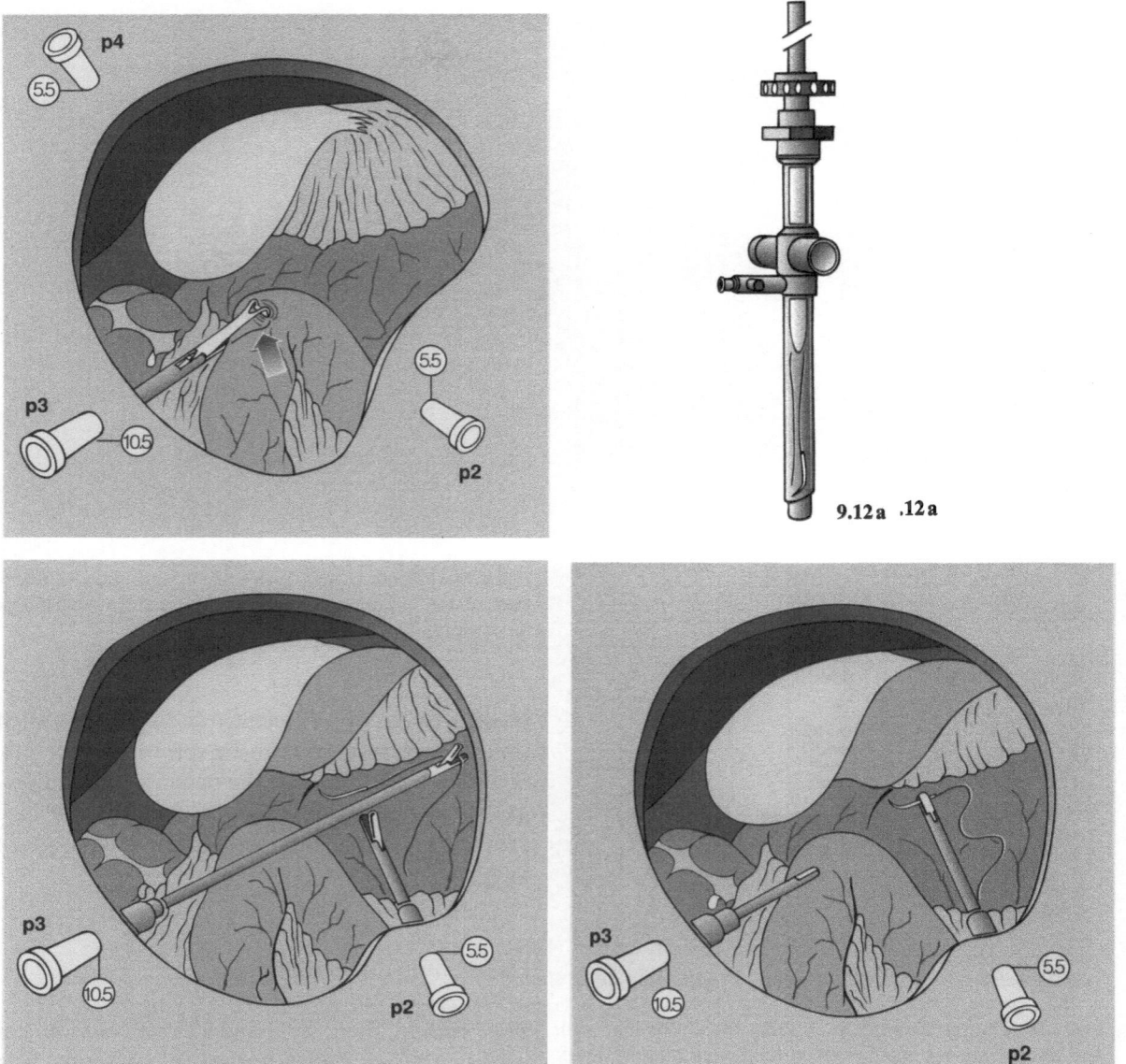

9.11

9.12a

9.12b

9.12c

Fig. 9.11. An upper jejunal loop, some 40 cm in length, is selected and its apex grasped and brought up antecolically to the gallbladder to ensure sufficient reach to enable the performance of a tension-free anastomosis between the two organs

Fig. 9.12a–c. Safe technique for introducing the atraumatic suture with needle inside the peritoneal cavity. Inserting one of the needle holders inside the reducer tube, withdrawing the needle holder and pulling the needle and suture inside the reducer tube (**a**), placing the suture on the anterior surface of the stomach by the left needle holder (**b**), and then grasping the endoski needle by the right needle holder on the distal part of the straight section (**c**)

geon's starter knot is preferred, the length of the suture should be 18–20 cm. One of the needle holders is inserted inside the reducer tube and grasps the suture half way along itws length. The needle holder is then withdrawn, pulling the needle and suture inside the reducer tube (Fig. 9.12a). The loaded reducer tube and needle holder are inserted down the right 10.5-mm suturing cannula and the suture placed on the anterior surface of the stomach by the left needle holder (Fig. 9.12b). The endoski needle is then grasped by the needle holder

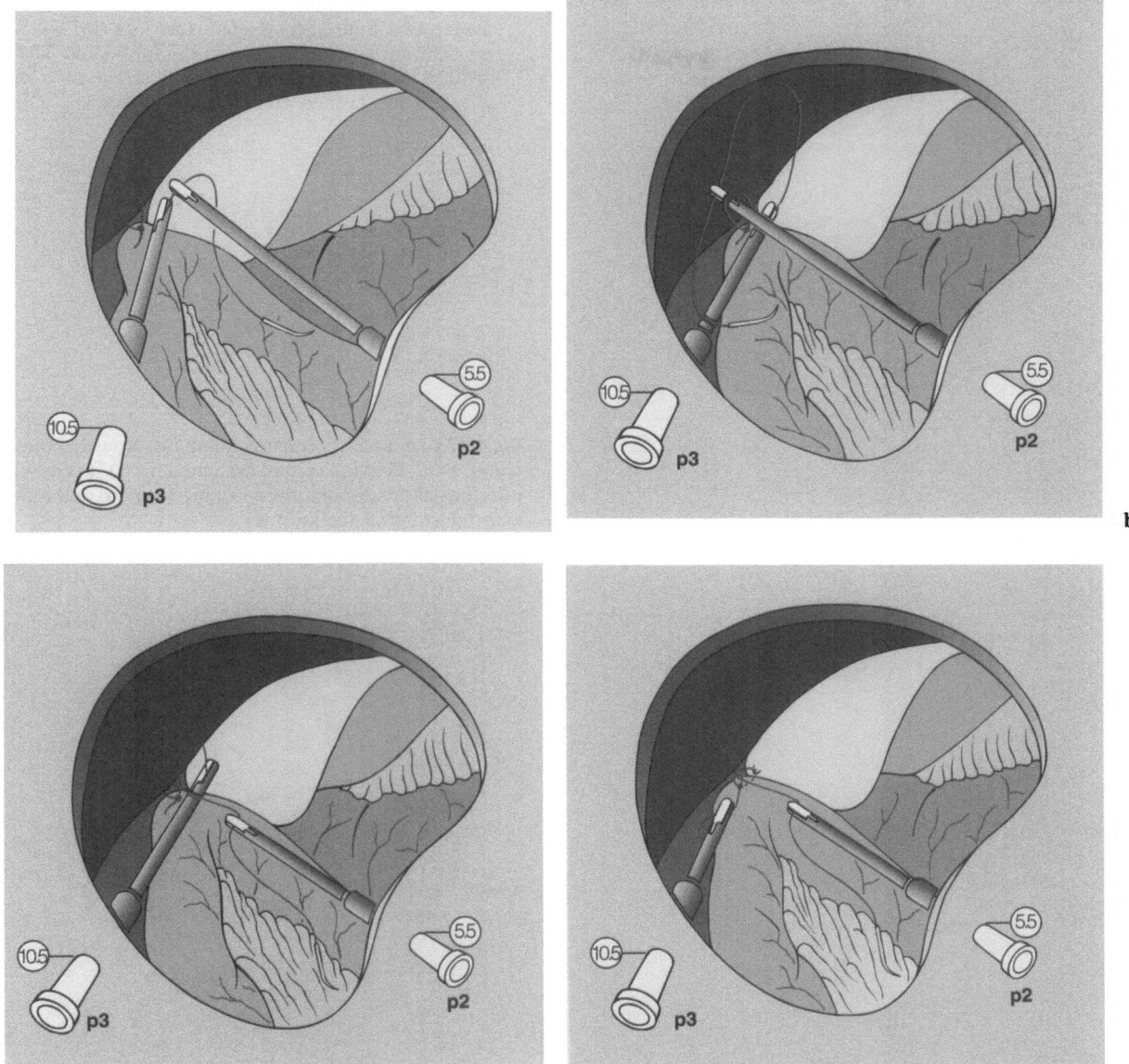

on the distal part of the straight section (Fig. 9.12c).

Posterior Suture Line with Jamming Loop Starter Knot. After passage through the seromuscular layer of the jejunum and the gallbladder, the suture is pulled until the jamming loop knot impinges on the jejunum. The two organs are approximated with further traction on the suture (Fig. 9.13a), and while tension is maintained on the suture, the right needle driver is passed through the loop

Fig. 9.13a–d. Starter Dundee jamming loop knot for commencement of the posterior continuous suture line. Approximating the two organs with further traction on the suture (**a**), passing the right needle driver through the loop to grasp the standing part of the suture (**b**), pulling it through the jamming loop (**c**), and then slipping (closing) the loop on the suture and locking the knot (**d**)

(Fig. 9.13b) and used to grasp the standing part of the suture, which is then pulled through the jamming loop (Fig. 9.13c). The loop is then slipped (closed) on the suture from the tail and the knot

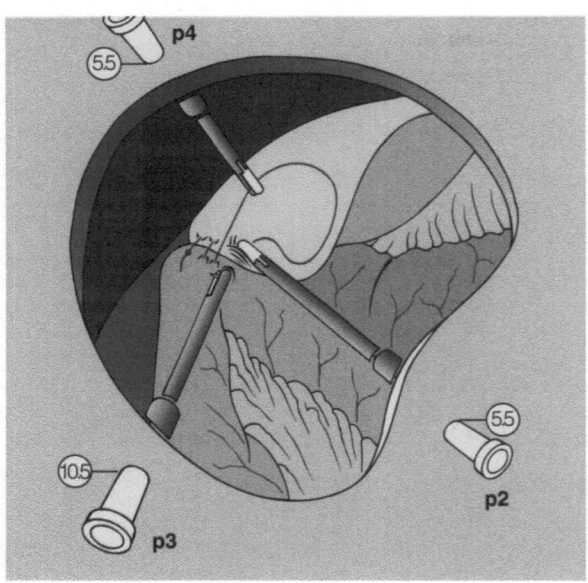

9.14

◄ Fig. 9.14. Continuous posterior seromuscular approximation over a distance of 3 cm is next carried out with the assistant holding tension on the suture line. The individual suture bites have to be inserted in a deep seromuscular fashion and be evenly spaced

Fig. 9.15 a – e. End of posterior suture line by use of the Aberdeen knot. First (**a**), second (**b**), and third (**c**) locking loop, inserting suture through third locking loop, (**d**) and locking and tightening of the knot (**e**) ►

▼

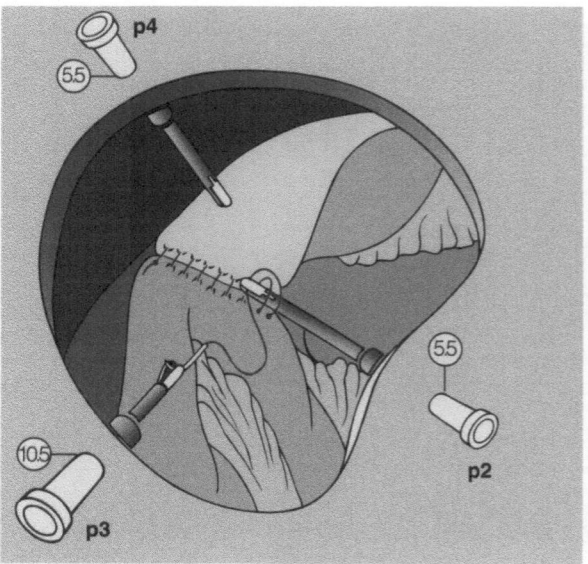

9.15 a

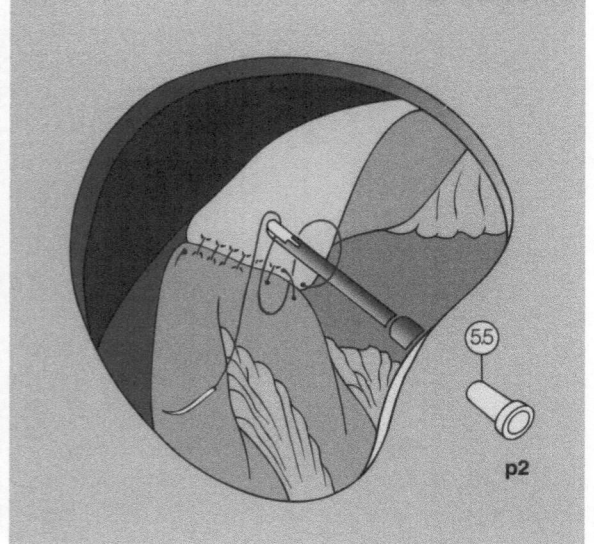

b

locked by pulling first the suture and then the tail against countertraction on the knot by the open jaws of the needle holder (Fig. 9.13d). A continuous posterior seromuscular approximation over a distance of 3 – 4 cm is next carried out with the assistant holding tension on the suture line (Fig. 9.14). The suturing technique involves use of the right needle holder as the active driver, with the left needle holder being used to apply countertraction on the tissue to facilitate needle passage and to pick up the needle after it emerges through the tis-

sues before transfer to the active needle holder. The individual suture bites have to be inserted in a deep seromuscular fashion and be evenly spaced. The last but one suture bite is locked and following a further passage of the needle through the two organs, the suture is tied using the Aberdeen knot (Fig. 9.15a–e). Once the posterior suture line is completed, the needle in left attached to the suture in case the anterior suture is too short or breaks during the performance of the final part of the anastomosis.

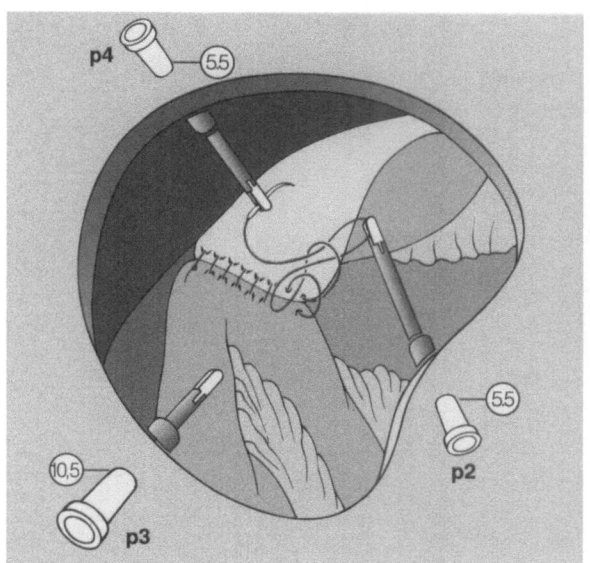

9.15 c

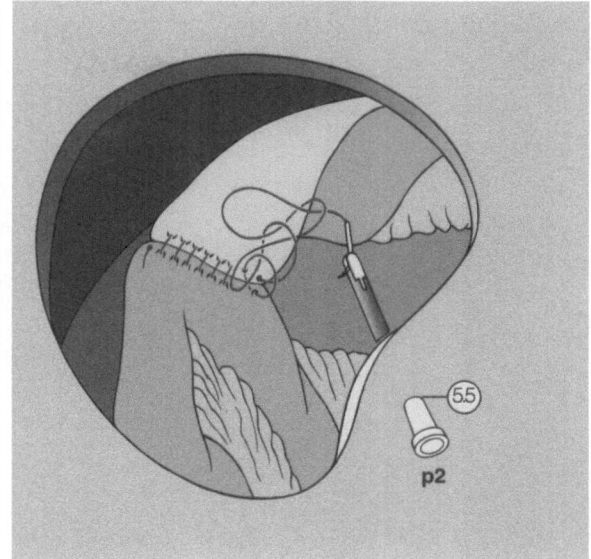

d

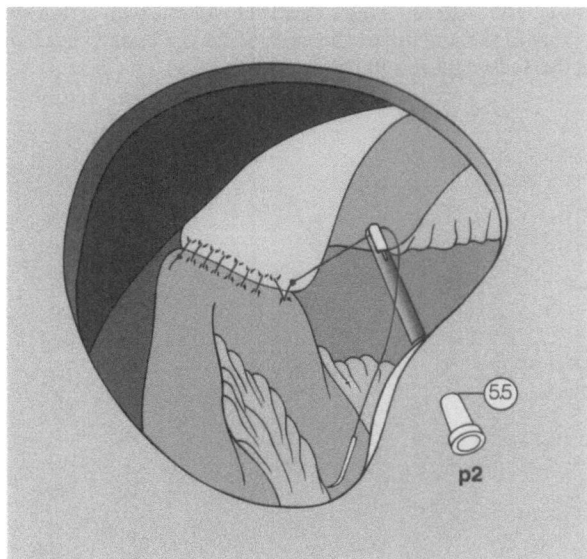

e

Posterior Suture Line With Starter Surgeon's Knot. In this situation, the apex of the jejunal loop is grasped by the assistant using an atraumatic Babcock's type forceps held in approximation to the gallbaldder while the surgeon passes the endoski needle through the seromuscular coats of the two organs and ties the microsurgical knot (double hitch followed by two single hitches). The principles underlining internal knotting are outlined in Vol. 1, Chap. 7. The suturing of the posterior layer is then conducted using the technique outlined above.

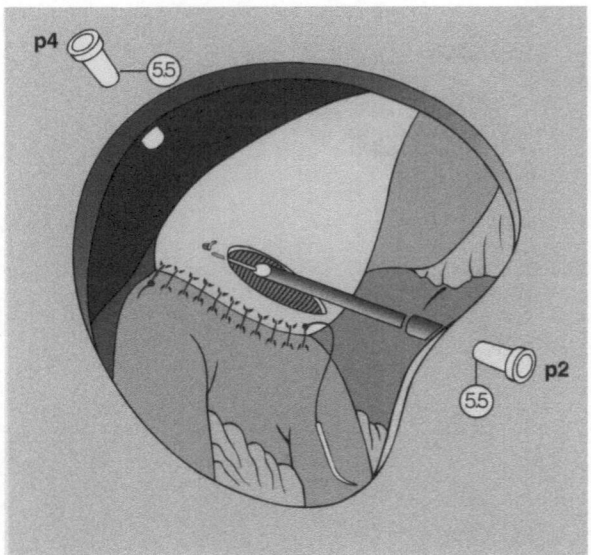

Fig. 9.16. Incising the seromuscular layer of the gallbladder

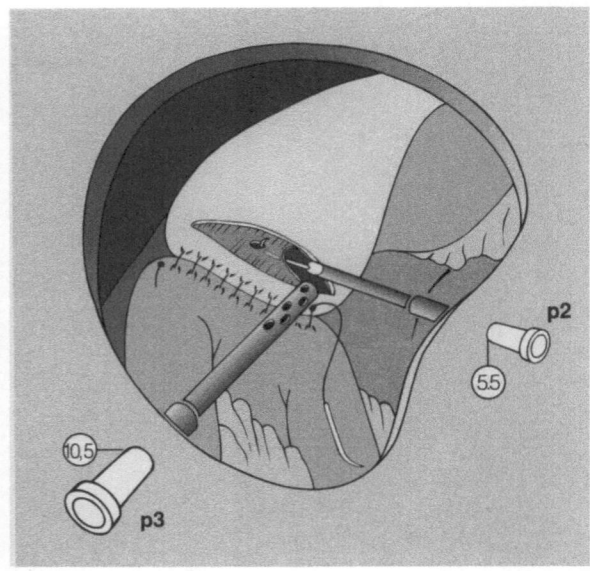

Fig. 9.17. After making a small cut with the twin action scissors in the mucosa of the gallbladder the hook is used and the sucker tip introduced

Opening of the Gallbladder and Enterotomy. The seromuscular layer of the gallbladder is then incised over a distance of 3.0 cm with the electrosurgical hook knife, using a blender monopolar current, 0.5 cm anterior and parallel to the completed posterior suture line (Fig. 9.16). With the sucker in place, a small cut is made with the twin action scissors in the mucosa, the sucker tip introduced into the gallbladder lumen and the bile aspirated (Fig. 9.17). The mucosal cut is then extended and the interior wall of the gallbladder inspected and irrigated thoroughly with Hartmann's solution to ensure removal of all debris and blood clots (Fig. 9.18). Any bleeding from the cut gallbladder wall has to be arrested by soft electrocoagulation. The enterotomy is fashioned to an equivalent length using the same technique, but the intraluminal irrigation step is avoided. With the jejunum attached to the gallbladder, which keeps it tented high up, leakage from the enterotomy does not occur.

Suturing of the Anterior Wall of the Anastomosis. The approximation of the anterior wall of the anastomosis is performed using a similar technique. Again, either a preformed starter jamming loop knot can be used or the anterior part of the anasto-

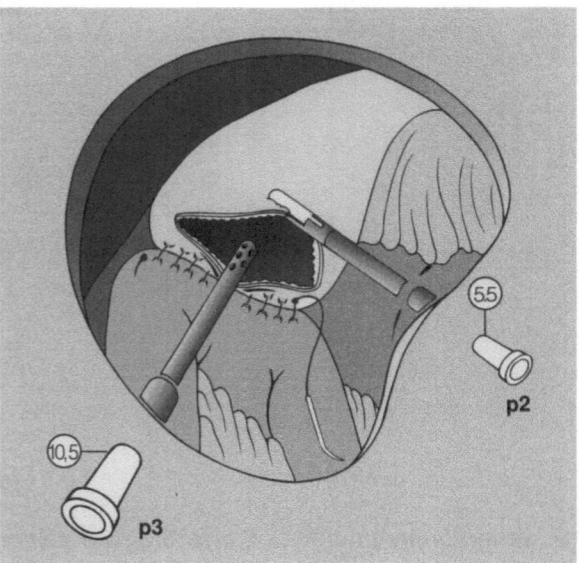

Fig. 9.18. Extending the mucosal cut, inspecting the interior wall of the gallbladder and irrigating it thoroughly with Hartmann's solution to ensure removal of all debris and blood clots

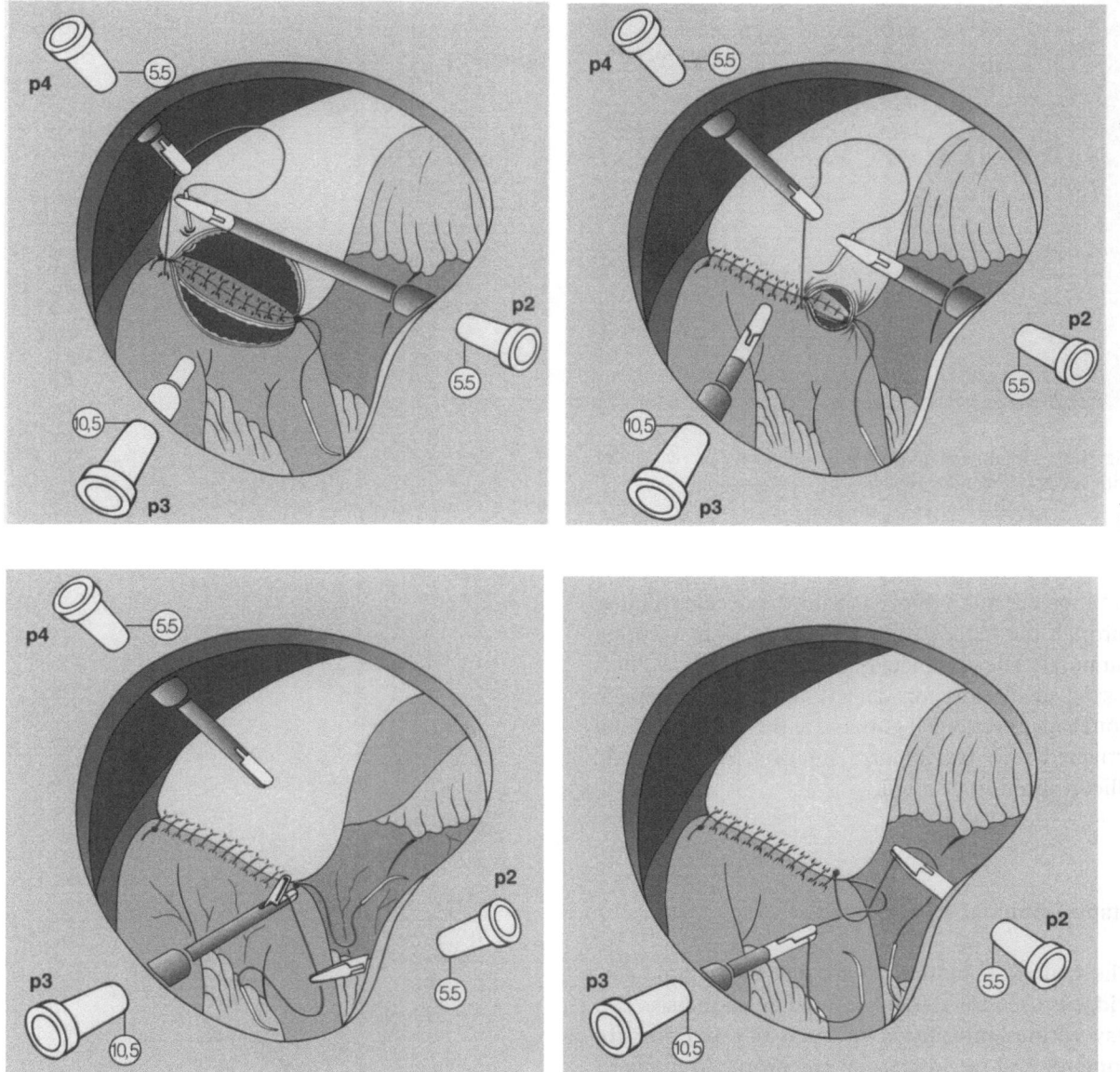

mosis is commenced with a surgeon's knot tied internally. In either event, the anterior suturing should be started close to but lateral to the extremity of the posterior suture line (Fig. 9.19a). Once the end of the anterior approximation has been reached (Fig. 9.19b), the needle is cut and removed. After adjusting the tension on the suture line (Fig. 9.19c), the anterior suture is tied to the tail of the posterior one using a standard microsurgical knot (Fig. 9.19d). The excess suture material beyond the knot together with the posterior needle

Fig. 9.19a–d. Approximation of the anterior walls of the anastomosis by continuous suturing. Approximating the anterior walls of the cholecystojejunostomy lateral to the extremity of the posterior suture line (**a**) and continously suturing to the opposite corner (**b**), adjusting the tension on the suture line (**c**) and tying the anterior suture to the tail of the posterior one using a standard microsurgical knot (**d**)

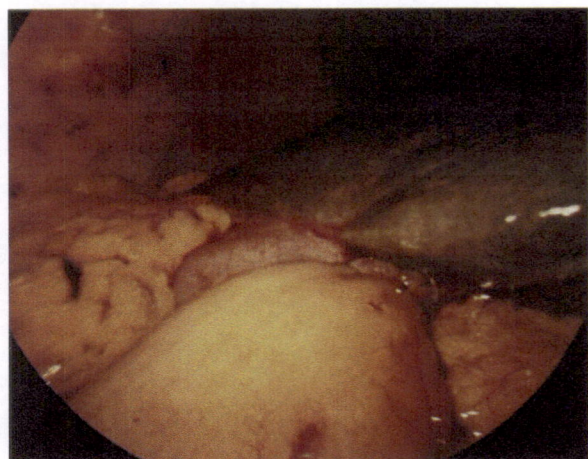

Fig. 9.20. Completed cholecystojejunostomy in a patient with advanced pancreatic cancer

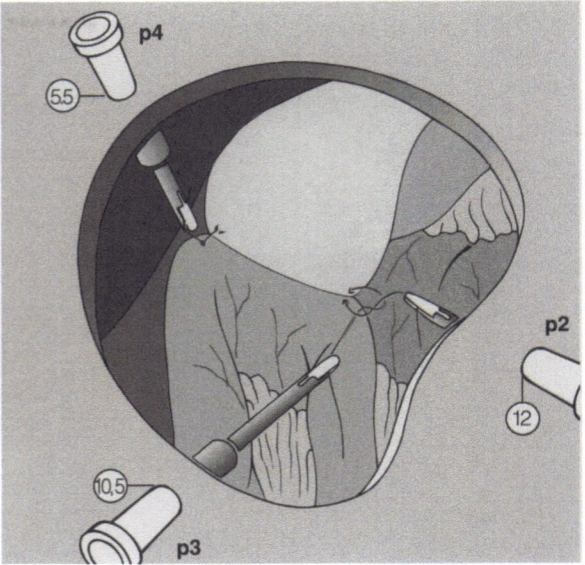

9.21

are then cut and removed (with the needle trailing) through the reducer tube (inside the right suturing cannula). The completed anastomosis (Fig. 9.20) is inspected closely for defects and the subhepatic pouch and peritoneal gutters are then aspirated and irrigated with Hartmann's solution. A subhepatic silicon drain is inserted.

Stapled-Sutured Anastomosis

The endoGIA mounted with the blue staple cartridge is used for stapled-sutured anastomosis. Two stay sutures introduced through the anterior abdominal wall are inserted at the proposed limits of the anastomosis between the two organs (Fig. 9.21). A small opening sufficient to admit the limbs of the stapler is then made on each organ at the right end of the approximated organs (Fig. 9.22). The endoGIA is introduced through the right suturing cannula (which has to be 12.5 cm) and the stapler limbs separated (Fig. 9.23 a). As the approximated organs are held stretched by pulling the right stay suture to the right, the two limbs of the stapler are introduced through the previously formed openings in the gallbladder and jejunum as far as the hilt of the instrument (Fig. 9.23 b). The stapler limbs are then tilted upwards (Fig. 9.23 b) before being approximated. A careful inspection is undertaken to

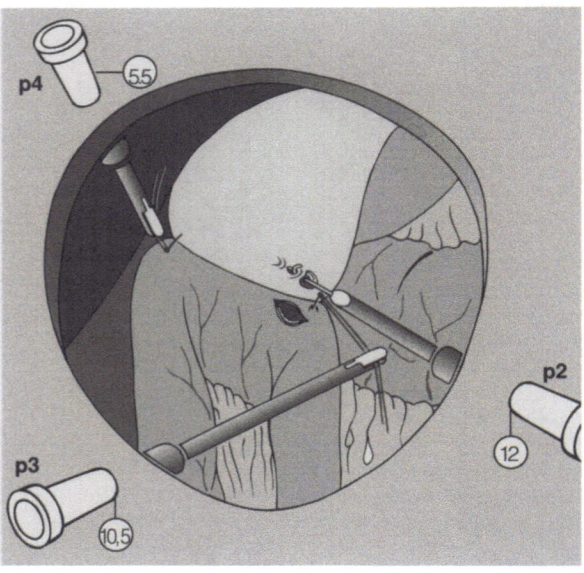

9.22

Fig. 9.21. Insertion of stay sutures prior to use of EndoGIA

Fig. 9.22. A small opening sufficient to admit the limbs of the stapler is made on each organ at their right extremity

ensure that no extraneous tissue has been caught between the two stapler limbs and that the line of the proposed anastomosis is correct. Once this is established, the instrument is fired, disengaged and removed. The stapled anastomosis is inspected

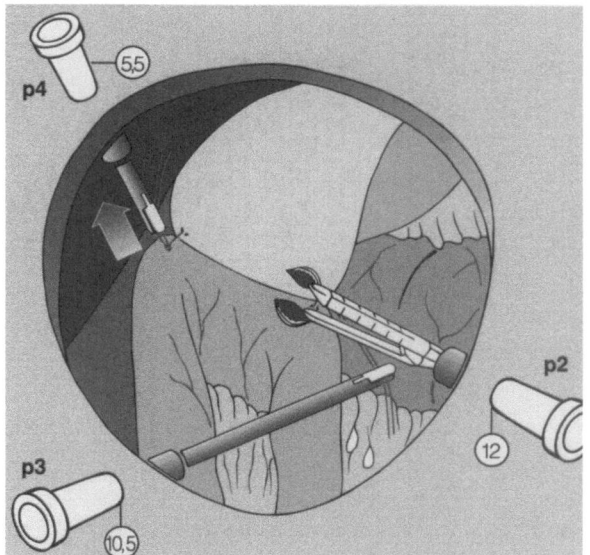

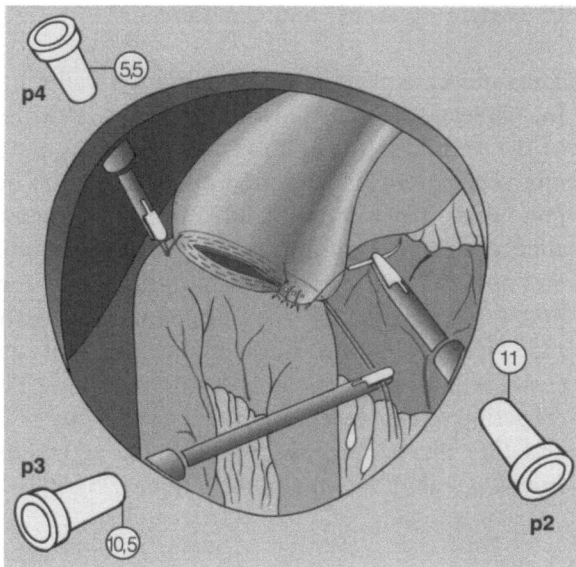

Fig. 9.24. Closing the anterior defect with a running suture with Polysorb as described above

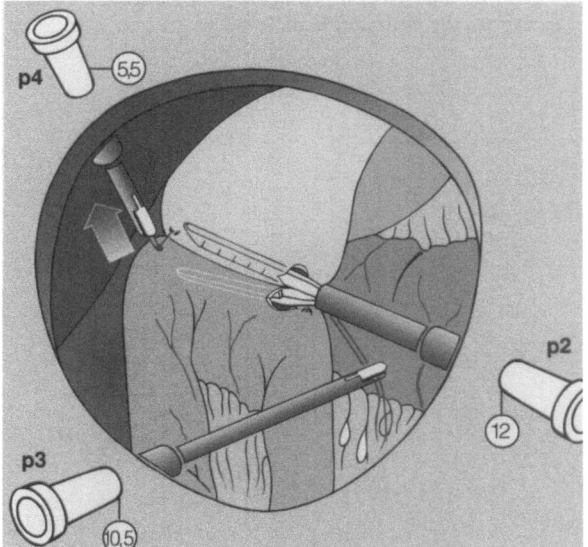

Fig. 9.23 a, b. Steps in the creation of the stapled cholecystojejunostomy. Opening the stapler limbs close to the openings in the gallbladder and jejunum (**a**), introducing the two limbs of the stapler into the gallbladder and jejunum as far as the hilt of the instrument and then tilting the stapler limbs upwards (**b**)

Operative Steps of Choledochojejunostomy

Choledochojejunostomy can only be performed by suturing and requires considerable experience in laparoscopic biliary surgery as it is undoubtedly more difficult than cholecystojejunostomy. It should only be attempted if a 2.5-cm section of the common hepatic/upper common bile duct is clearly visible between the hepatic parenchyma and the upper limit of the tumour mass. Choledochojejunostomy is contraindicated if there is evidence of portal hypertension caused by tumour involvement of the portal vein. This should be suspected if the hepatoportal pedicle is surrounded by large vessels and is best confirmed by use of laparoscopic ultrasound examination using the Aloka (Aloka, Japan) or Laparoscan systems (EndoMedix, Irvine, USA). These patients should be managed either by open surgical segment 3 bypass or by endoscopic stenting.

from the inside to establish its integrity and the absence of any tissue bridges. The anterior defect is closed with a running suture with Polysorb as described above (Fig. 9.24).

Placement of Trocar and Cannulae

The same cannulae sites and abdominal wall lift as for cholecystojejunostomy are used but retraction of the right lobe and gallbladder is essential to obtain exposure of the proximal dilated common hepatic duct. This is best achieved using the dipping endoretractor, which houses the 30° forward oblique optic. If this is not available, an extra 11-mm port is used for the insertion of a retracting plastic rod. This is positioned in the immediate right subcostal region along the anterior axillary line. The retracting rod is placed across the gallbladder neck and lifts this organ together with the right lobe from the common hepatic duct (Fig. 9.25).

Layout of Ancillary Equipment and Positioning of Staff

The surgeon operates from the left side of the patient and the disposition of the staff and layout of the ancillary equipment is identical to that used in cholecystojejunostomy. Good illumination and expert camera work are essential.

Procedure

The selected loop is held in an atraumatic Babcock forceps by the assistant. A 1.5-cm opening is made on its antimesenteric border using the cutting electrosurgical current (Fig. 9.26). It is important that bleeding from the cut edges of the enterotomy is controlled by electrocoagulation as a dry field is essential for creation of the anastomosis. As the common hepatic and upper common bile ducts are enlarged and prominent, dissection is not usually necessary unless there is an anomalous right hepatic artery crossing anterior to the duct. Stay sutures are not inserted. A 1.5-cm transverse or oblique incision is made with a retractable knife or curved microscissors on the anterior wall of the duct, midway between the hepatic parenchyma and the upper limit of the tumour mass (Fig. 9.27). Initially, the field is flooded and obscured with bile. This is aspirated and a specimen obtained for culture. If bile continues to flow in profuse amounts, a biliary balloon catheter (2-ml ballon) is inserted through the

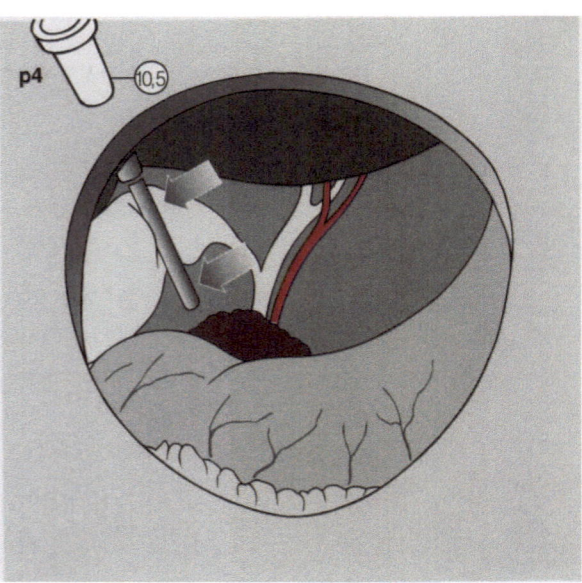

Fig. 9.25. Rod retractor lifting the gallbladder and right lobe to expose the common hepatic duct

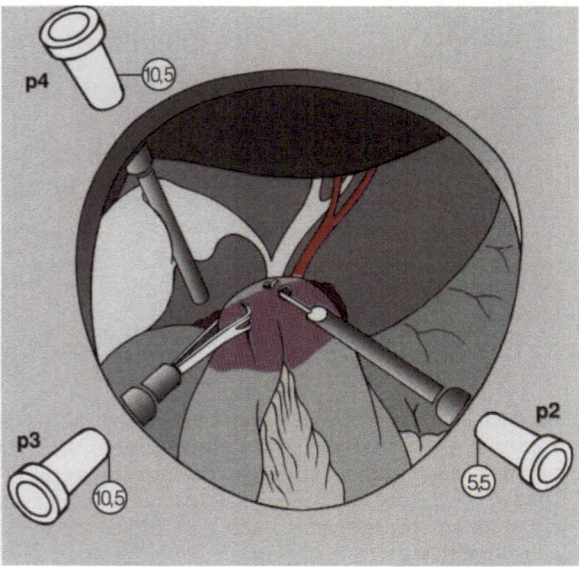

Fig. 9.26. As the selected loop is held by the assistant, a 1.5-cm enterotomy is made on its antimesenteric border

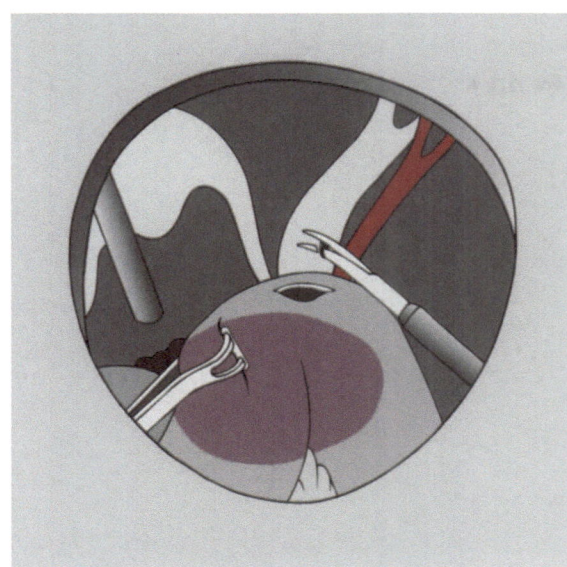

Fig. 9.27. Making 1.5-cm transverse or oblique incision with a retractable knife or curved microscissors on the anterior wall of the duct midway between the hepatic parenchyma and the upper limit of the tumour mass

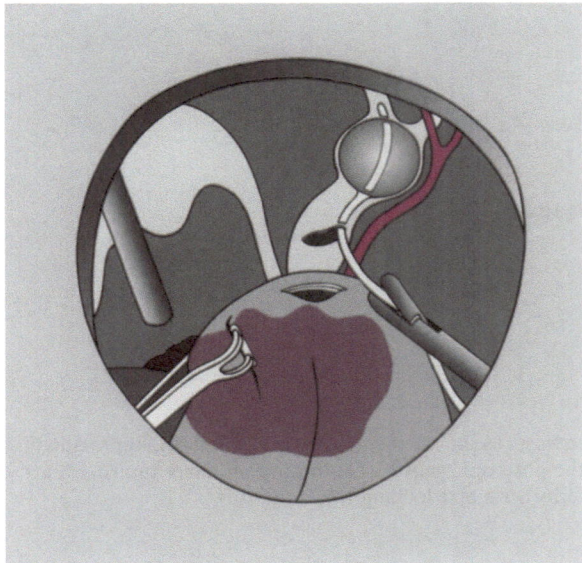

Fig. 9.28. Balloon catheter occlusion of the proximal common hepatic duct

choledochotomy and the balloon inflated with air. This occlusion of the proximal common hepatic duct just below the bifurcation (Fig. 9.28) is maintained until the choledochojejunostomy is nearing completion, at which time the balloon is deflated and the catheter removed.

The suturing is performed with 4/0 Polysorb or coated Vicryl and the technique consists of a single, all-coats layer with continuous or interrupted sutures. We currently prefer a continuous suture for the posterior wall of the anastomosis and interrupted sutures for the anterior approximation.

Posterior Continuous Suture. After passage (inside out) through the right corner of the enterotomy, the needle is reversed and made to enter the bile duct lumen (outside in) at the equivalent point (Fig. 9.29a). A standard internal microsurgeon's knot is used to achieve the approximation of the right end of the posterior wall of the anastomosis (Fig. 9.92b), after which the assistant releases the grasper holding the jejunal loop. Alternatively, a Dundee jamming loop knot is used as a starter knot (Fig. 9.29c). The approximation of the posterior walls of the anastomosis by continuous all coats suturing is conducted (Fig. 9.29d) until the left extremity is reached; then the suture is exteriorised through the bile duct side and locked after passage through the outside left extremity of the anastomosis. The needle is cut leaving a long tail.

Anterior Interrupted Sutures. Four interrupted sutures are used to close the anterior part of the choledochojejunostomy. The sutures are some 4-mm deep and equally spaced. When the first suture is tied, it is held by the assistant on tension; this automatically aligns the anastomosis and facilitates the insertion of the subsequent suture (Fig. 9.30a). This technique is continued until the left extremity of the choledochojejunostomy is reached (Fig. 9.30b). After the last interrupted suture is tied, one of the ends is tied to the tail of the posterior suture.

On completion, the anastomosis is checked for integrity, extravasated bile aspirated and the gutters irrigated by warm Hartmann's solution until clean. A subhepatic silicon drain is left.

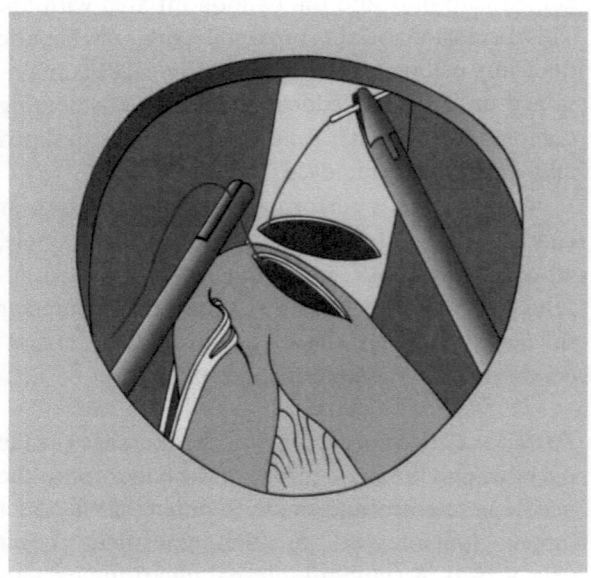

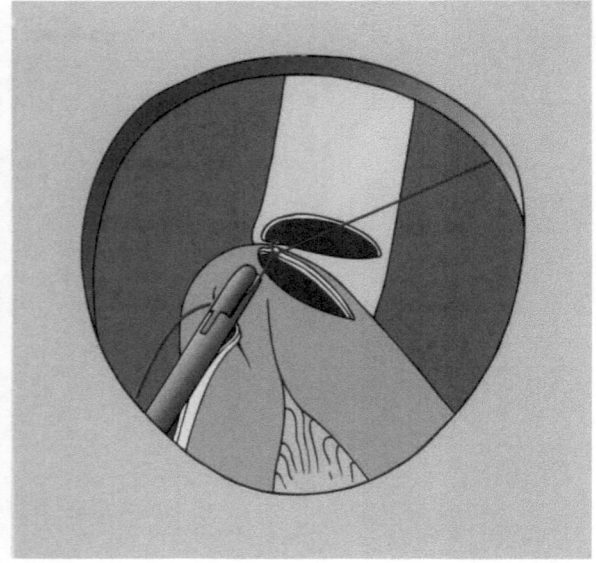

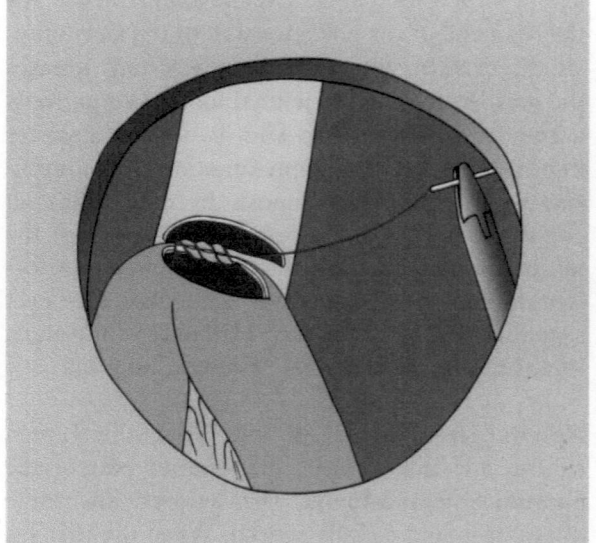

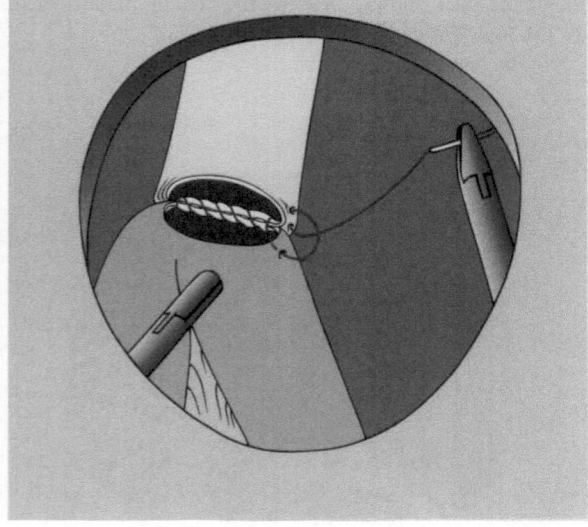

Fig. 9.29 a – d. Suturing of the posterior wall of the anastomosis. Inserting the suture through the right corners of the anastomosis (**a**), approximating the right corner of the anastomosis as the microsurgical knot is tied (**b**), approximating the posterior walls by continuous all coats suturing (**c**), exteriorising and locking the suture (**d**)

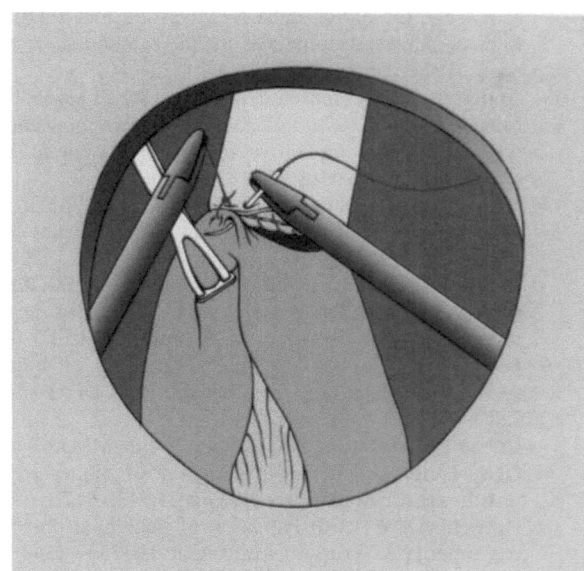

a

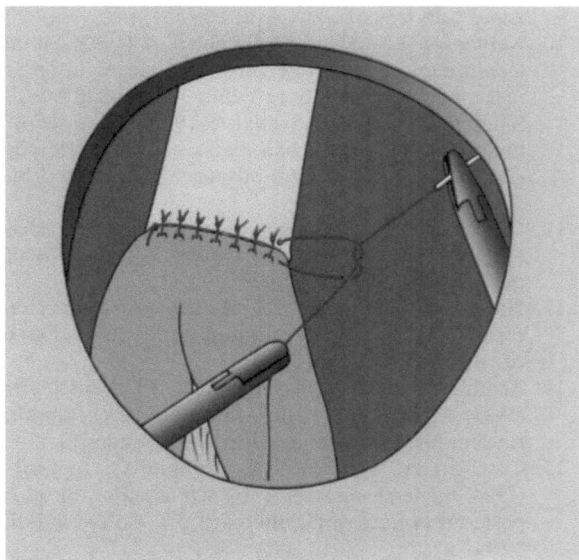

b

Fig. 9.30a, b. Approximation of the anterior walls of the choledochojejunostomy by interrupted sutures. The first suture is tied, held by the assistant on tension (a), completion of anterior interrupted suture line (b)

Gastrojejunostomy

If a double bypass is needed, the bilioenteric bypass (cholecystojejunostomy or choledochojejunostomy) is performed first and the anterior gastrojejunostomy second. In this fashion the first anastomosis results in automatic approximation of the jejunal loop to the anterior wall of the stomach. The selected loop has to be of sufficient length, usually with its apex some 50–60 cm from the ligament of Treitz. The technique of anterior gastroenterostomy is described in Chap. 13.

Postoperative Management

We do not leave a nasogastric tube after completion of the operation. The duration of ileus is short and seldom exceeds 24 h. An intravenous line for infusion of crystalloids is maintained until the patient is fully able to take fluids orally, usually within 72–36 h. A second dose of cephalosporin is administered at 12–24 h. However, if the bile cultuve is positive, a full course of antibiotics is indicated over a period of 5–7 days. In this situation, the choice of antibiotic is dependent on the results of the sensitivity tests. Pain is minimal and analgesic requirements are met by intramuscular opiates, usually during the first 12 h. The function of the bilioenteric anastomosis is confirmed by serial liver function tests. Biliary scintiscanning can also be used for this purpose and is indicated if there is bile leakage from the drain. If progress is satisfactory, discharge from hospital is usually on the day 5–7.

The postoperative period has been uncomplicated in 11 of 12 patients. In our third patient, after an initial fall, the bilirubin level remained elevated. Both a percutaneous transhepatic cholangiogram and a biliary scintiscan confirmed a nonfunctioning anastomosis. At reintervation, an otherwise intact anastomosis was found to be obstructed by a bolus of debris and blood clot. This was aspirated and the incision in the gallbladder closed. The patient made a speedy recovery with complete resolution of the jaundice after this minimal procedure. This patient demonstrates the importance of adequate irrigation of the lumen of the gallbladder and meticulous haemostasis during the creation of laparoscopic bilioenteric bypass.

Clinical Results

Our experience with laparoscopic bilioenteric bypass is limited to 18 patients in whom 19 procedures were attempted. Sixteen patients had cholecystojejunostomy and all but one of these have remained free of jaundice and itching until the time of death (3 to 9 months). Two patients required readmission 5 months later with recurrence of jaundice. At relaparoscopy, occlusion of the anastomosis by metastatic deposits on the gallbladder and small bowel was found. In this patient, a laparoscopic proximal hepaticojejunostomy was attempted but had to be abandoned because of portal bleeding from high pressure varices due to occlusion of the portal vein by the tumour. This was confirmed at open operation. Two patients has had a laparoscopic choledochojejunostomy as the primary palliative procedure because of the proximity of the tumour to the cystic duct. Five patients have received supervoltage radiotherapy and six have required a percutaneous coeliac plexus phenol nerve block for pain. A gastrojejunostomy was required in five. More recently, patients with interactable pain have been treated with bilateral thoracoscopic splanchnicectomy [15].

References

1. Connolly MM, Dawson PJ, Michelassi F, Moossa AR, Lowenstein F (1987) Survival in 1001 patients with cancer of the pancreas. Ann Surg 206:366–373
2. Manabe T, Ohshio G, Baba N, Miyashita T et al (1989) Radical pancreatectomy for ductal carcinoma of the head of the pancreas. Cancer 64:1132–1137
3. Andersen JR, Scorensen SM, Kruse A, Rokkjaer M, Matzen P (1989) Randomized trial of endoscopic endoprostheses versus operative bypass in malignant obstructive jaundice. Gut 30:1132–1135
4. Neuhaus H, Hagenmuller F, Classen M (1989) Self expanding biliary stents: preliminary clinical experience. Endoscopy 21:225–228
5. Gillams A, Dick R, Dooley JS, Wallsten H, El-Din A (1990) Self-expandable stainless steel braided endoprosthesis for biliary strictures. Radiology 174:137–140
6. Leung JWC, Banez VP (1990) Clogging of biliary stents: mechanism and possible solution. Dig Endosc 2:97–105
7. Coene PPLO, Groen AK, Cheng J, Out MMJ, Tytgat GNJ, Huibregste K (1990) Clogging of biliary endoprosthesis: a new perspective. Gut 31:913–917
8. Hatfield ARW (1990) Palliation of malignant obstructive jaundice: surgery or stent? Gut 31:1339–1340
9. Proctor H, Mauro M (1990) Biliary diversion for pancreatic cancer: matching the methods and the patient. Am J Surg 159:67–71
10. Nathanson LK, Shimi S, Cuschieri A (1992) Sutured laparoscopic cholecystojejunostomy evolved in an animal model. J R Coll Surg Edinb 37:215–220
11. Shimi S, Banting S, Cuschieri A (1992) Laparoscopy in the management of pancreatic cancer: endoscopic cholecystojejunostomy for advanced disease. Br J Surg 79:317–319
12. Cuschieri A (1993) Cholécysto-entérostomie per coelioscopique: une alternative au drainage biliare endoscopique. Acta Endosc 23:135–141
13. Hawsali A (1992) Laparoscopic cholecysto-jejunostomy for obstructing pancreatic cancer: technique and report of two cases
14. Banting S, Shimi S, Van der Velpen G, Cuschieri A (1993) Abdominal wall lift: low pressure pneumoperitoneum for laparoscopic surgery. Surg Endosc 7:57–59
15. Cuschieri A, Shimi SM, Crosthwaite G, Joypaul V (1994) Bilateral endoscopic splanchnicectomy through a posterior thoracoscopic approach. J R Coll Surg Edinb 39:44–47

10 Laparoscopic Treatment of Ductal Calculi

A. CUSCHIERI

Introduction

Although stones in the common duct may remain asymptomatic for varying periods or give rise to vague dyspepsia, patients with stones are prone to serious complications which are attended by a significant morbidity and an appreciable mortality. The majority of ductal calculi originate from the gallbladder (cholesterol and black pigment stones) by migration through the cystic duct, but some develop primarily in the common duct. Primary ductal calculi, also known as brown pigment stones, have a soft consistency and are caused by infection (bacterbilia) and obstruction of the bile duct [1].

In surgical practice, ductal calculi are encountered in four different clinical settings: (1) complicated group: obstructive jaundice, cholangitis and acute pancreatitis; (2) subclinical obstructive group: minor elevations of some of the parameters of the liver function tests, particularly elevated levels of alkaline phosphatase, transaminases or ultrasound-detected dilatation of the common duct; (3) unsuspected group: ductal stones discovered by intraoperative cholangiography (IOC) during cholecystectomy in patients with normal results of preoperative liver function tests (Lfts) and biliary ultrasound scanning; (4) Postcholecystectomy group: symptomatic stones after a previous cholecystectomy.

The stones found in the postcholecystectomy group are often ones which have been missed or retained (undetected though present at the time of cholecystectomy), but others may form subsequent to this operation (recurrent). In some patients, it may be difficult to determine whether the postcholecystectomy ductal calculi are retained or recurrent. A cut-off period of 2 years after cholecystectomy was suggested by Schein as a differentiat-

ing criterion between the two groups [2], although evidence for this assumption is lacking.

The unsuspected stone group, which accounts for 2% – 8% of cases, is important because such stones can always be detected by intraoperative cholangiography (IOC) and can be removed at the time of surgery. This, indeed, is one of the benefits of routine IOC during cholecystectomy. There is good evidence that routine preoperative tests (Lfts and ultrasound) do not reliably exclude all ductal calculi. Since the advent of laparoscopic cholecystectomy, there has been a resurgence of the routine use of preoperative infusion intravenous cholangiography to detect ductal calculi and duct anomalies [3] but subsequent experience has failed to confirm the reliability of this investigation [4]. Ductal calculi can only be diagnosed with certainty in the preoperative period by endoscopic retrograde cholangiopancreaticographic study (ERCP) which is indicated in patients with abnormal results of Lfts and ultrasound examination and in patients with a history of acute pancreatitis. However, the routine use of preoperative ERCP in patients undergoing laparoscopic cholecystectomy cannot be justified because of the inevitable increased morbidity [5] and poor yield [6]. The options for management of ductal calculi in patients with symptomatic gallstones are:

(1) Endoscopic sphincterotomy and stone extraction followed by laparoscopic cholecystectomy
(2) Open cholecystectomy and common duct exploration
(3) Laparoscopic cholecystectomy and ductal clearance.

In the author's view, the correct treatment in the individual patient depends on five factors: the clinical setting, the condition of the patient, the calibre of the common bile duct, extent of stone load, the level of local expertise in endoscopic treatment and the experience of the surgeon in laparoscopic biliary surgery.

In patients with retained stones after cholecystectomy, the generally favoured management is endoscopic sphincterotomy, although in patients with an indwelling T-tube percutaneous extraction via the T-tube tract is a viable and safe alternative.

Indications and Contraindications for Laparoscopic Ductal Clearance of Stones

Ductal Calculi Discovered Before Surgery

Severe, complicated calculous disease and poor condition of patients are contraindications to laparoscopic stone clearance. Thus patients who are deeply jaundiced with impaired renal function, those with cholangitis or severe pancreatitis due to ampullary impaction and poor-risk patients (cardio-respiratory disease) are best treated by endoscopic sphincterotomy and stone extraction in the first instance. Laparoscopic cholecystectomy (LC) is undertaken once the condition of the patient has improved. Another important contraindication to elective laparoscopic stone extraction is gross dilatation of the bile duct (>2 cm) and multiple ductal calculi. These patients need a drainage procedure: choledochoduodenostomy preferably by the transection technique [7] or adequate endoscopic sphincterotomy, in addition to ductal clearance and cholecystectomy.

By contrast, good-risk patients, even if jaundiced, can be managed by laparoscopic stone extraction during LC, provided the necessary surgical expertise is available. Another indication for laparoscopic management concerns those patients in whom endoscopic stone extraction has failed usually because of large occluding stones or the presence of duodenal diverticulum. An important practical point here is the need for a repeat fluorocholangiogram during the LC as occasionally, large stones which defy endoscopic extraction after sphincterotomy may pass into the duodenum during the interval between this procedure and the operation.

Ductal Calculi Discovered During Surgery

If the surgeon is experienced, the most appropriate treatment is laparoscopic stone extraction either through the cystic duct or via a limited supraduodenal choledocholithotomy. For small calculi, the success of cystic duct extraction now approaches 80% [8–11]. Although these procedures add an extra hour to the operating time, the benefits include completion of treatment in one procedure and negligible morbidity. The single-stage laparoscopic treatment is a more cost-effective option than postoperative endoscopic stone extraction and avoids the necessity for a sphincterotomy, which is an important consideration in young and middle-aged patients.

Laparoscopic extraction for unsuspected calculi at the time of cholecystectomy is inadvisable in patients with a narrow common bile duct. The risk of complications, particularly ductal damage and stricture, following any bile duct exploration (laparoscopic or open) in these patients is appreciable and for this reason they are better treated by postoperative endoscopic extraction or simply followed up. As these stones are small and nonoccluding, the chance of spontaneous passage is high. In patients in whom a ductal calculus is not dealt with at the time of LC, a small cannula inserted into the common duct through the cystic duct is recommended. In addition to providing an excellent access for postoperative cholangiography, a guidewire can be easily inserted through the cannula down the bile duct into the duodenum, thereby facilitating endoscopic sphincterotomy in the postoperative period.

Preoperative Work-up and Preparation

The standard preoperative work-up includes ultrasound examination and Lfts (bilirubin, transaminase, alkaline phosphatase). Although some add infusion intravenous tomographic cholangiography as a routine in all patients, this practice is not in widespread use, and there are doubts concerning its diagnostic reliability and the risk of hypersensitivity reactions. Patients with a history of jaundice or acute pancreatitis and those who exhibit abnormalities in the Lfts or suggestive ultrasound features should be considered as likely to harbour ductal calculi. In the author's view, these patients should be subjected to ERCP. Others maintain the view that ERCP is not necessary in those patients in whom laparoscopic stone clearance is intended at the time of LC, as cholangiographic documentation is obtained during surgery. These surgeons would restrict ERCP to those patients in whom preoperative stone extraction by endoscopic sphincterotomy is contemplated. Although, this policy appears logical and cost-effective, it overlooks a small but significant cohort of patients who have organic ductal disease (cancer or otherwise) rather than calculi or, indeed, dual ductal pathology.

Jaundiced patients require special prophylactic measures. Antibiotics are administered routinely starting with induction of anaesthesia. As the majority of these patients are elderly, chemoprophylaxis with heparin against deep venous thrombosis is wise. In addition, all our patients wear antithrombosis graduated elastic stockings.

Anaesthesia

Laparoscopic ductal clearance is conducted as an integral part of cholecystectomy under general endotracheal anaesthesia. A size 14-F Salem sump suction tube is inserted and positioned in the distal antrum/first part of the duodenum to ensure deflation of the duodenal bulb, which is essential for adequate laparoscopic exposure of the common bile duct. The patient's urinary bladder is catheterized before induction of the pneumoperitoneum. If the patient is jaundiced, the catheter is left for postoperative, hourly monitoring of urine output. Otherwise it is removed after the procedure is completed.

Patient Positioning and Skin Preparation

The same position is used as for LC: supine with a moderate head-up tilt. The skin of the abdomen from the lower chest to the suprapubic region is prepared with medicated soap and then disinfected with the antiseptic of choice. Draping is the same as in LC (Vol. 1, Chap. 16).

Layout of Ancillary Instruments and Positioning of Staff

The surgeon operates from the left side of the operating table. Unless a telescope holder is used, the camera person stands on the same side, with the first assistant and the scrub nurse on the opposite side of the operating table. Dual monitor display is essential and a "picture in picture" video set up is desirable. The light source, camera unit, insufflator, electrosurgical unit and suction/irrigation are placed on a stack behind the surgeon. The instrument trolley is placed beyond and behind the nurse on the right side. A separate sterile trolley is used for the flexible endoscope(s), guidewires, selection of Dormia baskets, balloon extraction catheters, angioplasty dilatation catheters, T-tube and infant feeding catheter or the Cuschieri cystic duct drainage cannula.

Details of Specific Instruments and Consumables

In addition to the basic set, the following instruments are needed:

- Portable C-arm fluorocholangiographic unit
- Cholangiograsper (for cholangiography)
- Pair of 5-mm needle holders
- Dipping endoretractor
- Flexible ureteroscope (visually guided, transcystic extraction)
- Flexible choledochoscope (common duct exploration)
- Dormia baskets (3- to 5-F)

Laparoscopic clearance of ductal stones, by whatever method, should be conducted using the 30° forward-oblique telescope.

The following consumables are required: 4/0 atraumatic absorbable sutures mounted on endoski needles (Polysorb, coated vicryl), balloon dilators, balloon extraction catheters (embolectomy type), guidewires, 14-F T-tube (common duct exploration), 7- to 8-F infant feeding tube or cystic duct drainage cannula (cystic duct drainage) and catgut (1.5-m lengths) mounted on push rods (cystic duct drainage).

Operative Steps of Transcystic Clearance

Small calculi in the distal common duct, which account for the vast majority, can be extracted through the cystic duct. This approach is unsuitable for proximal stones and multiple large occluding calculi, where laparoscopic supraduodenal bile duct exploration is indicated. Cystic duct clearance can be performed under radiological control or by direct visual guidance. *Irrespective of technique, the procedure must be performed before the cystic duct continuity is disrupted and before dissection of the gallbladder from the liver bed is commenced.*

Types and Placement of Trocar and Cannulae

Usually no ports other than those used in conducting LC are needed for laparoscopic transcystic extraction of ductal calculi. However, in cases where there is a floppy quadrate lobe, an extra 5.5-mm cannula below and to the right of the xiphoid (Fig. 10.1; p5) is used for retraction. This extra cannula is also advisable for the introduction of the flexible choledochoscope during direct exploration of the common bile duct (see below).

Radiologically Controlled Technique

The radiologically controlled technique has been popularized by Hunter [11]. It is quicker than the endoscopically guided method and avoids the need for dilatation of the cystic duct. Multiple stone evacuation per single basket passage constitutes a further advantage. The disadvantage is increased radiation exposure. The radiologically guided technique necessitates the availability of modern real-time fluorocholangiography. In this respect we have found the "road-mapping" mode of the OEC Diasonics (Utah, USA) C-arm Unit particularly useful as it shows in relief and with remarkable clarity the basket against the contrast background and filling defects caused by the calculi.

The procedure is performed with the patient in the head-down position.

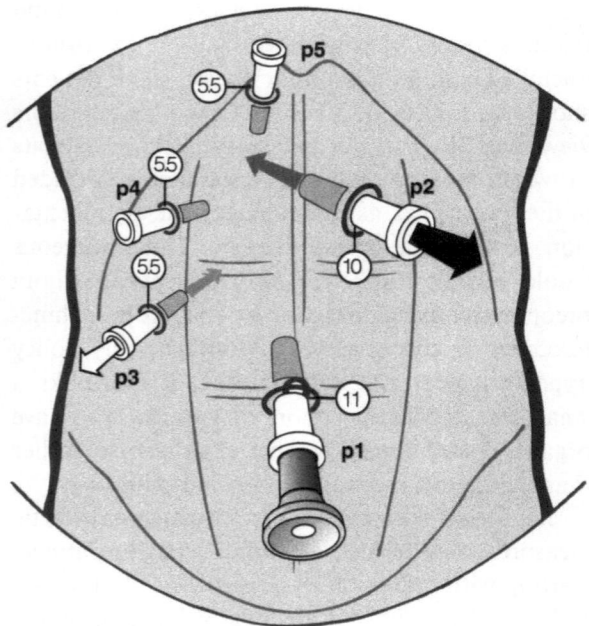

Fig. 10.1. Sites of trocar cannulae for laparoscopic ductal stone clearance. An extra 5.5-mm port below and to the right of the xiphoid may be needed for retraction of a floppy quadrate lobe (p5)

Initial Cholangiogram. An opening is made by the curved microscissors on the anterosuperior walls of the dissected cystic duct. The cholangiography catheter (5-F Cook ureteric catheter or substitute) loaded inside the cholangiograsper is introduced into the cystic for a distance of 1 cm and the jaws of the cholangiograsper closed, gripping the cystic duct walls over the cholangiocatheter (Fig. 10.2). The fully primed system is connected by a three-way tap to saline- and contrast-filled syringes (sodium diatrozoate). Resistance to the passage of the catheter tip may be due to the mucosal folds (Heister valve) or a small calculus in the cystic duct. When encountered, gentle saline injection assists in catheter insertion. If this measure fails, a cystic duct calculus should be suspected. In this case, the cystic duct should be massaged gently between the jaws of an atraumatic grasper in a mediolateral direction (Fig. 10.3). This will dislodge the stone, which then appears in the cystic duct opening (Fig. 10.4) and is removed before the cholangiography catheter is reintroduced. If small distal ductal calculi are encountered, warm saline irrigation together with the intravenous administration of a

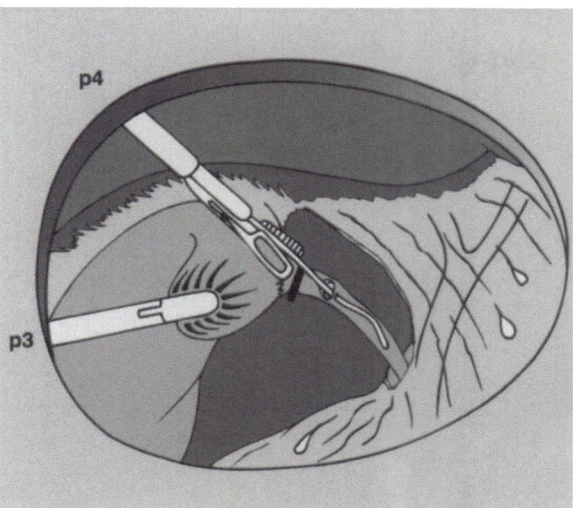

Fig. 10.2. Introducing the cholangiography catheter loaded inside the cholangiograsper into the cystic duct. The jaws of the cholangiograsper are then closed, gripping the cystic duct walls over the catheter

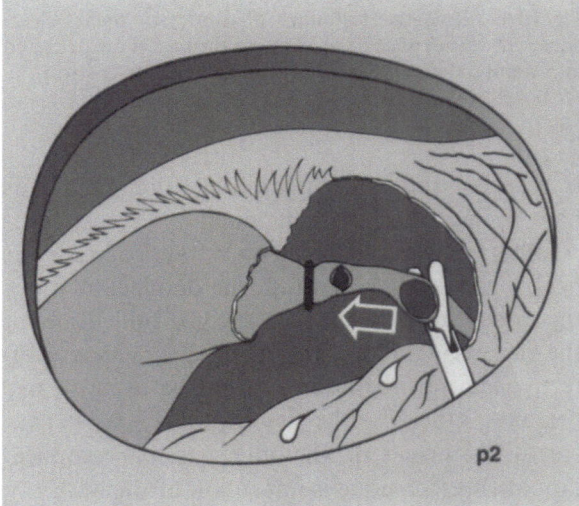

Fig. 10.3. Technique of massage of the cystic duct by the jaws of an atraumatic grasper in a mediolateral direction to dislodge cystic duct stones

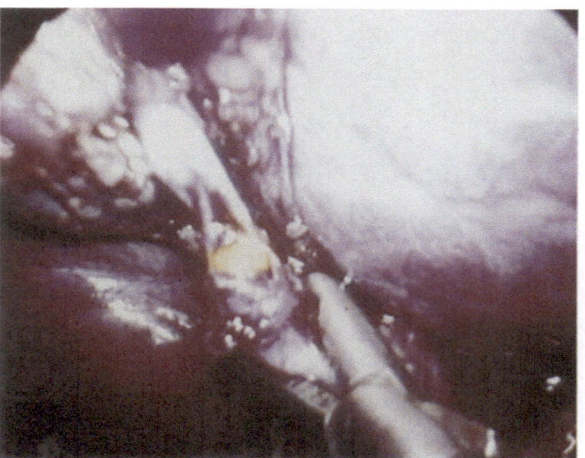

a

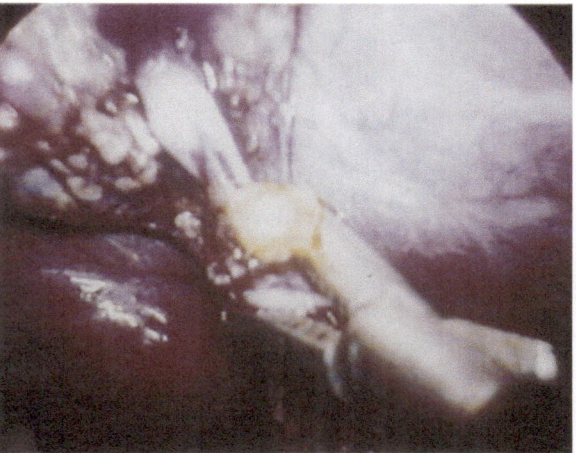

b

Fig. 10.4a, b. Stone in cystic duct dislodged by cystic duct massage (see 10.3)

spasmolytic agent (glucagon or secretin) may result in passage of the stones into the duodenum. If not, transcystic extraction is carried out.

Insertion of Dormia Basket and Stone Capture. The cholangiogram catheter is replaced by a 4-F Dormia or Segura basket preferably with a filiform

tip. Under screening control (preferably in the roadmapping mode) the basket (in the closed position) is passed down the cystic duct into the distal common bile duct such that its floppy tip lies in the duodenum.

Trawling and Extraction of the Stones. When this position is achieved, the wire basket is opened just above the lower choledochal sphincter (Fig. 10.5) and pulled back along the distal common bile duct into the cystic duct where the basket is closed over the stones caught in the troll. Careful closure of the basket to the appropriate extent, i.e. sufficient to ensnare without crushing the stones, is the desired objective. However, if the stones are larger than the cystic duct lumen, further closure of the basket is necessary to achieve crushing. The trawling process

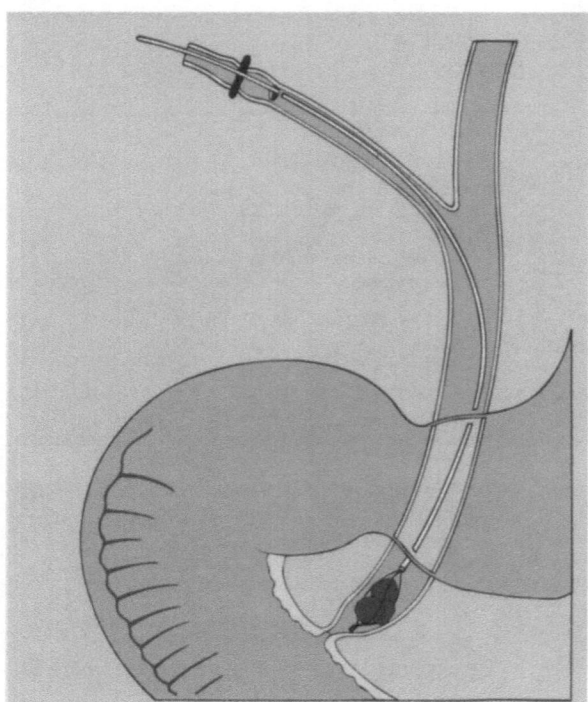

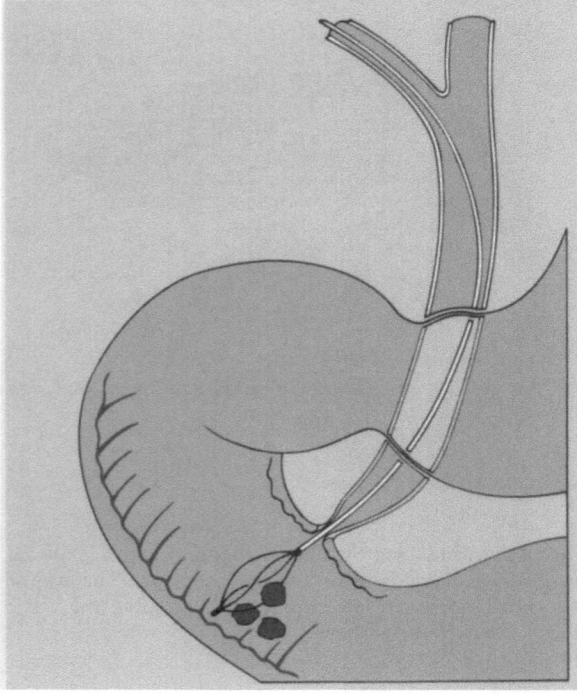

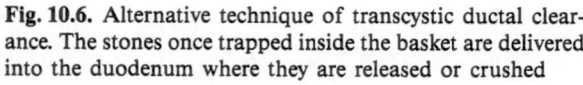

Fig. 10.6. Alternative technique of transcystic ductal clearance. The stones once trapped inside the basket are delivered into the duodenum where they are released or crushed

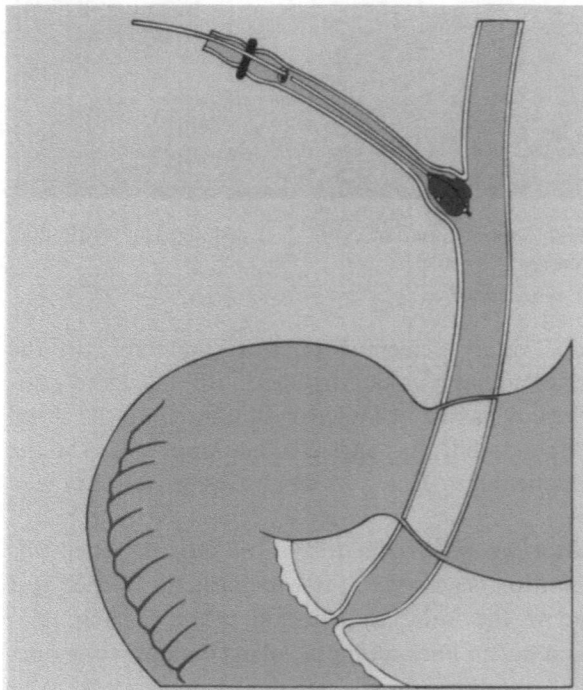

Fig. 10.5. a Wire basket just above the lower choledochal sphincter to trap the stones. **b** Pulling the basket back along the distal common bile duct into the cystic duct where it is closed over the stones caught in the troll

is repeated until all discernible stone fragments have been cleared from the duct.

Alternatively, the stones once trapped inside the basket can be delivered into the duodenum where the stones are released or crushed by full closure of the basket (Fig. 10.6). This method is quick and effective but must be limited to one or, at most, two passages, otherwise the risk of postoperative pancreatitis is increased. The other possible complication of this technique is impaction of the basket in the sphincter. It is less often used than transcystic extraction because of these perceived risks.

Flushing and Completion Cholangiography. The Dormia basket is withdrawn and replaced by the cholangiocatheter. The biliary tract is gently flushed and filled with saline. This washes out any debris and removes air bubbles. High-pressure injection must be avoided to reduce the risk of cholangiovenous reflux. The cholangiogram is then repeated and if ductal clearance is confirmed, the cholangiocatheter is removed and the cystic duct li-

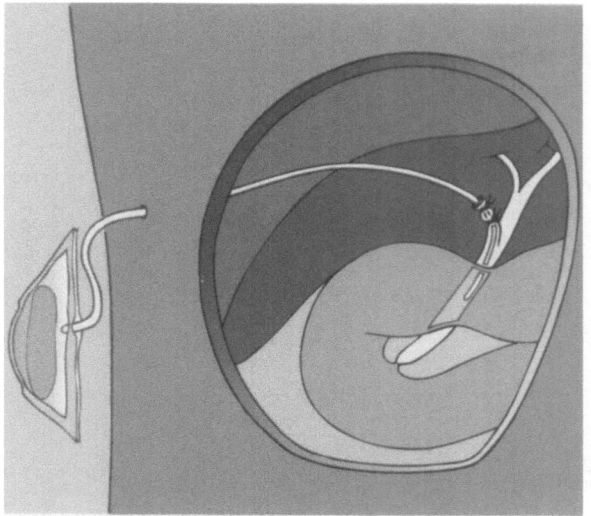
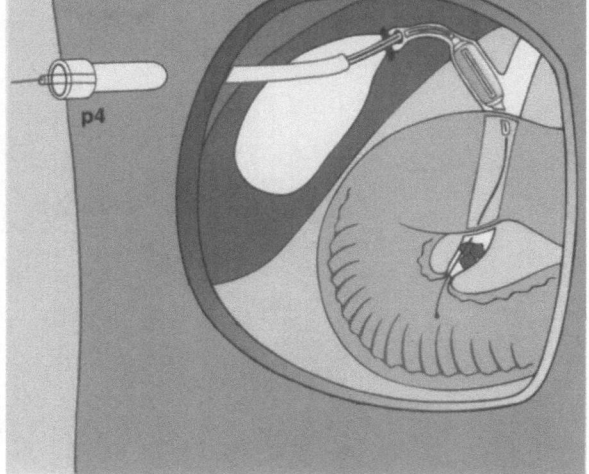

Fig. 10.7. Transcystic catheter drainage. The catheter is secured to the cystic duct stump by two catgut ligatures. Cholangiography can be performed and postoperative endoscopic sphincterotomy for residual calculi facilitated

Fig. 10.8. Balloon dilatation of the cystic duct. This is followed by the introduction of the flexible ureteroscope attached to a CCD camera for visually guided transcystic extraction of the ductal calculi

gated in continuity with catgut or transected and then secured with a preformed catgut endoloop.

Insertion of Cystic Duct Drainage Cannula. If the completion cholangiogram is equivocal (usually debris in the distal duct), the safest measure is to introduce a 7- to 8-F infant feeding tube through the cystic duct into the common bile duct. More recently, a specially designed cystic duct drainage cannula has been developed. The catheter is secured to the cystic duct stump by two catgut ligatures (Fig. 10.7). This cannula permits the performance of postoperative cholangiography. Further management is based on the findings of this investigation. In most instances, the postoperative cholangiogram proves to be normal.

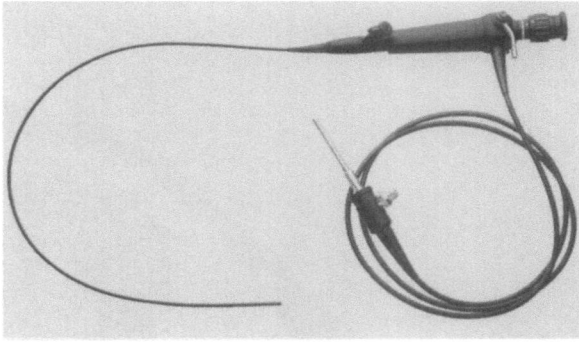

Fig. 10.9. Flexible ureteroscope for visually guided transcystic ductal clearance

Visually Guided Technique

The visually guided technique was pioneered by Dubois in France, Phillips et al. in Los Angeles and Petelin [8–10]. It necessitates the dilatation of the cystic duct followed by the introduction of the flexible ureteroscope (Fig. 10.8) attached to a charge-coupled device (CCD) camera for visually guided transcystic extraction of the ductal calculi. The

ureteroscope (Fig. 10.9) has a functional length of 30 cm, an outer diameter of 3.4–3.6 mm and an instrument channel of 1.2 mm. Finer endoscopes are available and can be used but these must have an instrument channel of at least 1 mm, otherwise irrigation is impossible once the basket is introduced. The other items of equipment needed are angioplasty balloon dilators and guidewires. The balloon dilators should be 6- to 7-F gauge with a balloon length of 40 mm and achieve maximal dilatation of 5 mm. They are insufflated with saline through a customized pressure gauge using a special syringe. Torque guidewires with soft pliable tips or J wires which fit the balloon catheters are used.

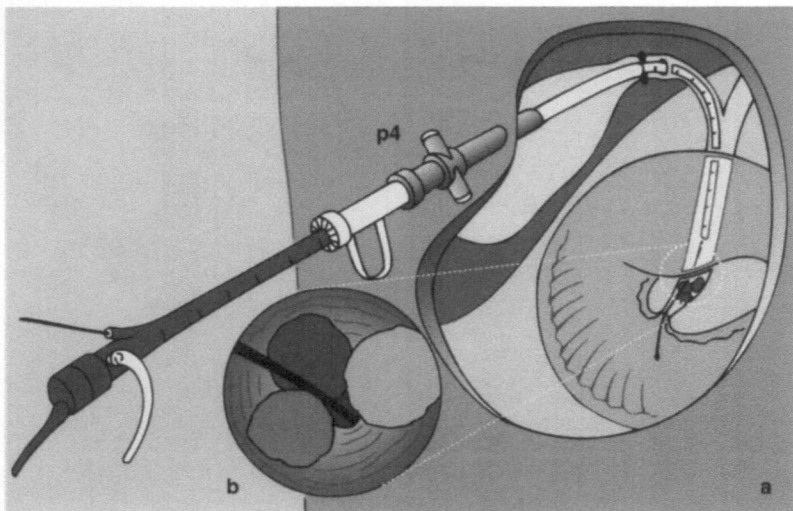

10.10

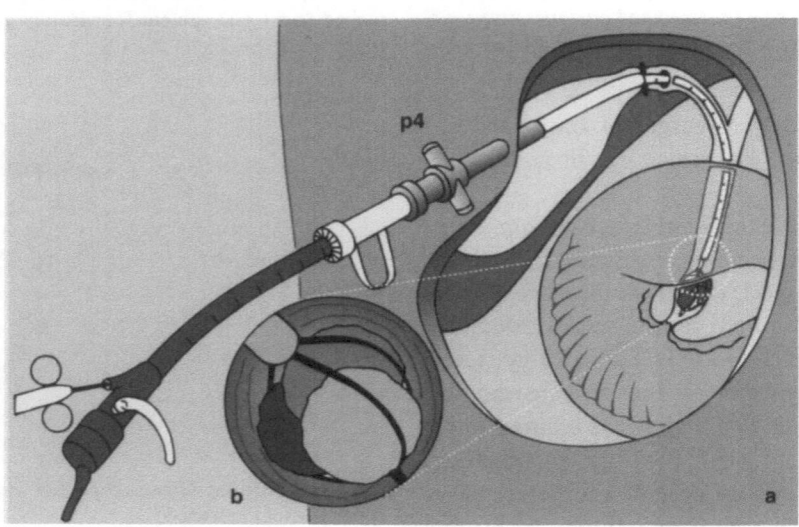

10.11

Fig. 10.10. a The flexible ureteroscope connected to the irrigation system and a CCD camera inserted through the midclavicular cannula and threaded over the guidewire into the common duct. **b** Endoscopic view

Fig. 10.11. a The guidewire being replaced by the Dormia basket which is used to trap and remove the stones under direct vision. **b** Endoscopic view

Initial Cholangiogram. The initial cholangiogram is performed as outlined previously.

Insertion of Guidewire. The guidewire is inserted under fluoroscopic control through the cholangiocatheter into the common bile duct and, if possible, into the duodenum. The cholangiocatheter is then removed and replaced by the balloon catheter which is threaded over the guidewire.

Dilatation. If the common bile duct is dilated, the balloon is positioned under fluoroscopic control across the choledochal sphincter and then inflated. Following dilatation of the sphincter, the balloon is deflated and the catheter withdrawn until the balloon lies in the cystic duct where it is reinflated to dilate this structure. The dilatation of the choledochal sphincter is omitted if the common bile duct is not dilated. At this stage an antispasmodic which relaxes the sphincter of Oddi is administered intra-

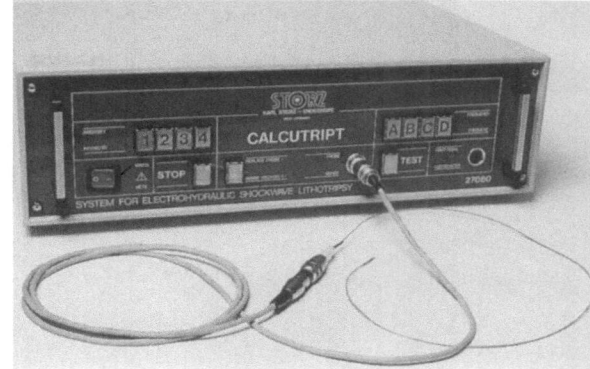

a

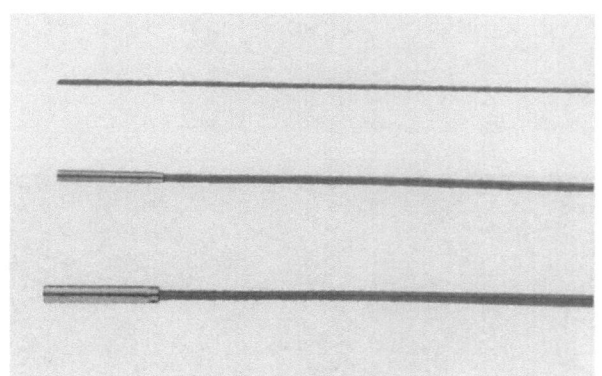

b

Fig. 10.12 a, b. Electrohydraulic lithotriptor (a) and lithotriptor probes (b)

Special measures are needed if the stone is impacted in the lower choledochal sphincter. The most useful is stone fragmentation by electrohydraulic lithotripsy (Fig. 10.12) using a 2.7-F probe. This requires accurate placement of the tip of the probe on the stone away from the duct wall, otherwise a small perforation may be induced when the electric spark is generated. Other methods of fragmentation, such as pulse dye laser (504 nm) transmitted through a thin quartz fibre (300 – 400 nm) can be used [12, 13]. The laser operates at 60 mJ per pulse at 10 Hz and achieves stone fragmentation within 1 – 2 min. The resulting fragments are extracted if large or flushed through the ampulla if small (< 2 m). A completion cholangiogram is made to establish stone clearance. The cystic duct is then ligated in continuity by means of a preformed endoloop. If the completion cholangiogram is equivocal, a cystic duct drainage cannula (7- to 8-F infant feeding tube) is inserted as described previously.

Operative Steps of Laparoscopic Exploration of the Common Duct

Laparoscopic exploration of the common duct is now the author's preferred technique if the common duct diameter is larger than 1 cm. It is essential in all patients with proximal stones. The dipping endoretractor (Storz, Tuttlingen, Germany) is very useful for elevating the quadrate lobe ahead of the optic and thereby provides excellent exposure of the common bile duct. If not available, the quadrate lobe and central part of the liver are elevated using the falciform/round ligament sling (Fig. 10.13). The use of the 30° forward-oblique telescope is essential. The flexible choledochoscope is best inserted through an extra 5.5-mm cannula placed below and to the right of the xiphoid process in line with the common bile duct.

Our technique of laparoscopic bile duct exploration has changed during the past 2 years. We used to conduct the stone extraction under endoscopic control with Dormia baskets (Fig. 10.14). Although undoubtedly effective and elegant, this method can be very time-consuming and is unnecessary, as the

venously. This is followed by irrigation of warm saline through the deflated balloon catheter in an attempt at flushing small calculi into the duodenum. The effect of this manoeuvre is ascertained by fluoroscopy and injection of contrast medium.

Insertion of Ureteroscope. If unsuccessful, the guidewire is reinserted through the lumen of the balloon catheter into the common duct and the catheter then removed. The flexible ureteroscope, connected to the irrigation system (Fenwall pressure cuff) and a CCD camera, is inserted through the midclavicular cannula and threaded over the guidewire into the common duct (Fig. 10.10). The guidewire is then replaced by the Dormia basket which is used to trap and remove the stones under direct vision (Fig. 10.11) either through the cystic duct or into the duodenum.

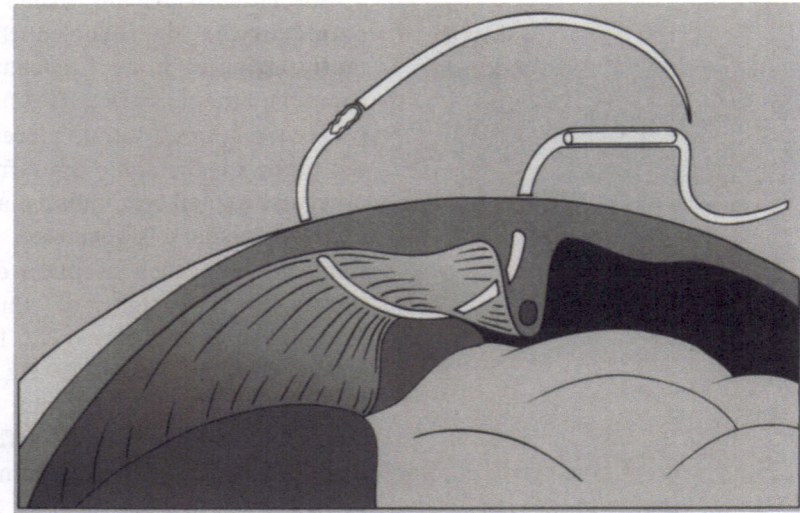

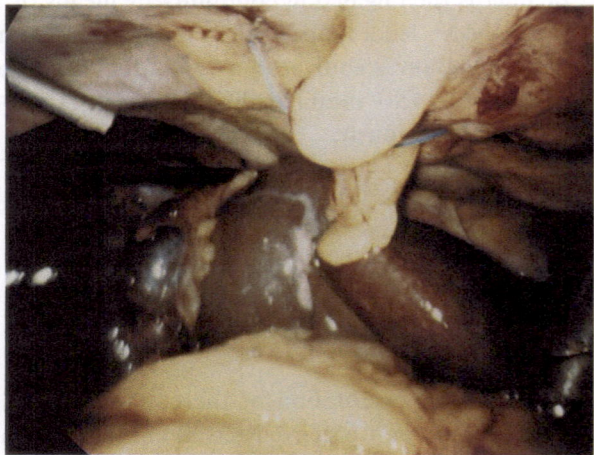

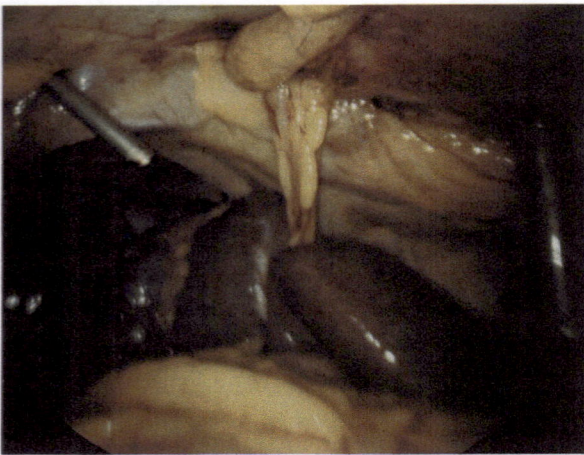

Fig. 10.13. a Diagrammatic representation of the falciform/round ligament sling. **b** Sling around falciform − round ligament before elevation (endophoto). **c** Elevation of central portion of the liver and quadrate lobe

vast majority of ductal calculi encountered during LC can be readily dislodged and brought to the choledochotomy by ductal massage or mild suction or blind trawling using embolectomy or biliary balloon catheters inflated with air.

Dissection of the Common Bile Duct and Choledochotomy. The catheter used for the cholangiogram is left in situ. Minimal dissection of the common duct is needed as only the anterior wall needs to be exposed. Stay sutures are unnecessary and use up ports. The incision of the anterior wall of the

common bile duct is made low down in a vertical oblique fashion and should initially not exceed 1 cm in length (Fig. 10.15). It may require extension if the stone is large but in practice we have observed that choledochotomy wounds (by virtue of the high elastin content of the bile duct) can be stretched to allow delivery of stones whose diameters are 30% − 50% greater than the size of the wound. The choledochotomy is made preferably with a retractable diamond knife. Otherwise sharp dissecting scissors are used. Bleeding from the cut edges is controlled by precise soft electrocoagulation. At this stage, saline is injected forcibly through the cystic duct cannula. This may result in escape of the stone, which is then picked by the spoon forceps and retrieved.

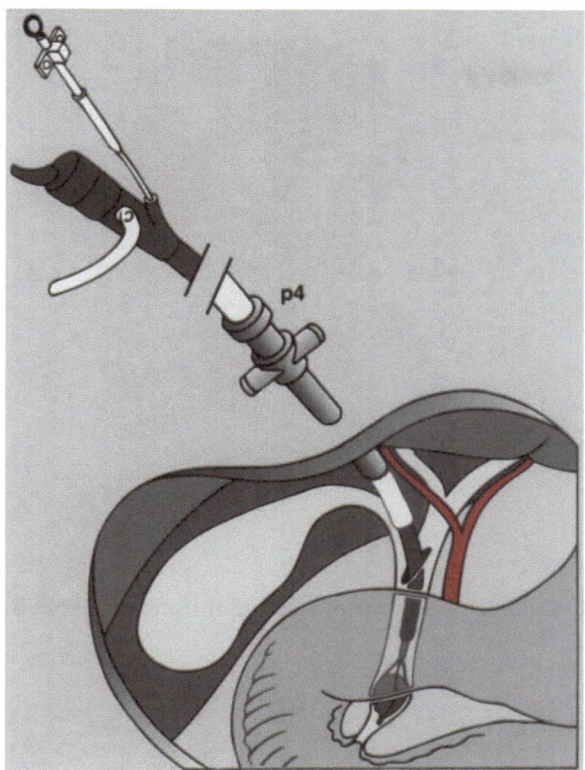

Fig. 10.14. Laparoscopic stone extraction by the flexible choledochoscope and Dormia basket introduced through supraduodenal choledochotomy. The flexible plastic tube (Rüsch, Germany) prevents damage to the endoscope

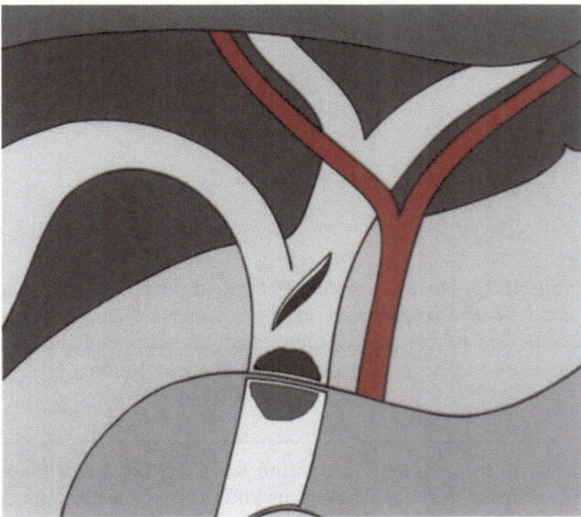

Fig. 10.15. The incision of the anterior wall of the common bile duct made low down in a vertical oblique fashion and initially not exceeding 1 cm in length

Suction Extraction. The next step consists of insertion of a suction device just inside the choledochotomy with the tip of the instrument pointing towards the choledochal sphincter (Fig. 10.16). Low suction is applied and used to adhere the stone to the tip of the suction instrument. Following delivery through the choledochotomy, the stone is transferred to a spoon forceps and removed. The duct can be often completely cleared by this simple technique.

Duct Massage. Two round-ended atraumatic graspers are used to straddle the common duct which is massaged between the two instruments in a proximal direction, starting at the lower end (Fig. 10.17). Once the stone has reached the choledochotomy, one of the graspers is used to compress the bile duct anteroposteriorly above the choledochotomy and the other to ease it out of the choledochotomy (Fig. 10.18). We have found this technique to be useful for large calculi (Fig. 10.19).

Extraction by Biliary Balloon Catheters. If the above methods fail, biliary balloon catheters (2 ml) are inserted through a large Medicut cannula into the common bile duct through the sphincter into the duodenum. After the balloon is inflated with air, the catheter is gently withdrawn until the resistance caused by the sphincter is encountered. The balloon is partially deflated while gentle traction is maintained until it negotiates the sphincter when the balloon is rapidly reinflated and the catheter then used to trawl the stones to the choledochotomy wound.

Visually Guided Extraction with Choledochoscope. In our experience, the above three methods used in the sequence outlined result in successful ductal clearance inside 30 min in 80% of patients. In these cases, the flexible choledochoscope is inserted to conduct a completion inspection. In the other 20%, visually guided Dormia basket extraction is performed.

The flexible choledochoscope connected to the irrigation system (Fenwall) and the CCD camera is introduced through a separate 5.5-mm cannula below and to the right of the xiphoid in line with the common bile duct. After placement of the distal 1 cm of the choledochoscope inside the bile duct

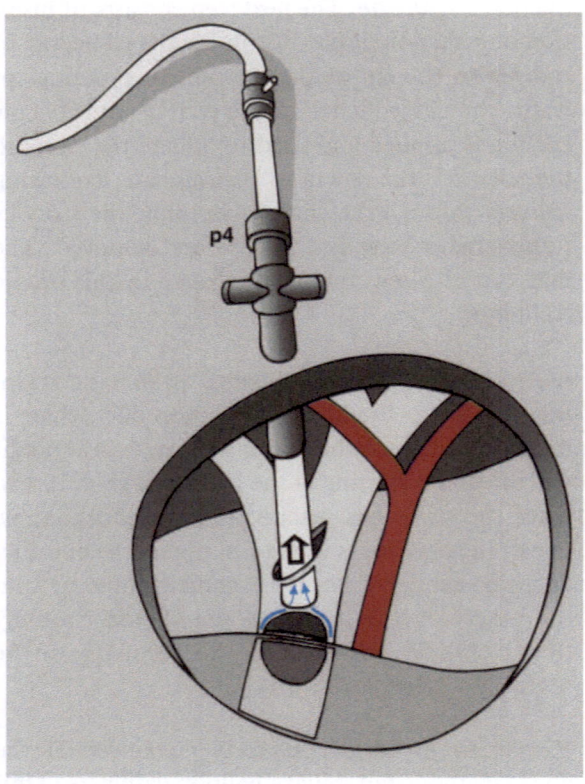

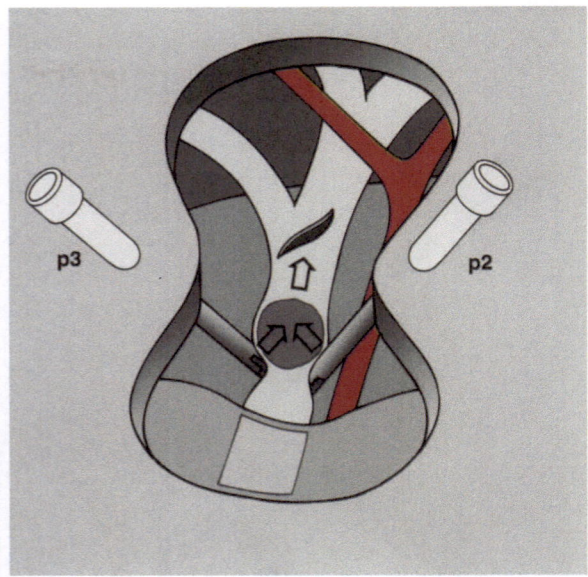

Fig. 10.17. Technique of massage of the common bile duct

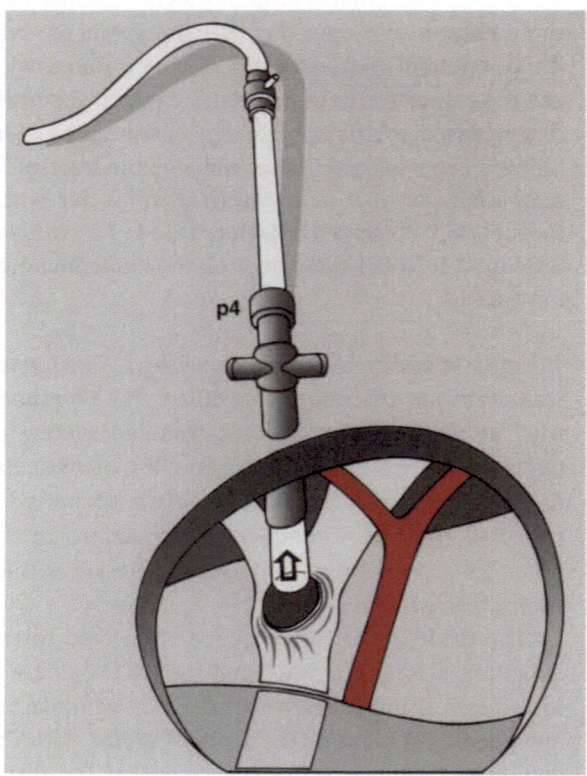

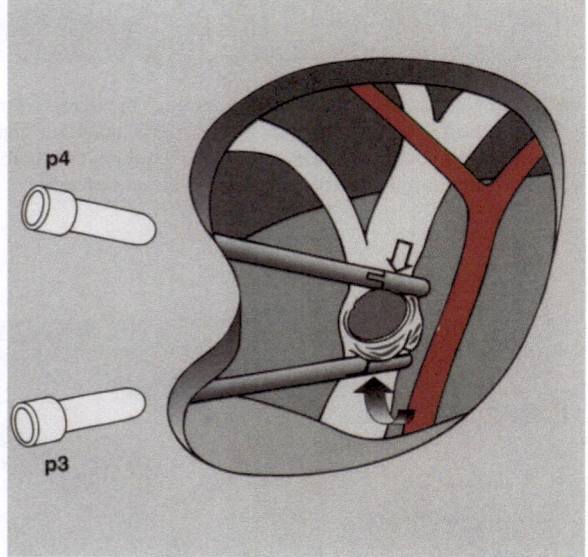

Fig. 10.18. Once the stone has reached the choledochotomy, one of the graspers is used to compress the bile duct anteroposteriorly above the choledochotomy and the other is employed to ease it out of the choledochotomy

Fig. 10.16. a Suction extraction with suction device placed just inside the choledochotomy and the tip of the instrument pointing towards the choledochal sphincter. **b** Stones adhere to the tip of the activated sucker and are thereby delivered through the choledochotomy

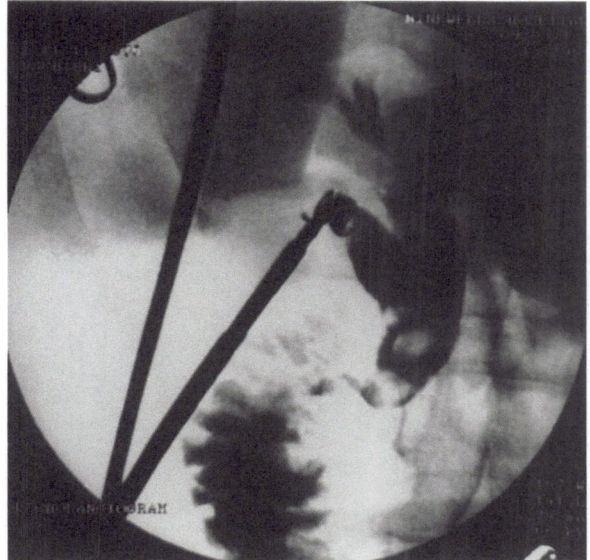

a

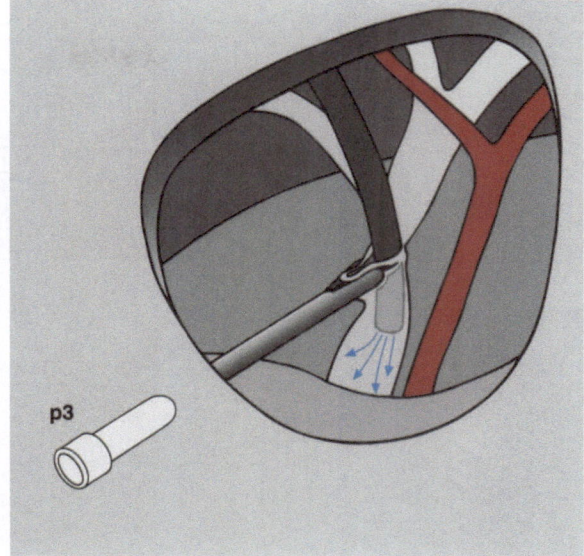

Fig. 10.20. After placing the distal 1 cm of the choledocho-scope inside the bile duct lumen, the walls of common bile duct are gathered around the flexible endoscope by an atraumatic forceps and irrigation commenced

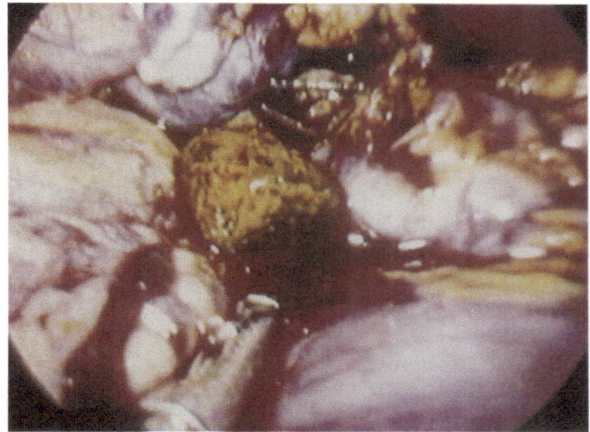

b

Fig. 10.19a, b. Large occluding stone (**a**) dislodged by stone massage and then delivered through the choledochotomy (**b**)

Common Duct Drainage. Drainage of the bile duct is essential after supraduodenal bile duct explora-tion as hold up due to oedema is encountered for several days after this procedure [14]. In addition, the drainage tube provides a ready access for post-operative cholangiography as a final check against retained stones. There are two techniques which can be used for biliary drainage: insertion of T-tube and cystic duct decompression.

lumen, the walls of common bile duct are gathered around the flexible endoscope by an atraumatic forceps and irrigation commenced (Fig. 10.20). The entire biliary tract is inspected (proximally and dis-tally) and any stones are trapped and removed un-der vision through the choledochotomy by means of a Dormia basket. Once outside the bile duct, the stones are transferred on each occasion to a spoon forceps and retrieved. After the bile duct is clear, choledochoscopic inspection of the biliary tract is repeated.

1. T-tube method: This is the standard technique. The horizontal limb of a 14-F latex tube is trimmed to a total length which does not exceed 1.5 cm and is filleted. These modifications greatly facilitate the insertion of the horizontal part inside the common bile duct. The tube is in-serted into the peritoneal cavity through a stab wound in the right flank such that the long limb runs a straight course to the choledochotomy. This straight alignment of the long limb of the T-tube is important should any residual stones be discovered postoperatively, as a straight tube tract facilitates percutaneous stone extraction by this route. In this respect, it is a mistake to use one of the cannula sites for the insertion of the T-tube, as more often then not, these do not pro-

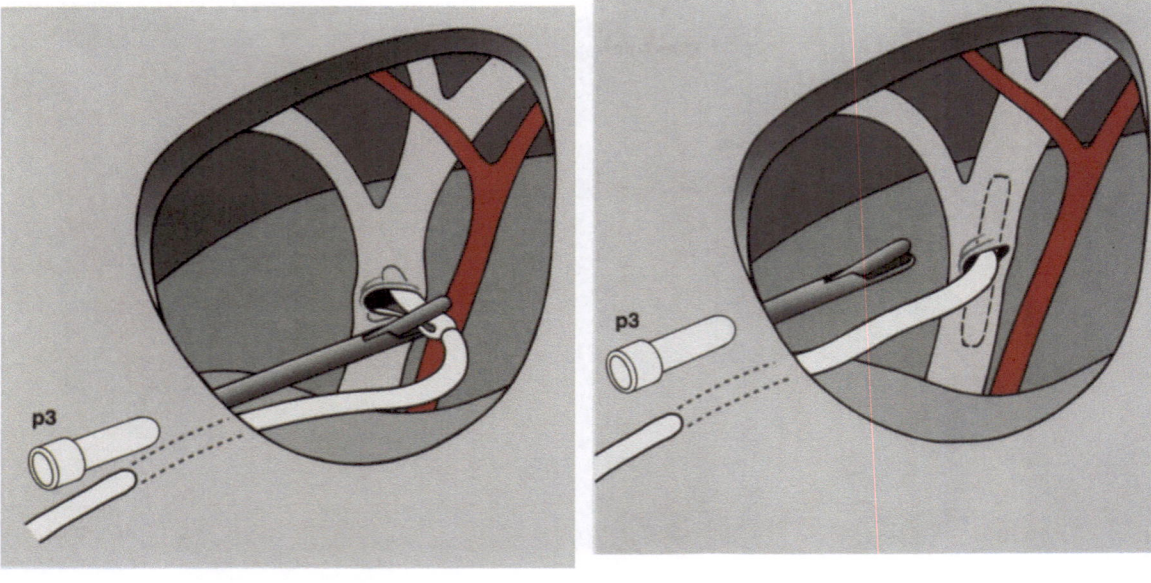

10.21a   b

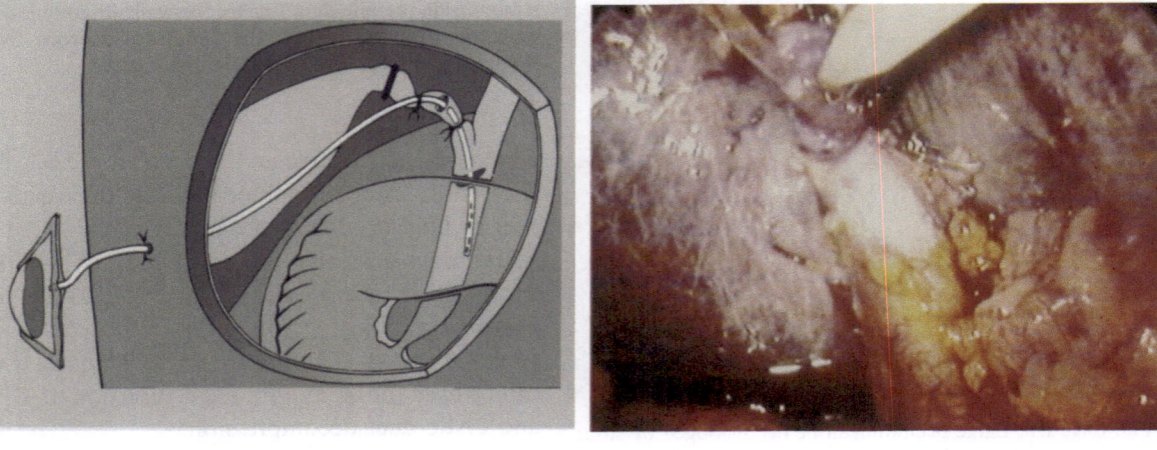

10.22a   b

Fig. 10.21a, b. The T-tube horizontal limbs are compressed together by means of an atraumatic forceps and then fed into the common bile duct (**a**), and then the forceps are released (**b**)

Fig. 10.22. a Infant-feeding tube being inserted through the cystic duct well into the common bile duct and then tying the cystic duct over the tube in continuity using a Roeder slip catgut knot. A second Roeder knot is applied a few millimetres further laterally but medial to the clip on the gallbladder end of the cystic duct. **b** Cystic duct cannula in situ

vide the ideal location. Once the tube is in the peritoneal cavity, its short horizontal limbs are compressed together by means of an atraumatic forceps and then fed into the common bile duct, at which time the forceps is released (Fig. 10.21). When the T-tube is in place, saline is instilled to irrigate the extrahepatic biliary tract.

2. Cystic duct drainage: We now prefer this technique [15], because the patient recovers quicker. Initialy an infant feeding, soft polyethylene tube (7–8 F) is used. It provides adequate drainage (average 300 ml/day) and excellent access for postoperative cholangiography. The cholangio-catheter is replaced by the infant feeding tube. This is introduced in the right flank via a large

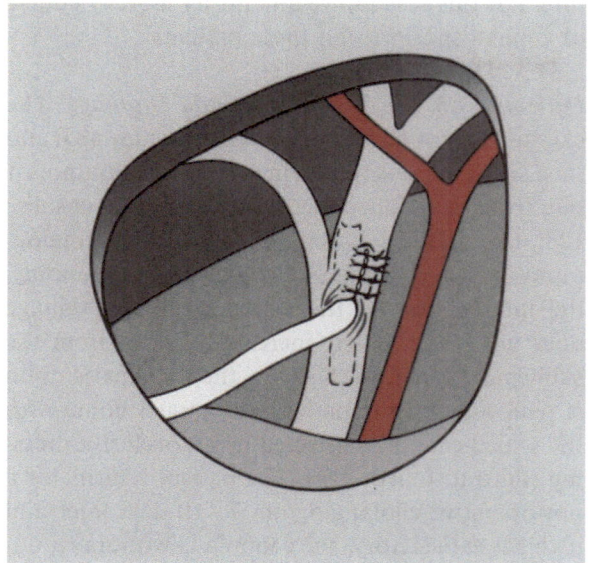

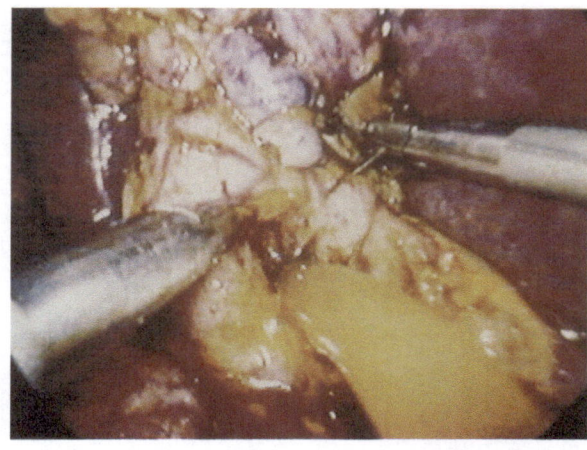

Fig. 10.23. a Closure of choledochotomy after placement of T-tube. The incision is closed above the long limb which then comes to lie at the bottom of the closed incision. **b** Closed T-tube choledochotomy

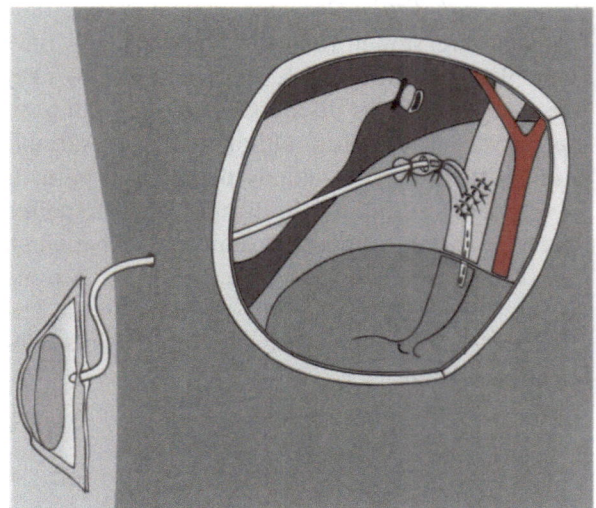

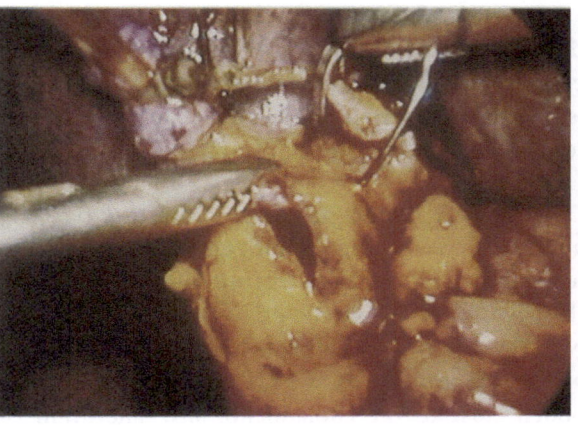

Fig. 10.24. a Primary closure of the common bile duct after placement of cystic duct cannula. **b** Suture closure of the common bile duct

Medicut cannula and then is inserted through the cystic duct well into the common bile duct (Fig. 10.22). More recently we have designed and now use a cystic duct drainage catheter with a terminal "S" configuration. This catheter (Cook, USA) is available in two sizes (7.5 F, 8.5 F) and has its own introducer hit. The cystic duct is then tied over the tube in continuity using a Roeder slip catgut knot. A second Roeder knot is applied a few millimetres further laterally but medial to the clip on the gallbladder end of the cystic duct. The cystic duct is then divided

with hook scissors between the lateral ligature and the clip. Saline is infused through the cystic duct cannula to ensure patency.

Suture Closure of the Common Bile Duct. The incision in the common bile duct is then closed by two to three interrupted 4/0 absorbable sutures (Polysorb, coated Vicryl). If a T-tube is placed, the choledochotomy is closed above the long limb, which then comes to lie at the bottom of the closed incision (Fig. 10.23). If cystic duct cannula drainage is used, primary complete closure of the chole-

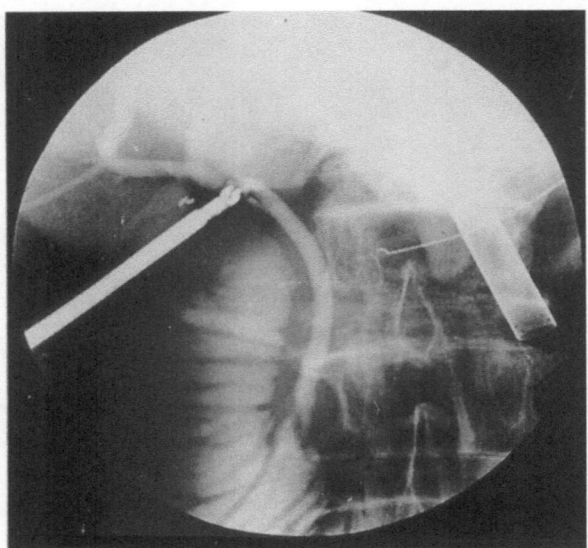

Fig. 10.25. Completion cholangiogram confirming total ductal clearance

dochotomy is performed (Fig. 10.24). In either case, when the suturing has been completed, saline is injected through the cystic duct cannula or T-tube to ensure a watertight seal.

Completion Cholangiogram and Insertion of Subhepatic Drain. A completion contrast study is performed in all cases to ensure ductal clearance (Fig. 10.25). A subhepatic drain is inserted routinely in these patients. This is introduced through the midclavicular cannula and placed in the subhepatic pouch close to the choledochotomy. The drain is connected to a closed drainage system. Thereafter, the peritoneum is desufflated and the drain and T-tube or cystic duct cannula are fixed by sutures to the skin.

Postoperative Management

The nasogastric tube is removed after recovery from anaesthesia since postoperative ileus has not been a common problem in these patients. In the presence of jaundice hourly monitoring of the urinary output is maintained for the first few days after surgery. In our experience about 30% of patients undergoing laparoscopic exploration have bacteria (gram-negative aerobes) in the bile on cul-

ture. For this reason, we administer a 5-day course of cephalosporin to all these patients.

Patients with Cystic Duct Cannula Drainage. The cannula is kept on free closed drainage for 48 h and then sealed. If this results in an increased output of bile from the subhepatic drain during the ensuing 12 h, free drainage is reestablished and cholangiography arranged within 24 h. Much more commonly, the interruption of the external biliary drainage does not result in any increased output from the subhepatic drain. In this case, the subhepatic drain is removed and the patient discharged home with the sealed cannula protected by an occlusive dressing (third to fourth day). The patient returns for a postoperative cholangiogram 7 – 10 days later and if this is satisfactory, the cannula is withdrawn under intravenous sedation.

Patients with T-tube Drainage. Patients with T-tube drainage are slower to recover and usually have some ileus, which resolves, however, by 48 h. They are usually ready for discharge from the sixth postoperative day onwards, although this is variable and is often longer in elderly patients. In patients in whom maturation of the T-tube tract is impaired (elderly, diabetics, immunosuppressed patients), the T-tube is left spigotted for at least 2 more weeks. Otherwise it is usually removed on the seventh to tenth day, provided the T-tube cholangiogram is normal.

Clinical Results

Although little experience has been reported, the results to date have been most encouraging, with a low postoperative morbidity and retained stone rate. Splitting of the cystic duct may result from balloon dilatation, which is often needed to insert the flexible ureteroscope. This complication is recognized immediately at operation and is easily treated by laparoscopic suture closure of the cystic duct stump. Hyperamylasaemia is common after transcystic removal (20%) but clinically significant pancreatitis is rare. The other complication is bile leakage. This has been encountered in 4% of our patients after supraduodenal common bile duct exploration and always resolves, provided a sub-hepatic drain is left at the time of surgery. In our series of 40 patients none died. One patient developed intestinal obstruction caused by a twist of an upper jejunal loop around the long limb of the T-tube.

In those patients with retained stones who have access to the biliary tree (T-tube), endoscopically guided percutaneous stone extraction via the T-tube tract is the preferred option. A few weeks are allowed for maturation of the tract before the procedure is undertaken. After the insertion of a guidewire, the T-tube is removed and the tract dilated. An Amplatz sheath is then inserted before passage of the flexible choledochoscope over the guidewire into the common bile duct. Good fluoroscopic imaging is also needed for this procedure.

In patients without a T-tube, endoscopic sphincterotomy and stone extraction remain the treatment of choice. In experienced hands this has a success rate of 90%. If a cystic duct cannula drainage is in situ, the passage of a guide-wire down the cannula through the bile duct into the duodenum virtually guarantees successful endoscopic stone extraction in all patients.

References

1. Cetta F (1991) The role of bacteria in pigment gallstone disease. Ann Surg 213:315–326
2. Schein CJ (1978) Postcholecystectomy syndromes. Harper and Row, Hagerstown
3. Dubois F, Icard P, Berthelot G, Levard H (1990) Coelioscopic cholecystectomy. Ann Surg 211:60–62
4. de Watteville JC, Gailleton R, Gayral F, Testas P (1992) Is routine intravenous cholangiography before laparoscopic cholecystectomy useful? Eurosurgery Congress, Brussels, June 1992 (Abstr)
5. Neoptolomos JP, Carr-Locke DL, Fossard DL (1987) Prospective randomized study of preoperative endoscopic sphincterotomy versus surgery alone for common bile duct stones. Br Med J 294:470–474
6. Southern Surgeons Club (1991) A prospective analysis of 1518 laparoscopic cholecystectomies. N Engl J Med 324:1073–1078
7. Cuschieri A, Wood RAB, Metcalf MJ, Cumming JGR (1983) Long term experience with transection choledochoduodenostomy. World J Surg 7:502–504
8. Sackier JM, Berci G, Paz-Partlow M (1991) Laparoscopic transcystic choledocholithotomy as an adjunct to laparoscopic cholecystectomy. Am Surg 57: 323–326
9. Sackier J, Berci G, Phillips E et al (1991) The role of cholangiography in laparoscopic cholecystectomy. Arch Surg 126:1021–1026
10. Petelin JB (1991) Laparoscopic approach to common duct pathology. Surg Lap Endosc 1:33–41
11. Hunter JG (1992) Laparoscopic transcystic common duct exploration. Am J Surg 163:53–58
12. Berci G, Hamlin JA, Daykhovsky L, Sackier J, Paz-Partlow M (1990) Common bile duct lithotripsy. Gastrointest Endosc 36:137–139
13. Shapiro SJ, Gordon LA, Daykhovsky L, Grundfest W (1991) Laparoscopic exploration of the common bile duct. J Laparosc Endosc 1:333–341
14. Holdsworth RJ, Sadek SA, Ambikar S, Baker PR, Cuschieri A (1989) Dynamics of bile flow through the human choledochal sphincter following exploration of the common bile duct. World J Surg 13:300–306
15. Shimi S, Banting S, Cuschieri A (1992) Cystic duct drainage after laparoscopic exploration of the common bile duct. Min Invas Ther 1:273–276

11 Laparoscopic Splenectomy

A. CUSCHIERI

Introduction

Nowadays, the need for splenectomy is indicated for trauma, in the management of patients with certain haematological disorders and in the staging of some patients with Hodgkin's disease. In trauma, the tendency in recent years has been towards splenic preservation with repair or segmental resection as indicated by the nature of the injury, with splenectomy being reserved for severe grade 4 lesions, including splenic hilar disruption [1]. The argument for splenic preservation is based on the risk of severe postsplenectomy sepsis due to encapsulated organisms, predominantly *Streptococcus pneumoniae* [2, 3]. However, a recent collective review of the literature has shown that the risk is mainly confined to infants and children and is significantly influenced by the nature of the underlying disease for which the splenectomy is performed [4]. Thus the lowest incidence of postsplenectomy sepsis is encountered when the spleen is removed for trauma.

In elective surgery, vaccination with polyvalent pneumococcal vaccine is practised although the evidence for effective protection by this measure is lacking [5, 6] and on immunological grounds, vaccination is likely to stimulate the memory T-independent lymphocytes only if commenced before the spleen is removed. The use of prophylactic penicillin therapy is advisable in infants and children.

Indications and Contraindications for Laparoscopic Splenectomy

Although minor injuries of the splenic poles can be repaired laparoscopically by the use of omentum and fibrin glue, laparoscopic splenectomy has been undertaken to date only in the elective situation. The assessment of splenic size, which determines the feasibility of laparoscopic splenectomy, is conducted by physical examination and splenic ultrasonography. The ideal patients for elective laparoscopic splenectomy are those suffering from idiopathic thrombocytopenic purpura (ITP) for two reasons. In the first instance, the splenic enlargement in these patients is only moderate, and secondly, the risk of postsplenectomy sepsis is minimal [4]. Laparoscopic splenectomy is also indicated for acquired haemolytic anaemia Hodgkin's disease (>15 cm), splenic cysts and tumours. Massive splenomegaly (>20 cm) of any cause is considered by the author to be a contraindication to the laparoscopic approach.

Preoperative Work-up and Preparation

In addition to full haematological testing including platelet count and bleeding time, it is advisable to perform an splenic ultrasound examination to determine exact splenic size, as this influences the need for interventional arteriography and the operative approach. Most patients with ITP have spleens which seldom exceed 12 cm along their longitudinal axis (Fig. 11.1). For larger spleens (>15 cm), splenic arteriography with embolization (gel foam, coils, etc.) of the splenic artery the day before surgery reduces splenic size and facilitates the laparoscopic procedure. Alternatively, primary ligature of the splenic artery at the start of the operation is performed (see below).

As all the patients with ITP have usually been exposed to long periods of steroid therapy in the form of oral prednisolone, the perioperative period is covered by parenteral hydrocortisone. Provided the platelet count is 50000 or more, there is no indi-

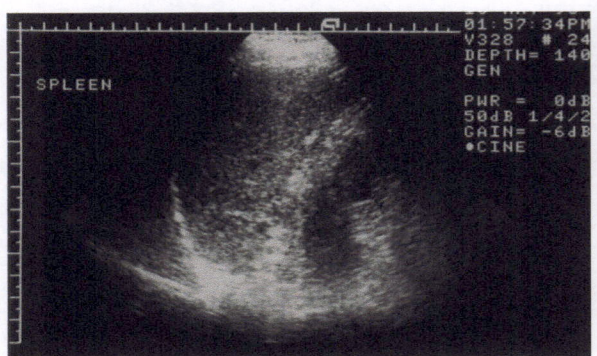

Fig. 11.1. Splenic ultrasound examination

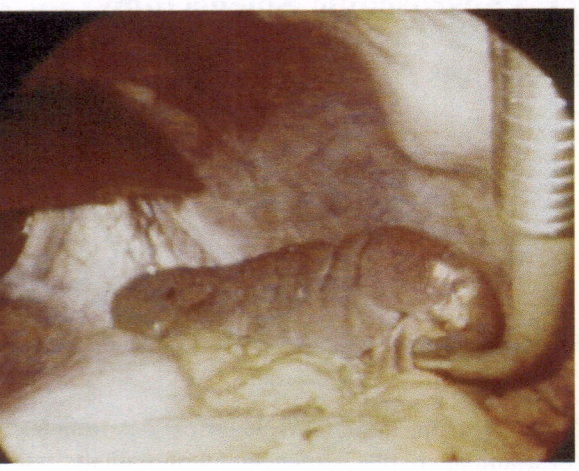

Fig. 11.2. Exposure of the spleen by positioning of the patient and operating table as described in the text

cation for preoperative platelet transfusions and preoperative administration of purified human IgG is sufficient. Chemoprophylaxis against deep venous thrombosis with subcutaneous administration of heparin is recommended in all patients undergoing laparoscopic splenectomy because of the rebound thrombocytosis encountered in the vast majority of patients in the postoperative period. The first subcutaneous dose (5000–8000 units) is administered with induction of anaesthesia. Antithrombosis graduated elastic stockings are also used in all patients.

Anaesthesia

Laparoscopic splenectomy is performed under general anaesthesia with endotracheal intubation. The exact details and premedication vary with the practice of the anaesthetist. Antibiotic prophylaxis is administered routinely, using a single-dose injection of a cephalosporin given after induction of anaesthesia. A size 14-F Salem sump nasogastric tube is inserted and kept on continuous low suction to ensure total and continued deflation of the stomach throughout the procedure. The patient's urinary bladder is catheterized before induction of the pneumoperitoneum. The catheter is withdrawn after the operation is completed.

Patient Positioning and Skin Preparation

The patient is operated upon in the half-lateral position with a 6-cm deep sand bag placed underneath the left rib cage – semi-lateral position –

and with a moderate (15°–30°) head-up tilt. In addition, a slight lateral tilt of the operating table to the right further improves the exposure of the spleen by elevation of the left subdiaphragmatic recess (Fig. 11.2). The skin of the abdomen and lower chest is prepared with medicated soap (Hibiscrub; ICI, UK) and then disinfected with the antiseptic of choice. The area prepared in this fashion extends from the nipple line to the pubis and laterally well into the flanks. Draping is such as to leave exposed the abdomen from the costal margins to the suprapubic region and extending well laterally in the left flank (Fig. 11.3).

Layout of Ancillary Instruments and Positioning of Staff

The surgeon operates from the right side of the operating table. Unless an adjustable vacuum-lock laparoscope holder (First Assistant, Leonard, Philadelphia) is used, the camera person and the first assistant both stand on the left side of the patient. The scrub nurse stands on the right side by the surgeon and her sterile instrument trolley is situated beyond and behind her (Fig. 11.4).

Fig. 11.3. Draping. The exposed area of the abdomen extends from the costal margins to the suprapubic region and laterally to the left flank

Fig. 11.4. Layout of staff and equipment; *S* Surgeon

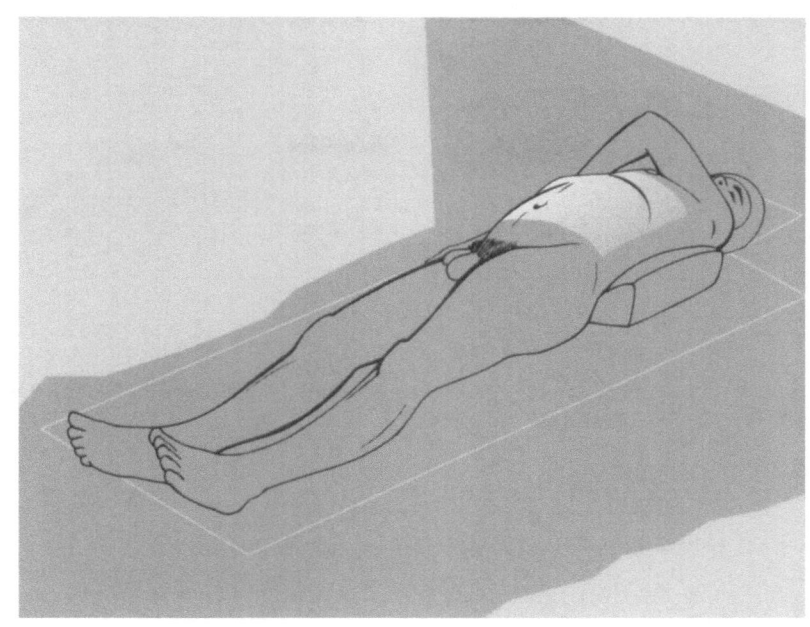

11.3

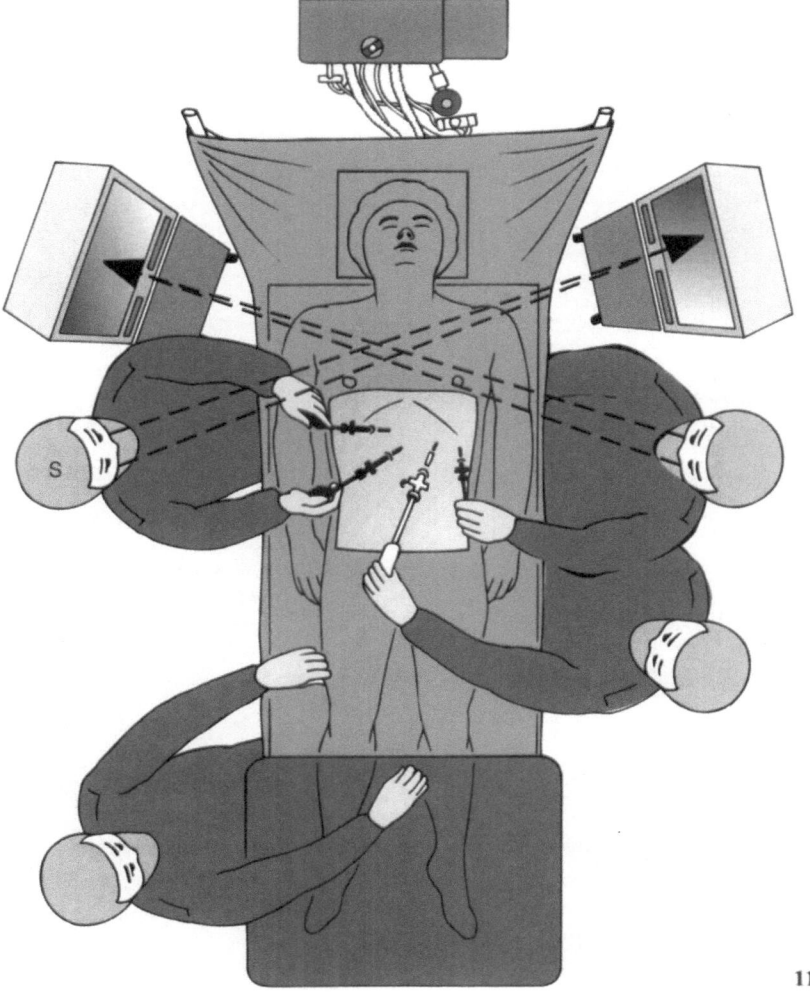

11.4

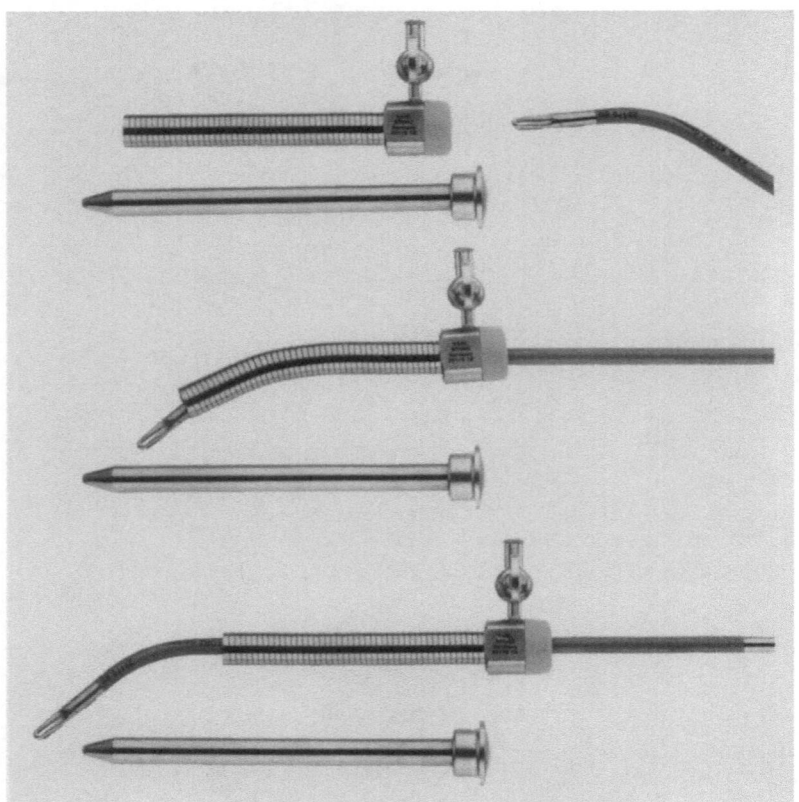

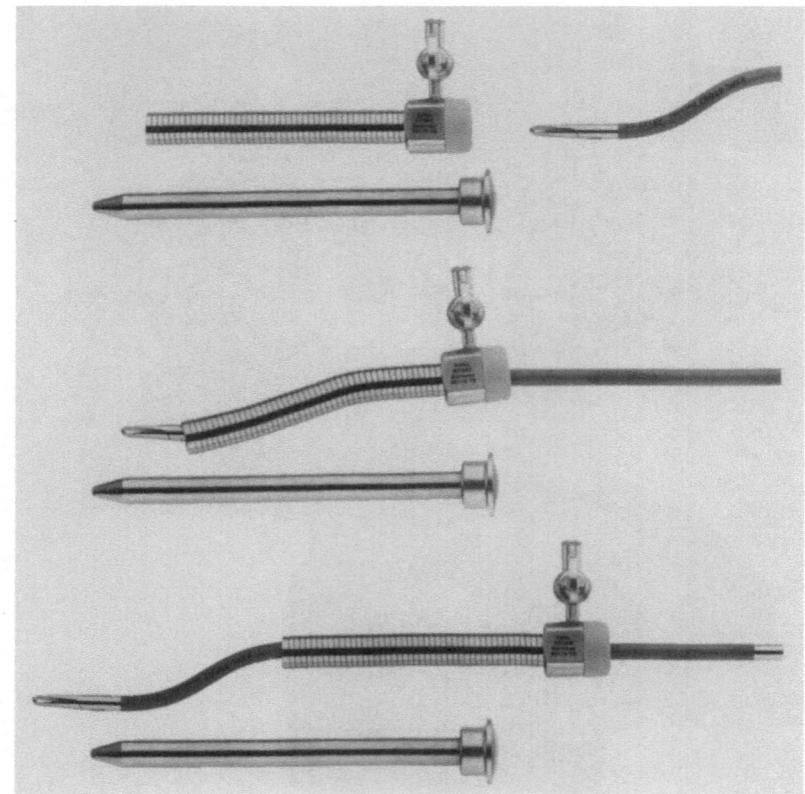

A two-monitor visual display is essential as the first assistant plays a very active part in the ligation of the short gastric vessels and during the dissection and securement of the splenic hilar vessels. The electrosurgical unit, preferably of the microprocessor controlled type (Erbe, Tübingen, Germany), suction irrigation, insufflator and camera unit are placed on a stack behind the surgeon. The use of a pulsed irrigation system is desirable to enable dispersal of clots during the dissection of the splenic hilium.

Details of Specific Instruments and Consumables for the Procedure

In addition to the basic instrumentation, the following special equipment is necessary for laparoscopic splenectomy:

- 10-mm 30° forward oblique telescope
- Curved coaxial instruments and flexible trocar cannulae (Fig. 11.5 a, b)
- Liver retractor rod
- Consumables
  Dacron or black silk ligatur (120–150 cm) mounted on a push rod (USSC, Norwalk, USA; Ethicon, Edinburgh, UK)
  EndoGIA* with vascular cartridges (USSC, Norwalk, USA)

The use of curved and bayonet coaxial instruments which can be introduced through reusable flexible cannulae and allow change of direction of the functional tip by rotation of the longitudinal axis of the instrument [7] greatly facilitates dissection around the splenic poles and behind the spleen (Fig. 11.6). The dissection of the splenic hilar vessels from the tail of the pancreas and separation of the posterior surface of the spleen from the retroperitoneum, perirenal fat and adrenal gland is considerably expedited by the use of ultrasonic dissection [8] using the Selector probe (Surgical Technology Group, Andover, UK) (Fig. 11.7).

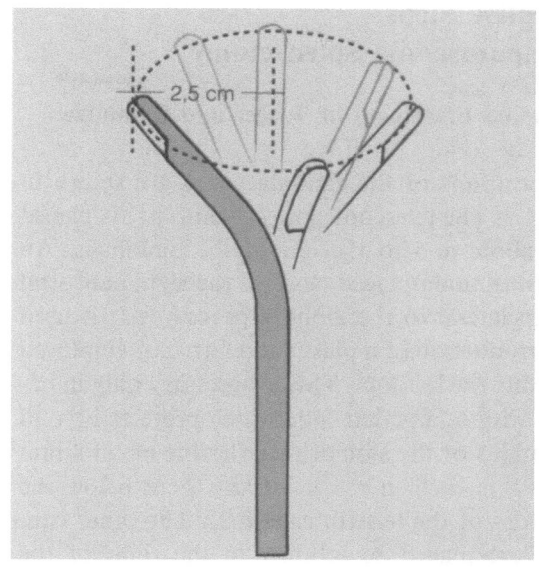

11.6

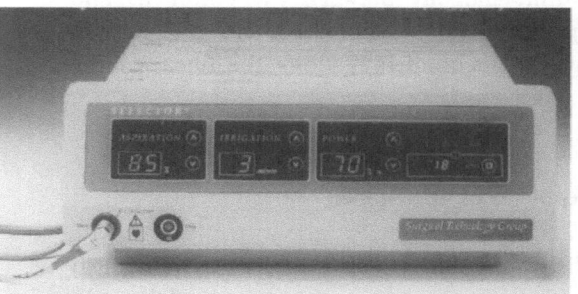

11.7a

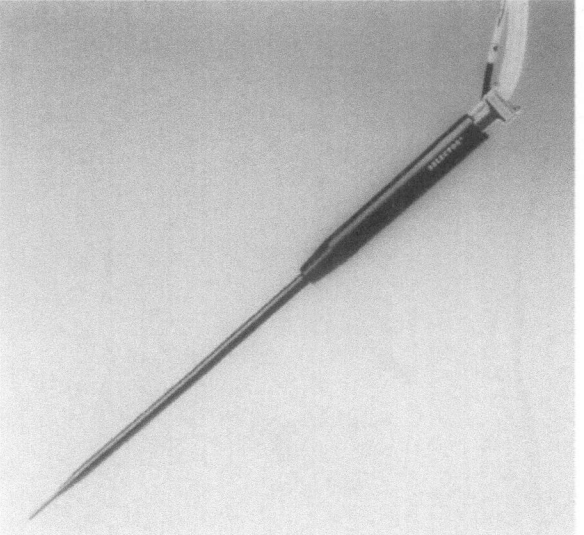

b

Fig. 11.6. Range of movement of the functional tip of the curved coaxial instrument as it is rotated longitudinally through 360°

Fig. 11.7 a, b. Selector ultrasonic dissector system with probe (Surgical Technology Group, Andover, UK)

◄───────────────────────────

Fig. 11.5. a Coaxial curved instruments which are introduced through reusable metal flexible cannulae (Storz, Tuttlingen, Germany). **b** Coaxial bayonet instruments using the same flexible cannula for their insertion

Operative Steps
of Laparoscopic Splenectomy

Types and Placement of Trocar and Cannulae

The positions of the cannulae used are shown in Fig. 11.8. The telescope port (11-mm, p1) is placed 2 cm above and to the left of the umbilicus. An 11-mm cannula placed close to the right subcostal margin lateral to the xiphoid process (p5) is used for introduction of a plastic rod retractor employed to elevate the left lobe. This is necessary only in patients with a large left lobe which projects beyond the fundus of the stomach. A flexible metal 8-mm cannula is sited in the left flank 2 cm below the convexity of the left rib cage (p2). The other cannulae are placed as follows: to the right of the midline halfway between the umbilicus and the xiphoid process (8-mm; p3, flexible) and in the right hypochondrium along the linea semilunaris (5.5 mm; p4).

Exposure of the Spleen

With positioning of the patient as previously described, the lower anterior aspect of the spleen is exposed in the majority of patients. In some, the greater omentum is seen rolled up, obscuring the organ. In this situation, the omentum is grasped with an atraumatic forceps and pulled down into the infracolic compartment. A coaxial-curved Babcock's type grasper is placed on the proximal body of the stomach near the greater curve and used to retract this organ downwards and to the right. This results in excellent exposure of the anterior aspect and lower pole of the spleen. At this stage the lower pole is seen attached to the splenic flexure of the colon by a vascular peritoneal fold (suspensory ligament).

Division of Splenocolic Attachments
and Devascularization of the Lower Pole

The first step of the operation is to divide the splenocolic attachments and devascularize the lower pole. Prior to scissors division of the splenocolic attachment, the leash of fine blood vessels in this peritoneal fold are electrocoagulated (Fig. 11.9) preferably in the soft coagulation mode (absence of electric arcing) using the ACC H-F electrosurgical unit (Erbe, Tübingen, Germany). This is an important practical point in view of the immediate proximity of the left colonic flexure. The peritoneum is then incised with the curved coaxial scissors (p3)

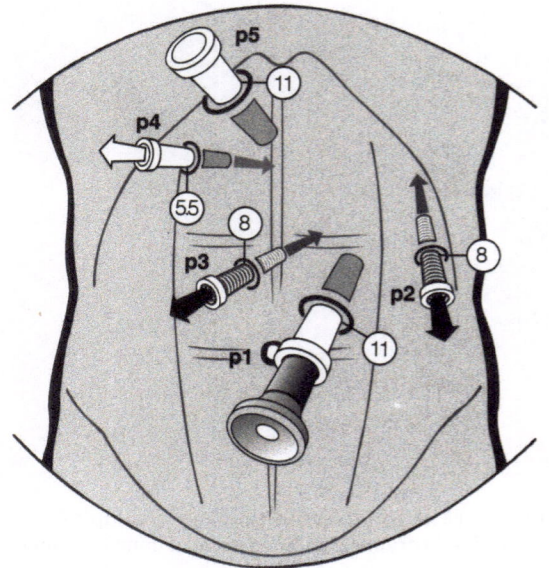

Fig. 11.8. Positions of the cannulae

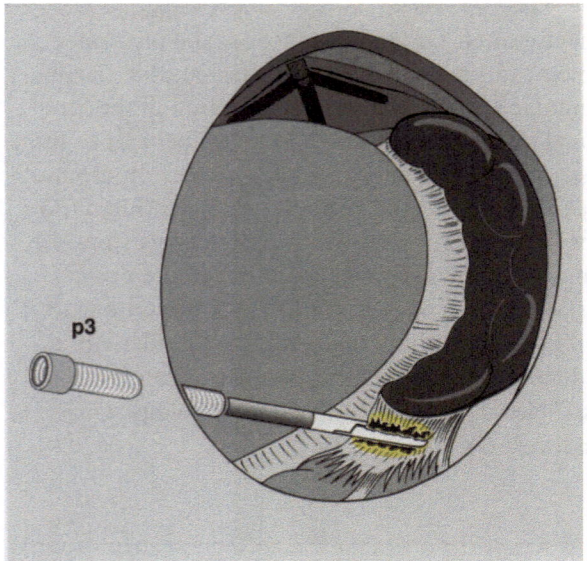

Fig. 11.9. Electrocoagulation of the splenocolic (suspensory) ligament prior to division by scissors. This must be performed in the soft coagulation mode

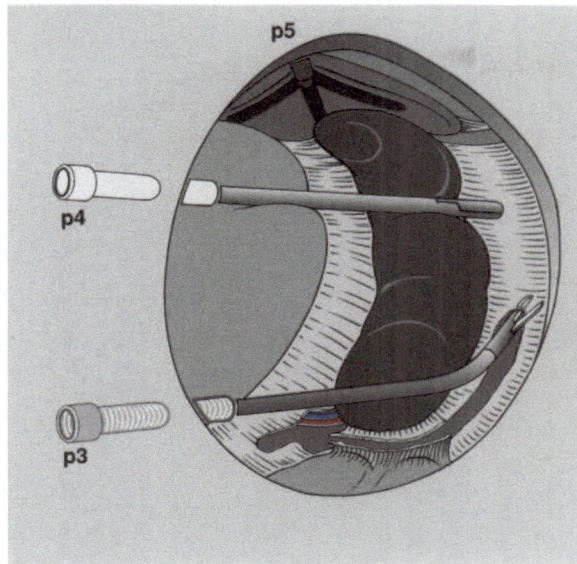

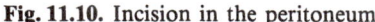

Fig. 11.10. Incision in the peritoneum

Fig. 11.12. Clipping the distal (splenic) ends

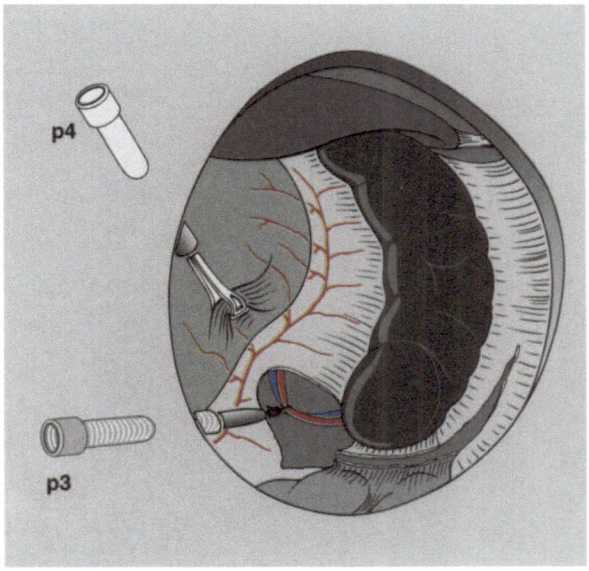

Fig. 11.11. Ligation of vessels to the lower pole (often double) proximally in continuity using Dacron or black silk mounted on a push rod and an external slip knot which is tightened and locked in placed

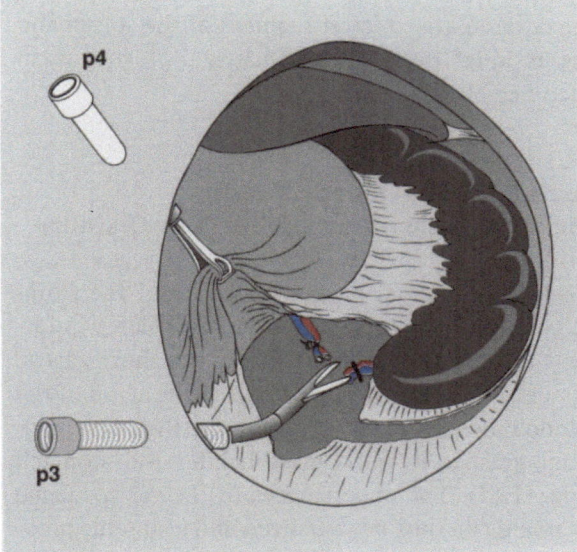

Fig. 11.13. Dividing the vessels with scissors

around the lower pole of the spleen to the back of the organ until the lower limit of the lienorenal ligament and underlying fascia are reached (Fig. 11.10). The vessels to the lower pole (often double) are best individually ligated proximally in continuity using Dacron or black silk mounted on a push rod and an external slip knot (Fig. 11.11): either the Tayside or the Melzer type. The distal (splenic) ends are clipped (Fig. 11.12) and the vessels then divided with scissors (Fig. 11.13). Following division, a clear line of demarcation between

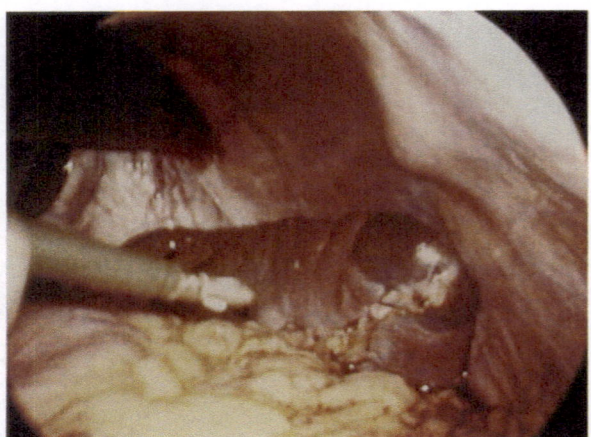

Fig. 11.14. Clear line of demarcation between the devascularized lower segment of the spleen and the residual perfused parenchyma of the organ after division

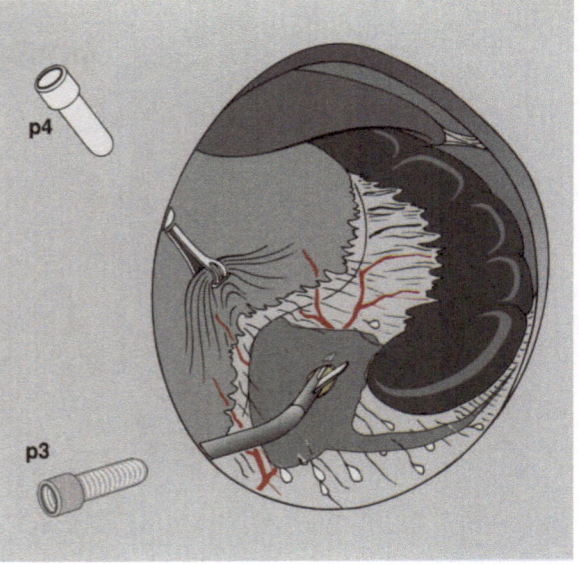

Fig. 11.15. Lifting the proximal greater curvature of the stomach to identify an avascular window near the greater curvature below the short gastric vessels and dividing the peritoneum by the curved coaxial scissors

the devascularized lower segment of the spleen and the residual perfused parenchyma of the organ becomes obvious (Fig. 11.14).

Stapling of Short Gastric Vessels and Detachment of the Gastrosplenic Omentum

Next, the proximal greater curvature of the stomach is lifted up to identify an avascular window near the greater curvature below the short gastric vessels. Following division of the peritoneum of the window by curved coaxial scissors, the curved coaxial grasper is introduced behind the stomach (Fig. 11.15). The undersurface of the gastrosplenic ligament can thus be visualized and a suitable proximal avascular window selected and opened by the coaxial curved scissors (Fig. 11.16). Often avascular adhesions between the posterior surface of the stomach and the pancreas are encountered. These are divided by the scissors until sufficient clearance is achieved. The EndoGIA* with vascular cartridge (USSC, Norwalk, USA) is then introduced with the thinner limb below and the thicker limb above the pedicle which is then stapled and cut as the device is activated (Fig. 11.17). Usually only one application of the Endo GIA* is necessary. Proximally there are deeper short gastric and phrenic vessels (usually two). These should not be included in the endoGIA but are best ligated medially and clipped laterally before being divided (Fig. 11.18).

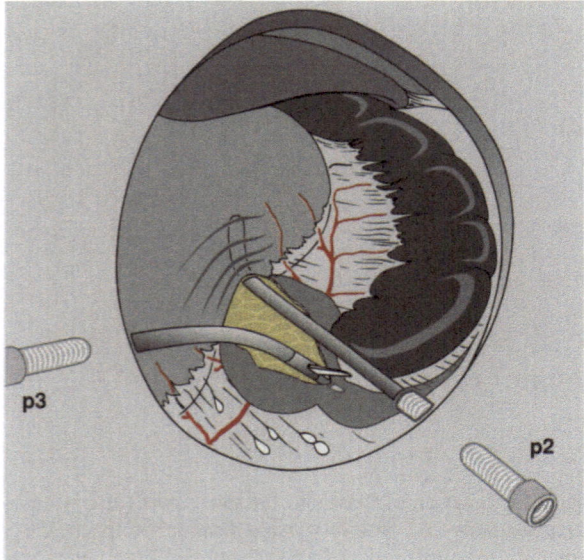

Fig. 11.16. Introducing the curved coaxial grasper (p2) behind the stomach to visualize the undersurface of the gastrosplenic ligament and selecting a suitable proximal avascular window which is opened by the coaxial curved scissors (p3)

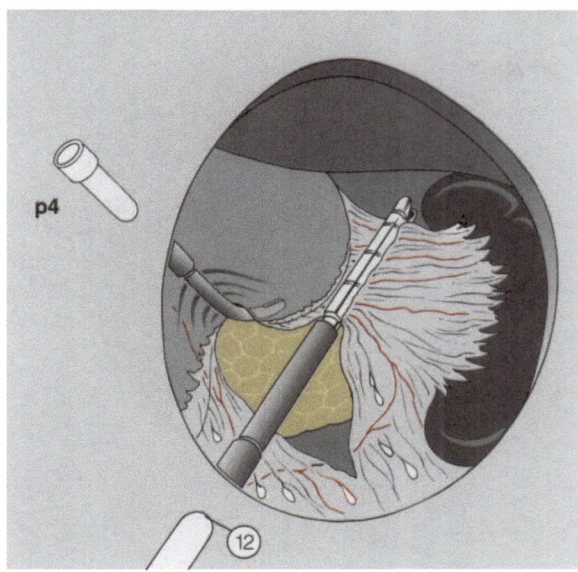

Fig. 11.17. The EndoGIA* with vascular cartridge (USSC, Norwalk, USA) being introduced and the pedicle stapled and cut

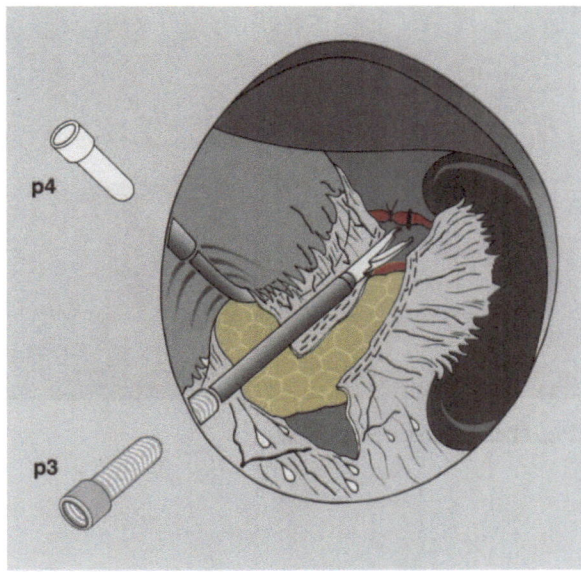

Fig. 11.18. Proximally the deeper short gastric and phrenic vessels are best ligated medially and clipped laterally before being divided

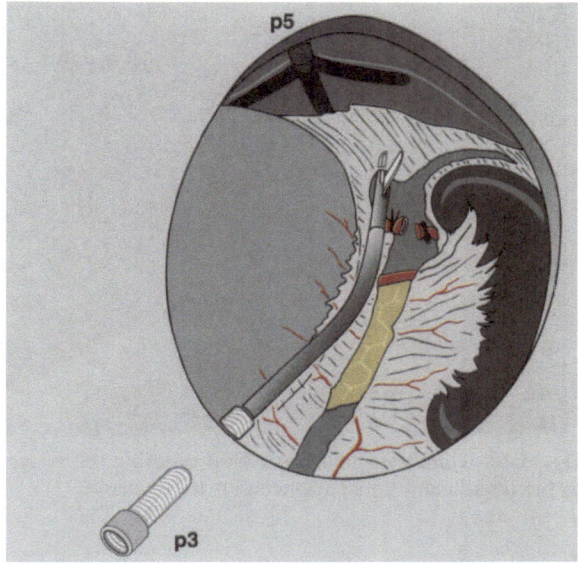

Fig. 11.19. Dividing the peritoneal reflection between the spleen and the oesophagogastric junction and between the upper pole of the organ and the diaphragm by the coaxial curved scissors and extending it around the upper pole exposing the tail of the pancreas and the splenic hilium, and dissecting the tail of the pancreas from the hilium of the spleen to identify the vascular pedicles to the middle and upper splenic segments

Division of the Proximal Gastrosplenicphrenic Peritoneal Reflection and Underlying Fascial Layer with Mobilization of the Upper Pole of the Spleen

The peritoneal reflection between the spleen and the oesophagogastric junction and between the upper pole of the organ and the diaphragm is then divided and extended around the upper pole (Fig. 11.19). The use of the coaxial curved and bayonet scissors is particularly useful during this stage of the operation. The division of the peritoneal fold exposes the fascial layer which binds the spleen to the retroperitoneum. This, too, requires division with scissors. At this stage the right adrenal gland is often identified.

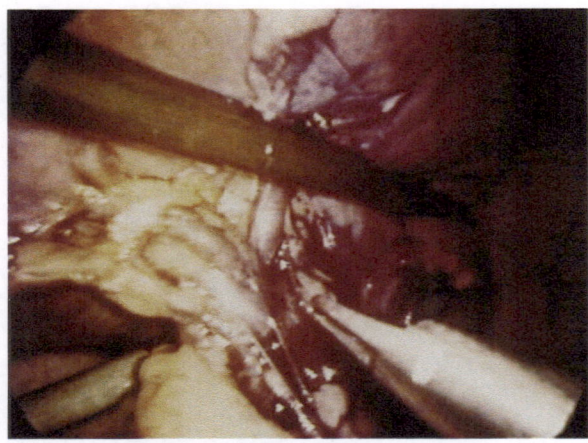

Fig. 11.20. Completed hilar dissection exposing the vessels to the middle and upper segments of the spleen

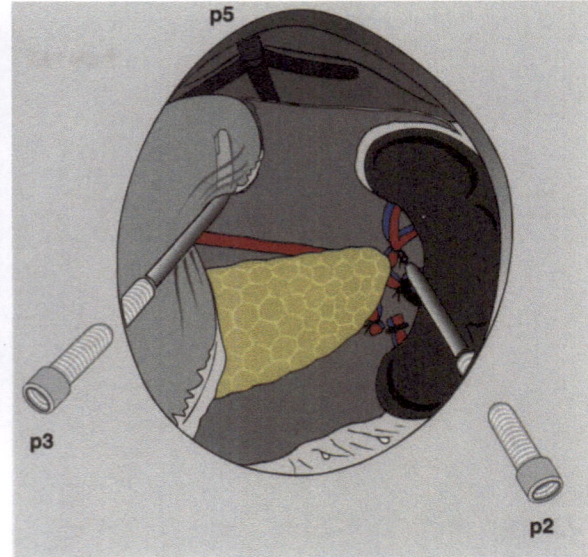

Fig. 11.21. Proximal ligature of the vascular pedicles to the middle and upper segments

Dissection of the Pancreatic Tail to Expose the Vascular Pedicles to the Middle and Upper Splenic Segments

The detachment of the short gastric vessels is followed by retraction of the mobilized upper part of the greater curvature of the stomach upwards and to the right by the assistant. This exposes the tail of the pancreas and the splenic hilium (Fig. 11.19). The dissection of the tail of the pancreas from the hilium of the spleen is necessary to avoid pancreatic injury and to identify the two remaining vascular pedicles to the middle and upper splenic segments (Fig. 11.19). This dissection has to be carried out with extreme care as inadvertent traction avulsion injury to small branches from the splenic vein and artery to the tail of the pancreas may result in substantial bleeding. The dissection of the splenic tail is best carried out by blunt scissors (Fig. 11.20) or ultrasonic dissection. If the latter is used, the machine should be set to deliver a low vibration energy. A combination of both is ideal.

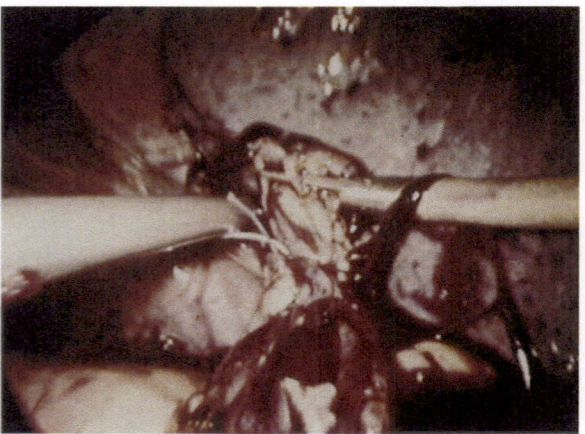

Fig. 11.22. Devascularized spleen

Ligature of Splenic Vessels to Middle and Upper Splenic Segments

Once the vessels to the middle and upper segments have been separated from the tail of the pancreas, they are ligated proximally in continuity using Dacron or black silk mounted on a push rod using an external slip knot (Tayside or Meltzer). If adequate dissection has been carried out, the proximal ligature of these vascular pedicles is straightforward (Fig. 11.21) and when complete, results in uniform dark discolouration of the entire spleen (Fig. 11.22). The distal splenic end of these vascular pedicles is left intact to enable splenic bleeding (see below).

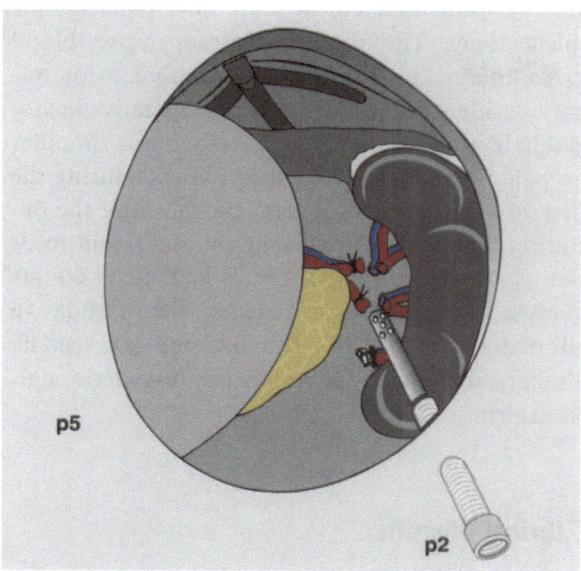

Fig. 11.23. Dividing the vascular pedicles to the middle and upper segments by scissors 1-cm distal to the proximal ligature. The sequestered blood in the splenic parenchyma is sucked from the splenic fossa, which is also irrigated with warm heparinized Hartmann's solution

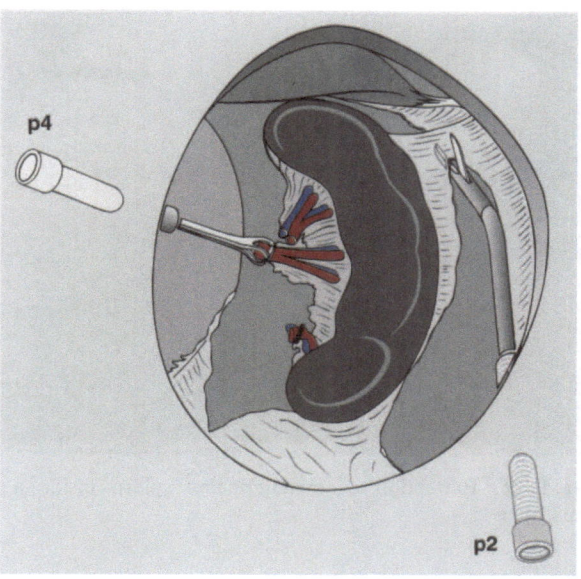

Fig. 11.25. Displacing the shrunken spleen to the right by a Babcock's grasper placed on the splenic hilar vessels and dividing the lienorenal ligament and underlying splenic fascia by scissors, with coagulation of any small bleeders

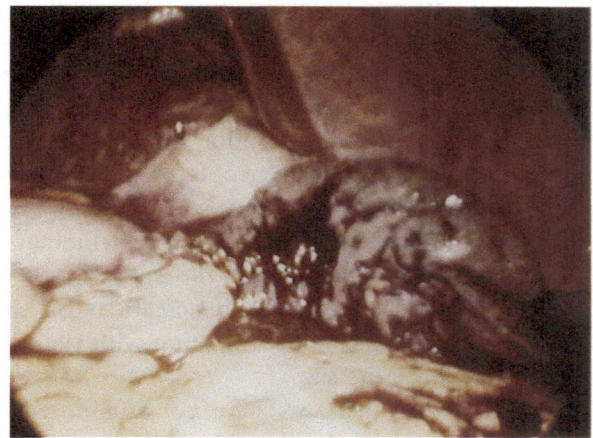

Fig. 11.24. Exsanguinated spleen

Bleeding of the Spleen After Vascular Isolation

A suction/irrigation device is placed in the left hypochondrium in the lateral splenic gutter. The vascular pedicles to the middle and upper segments are then divided by scissors 1 cm distal to the proximal ligature (Fig. 11.23). As the sequestered blood in the splenic parenchyma escapes it is sucked from the splenic fossa. This is also irrigated with warm heparinized Hartmann's solution to prevent clot formation during this process, which is continued until the splenic bleeding has ceased and the area is dry. A 50% reduction of splenic size is obtained by this simple measure (Fig. 11.24). This splenic bleeding is permissible whenever the splenectomy is being carried out for benign disease but is contraindicated if the procedure is being conducted for Hodgkin's lymphoma or other tumours.

Detachment of the Lienorenal Peritoneum and Fascia

The lienorenal ligament and underlying splenic fascia are then divided by scissors with coagulation of any small bleeders. During this stage, the spleen, which is now considerably reduced in size, is displaced to the right by a Babcock's grasper placed on the detached splenic hilium (Fig. 11.25). Separation of the posterior surface of the spleen form the perinephric fat completes the procedure.

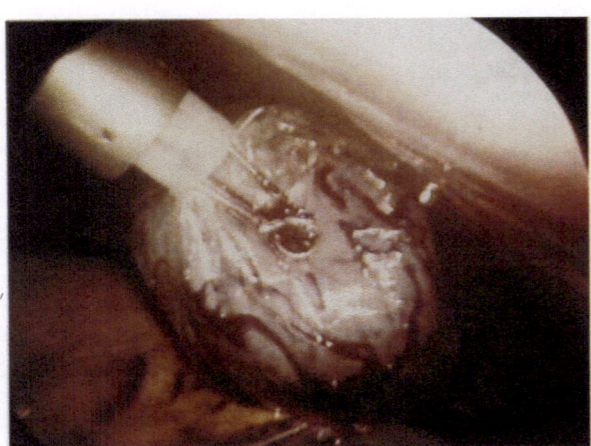

Fig. 11.26. Extraction of exsanguinated spleen inside a laparobag

Prior to extraction, a careful inspection is performed to ensure complete haemostasis and exclude any splenunculi. This is particularly important in patients suffering from ITP.

Extraction of Specimen

The shrunken detached spleen is grasped by the hilar vessels and placed inside a laparobag (Fig. 11.26). The neck of the bag is then exteriorized and the spleen sliced inside the transparent bag using McIndoe scissors, before extraction through a 2.5-cm incision (enlargement and retraction of the left subcostal port). More recently we prefer to use a superelastic shape memory alloy slicer. The mobilized spleen is first gripped inside the wire cage of the slicer and then placed in a sheathed retrieval system manufactured from rip-stop nylon (Cameron Balloons, Bristol, UK). Activation of the slicer results in splenic fillets which are extracted individually through the exteriorized neck of the retrieval system.

Postoperative Management

The patients have done well with no postoperative complications or deaths. Bleeding from traction avulsion of a small venule supplying the pancreatic tail was encountered in our first laparoscopic splenectomy. The resulting intraoperative blood loss amounted to 500 ml and blood transfusion was not considered necessary. The postoperative hemoglobin level in this patient was 10 g. Some shoulder tip pain is experienced by most patients during the first 24 h but all are ambulant the day after the operation. Significant ileus is absent and liquid feeds can usually be started within 24 h. Platelet counts in excess of 300000 are reached by the third day in all patients with ITP. The patients are usually discharged home on the fourth day on enteric coated aspirin.

Clinical Results

Our initial experience has been favourable and free of significant complications. Undoubtedly, the dissection is facilitated by the use of the distally curved coaxial instruments and the ultrasonic dissector. Provided an orderly approach to the operation is adopted, no great technical problems are encountered and with the right instrumentation and endoscopic experience the procedure is straightforward [9]. The most taxing part of the operation is the dissection of the pancreatic tail. The technique of hilar splenic devascularization described above is similar to that used by Carrol et al. [10, 11] and needs to be modified in patients with large spleens. The most important change consists of preliminary identification and ligature of the splenic artery above the upper border of the pancreatic tail. This should result in splenic decongestion with significant reduction in its size.

Contrary to others, we have not administered the pneumococcal polyvalent vaccine in adult patients with ITP as studies from this department have shown minimal if any risk from postsplenectomy sepsis in this group of patients, in contrast to infants, children with thalassaemia, adults with liver disease and lymphomas [4]. Our patients simply carry splenectomy cards and are advised to contact their general practitioners if they develop any fever.

References

1. Oakes DD, Charters AC (1981) Changing concepts in the management of splenic trauma. Surg Gynec Obstet 153:181–185
2. King H, Shumacker HB Jr (1952) Susceptibility to infection after splenectomy performed in infancy. Ann Surg 136:239–242
3. O'Neal BJ, McDonald JC (1981) The risk of sepsis in the asplenic adult. Ann Surg 194:775–778
4. Holdsworth RJ, Irving AD, Cuschieri A (1991) Postsplenectomy sepsis and its mortality rate: actual versus perceived risks. Br J Surg 78:1031–1038
5. Schlaeffer F, Rosenbeck S, Baumgarten-Kleinen A, Crieff Z, Alkan M (1985) Pneumococcal infections among immunized and splenectomized patients in Israel. J Infect 10:38–42
6. Giebink GS, Schiffmann G, Krivit W, Quie PG (1979) Vaccine-type pneumococcal pneumonia. Occurrence after vaccination in an asplenic patient. JAMA 241: 2736–2737
7. Cuschieri A, Shimi S, Banting S, Van Velpen G, Dunkley P (1993) Coaxial curved instruments for minimal access surgery. Surg Endosc (in press)
8. Cuschieri A, Shimi S, Banting S, Van Velpen G (1993) Endoscopic ultrasonic dissection for thoracoscopic and laparoscopic surgery. Surg Endosc (in press)
9. Cuschieri A (1992) Technical aspects of laparoscopic splenectomy: hilar segmental devascularization and instrumentation. J R Coll Surg Edinb (in press)
10. Carroll BJ, Phillips EH, Semel CJ, Fallas M, Morgenstern L (1992) Laparoscopic splenectomy. Surg Endosc 6:183–185
11. Gossot D, Debiolles M, El Meteini M et al (1992) Laparoscopic splenectomy: an experimental study (abstr). Second European Congress of Viscero-synthesis, Luxembourg, 1992

12 Laparoscopic Gastric Procedures

A. CUSCHIERI

Introduction

Elective surgery for peptic ulcer disease has decreased markedly in the last two decades with the introduction of H_2 receptor antagonists [1], although there is now clear evidence that prepyloric ulcers are not controlled by this medication and require surgical treatment [2, 3]. The vast majority of ulcer surgery undertaken nowadays is for acute (perforation and haemorrhage) and chronic complications (stenosis) of ulcer disease although it appears that the number of patients with uncomplicated ulcer disease referred for elective surgical treatment has increased in the last few years due to long-term noncompliance with medication and the advent of laparoscopic surgery. The endoscopic vagotomy procedures of truncal vagotomy, highly selective vagotomy and posterior truncal vagotomy and anterior seromyotomy are covered in Vol. 1, Chap. 20 and 21. The laparoscopic surgical treatment of perforated ulcer disease is outlined in Chap. 22 of the same volume.

Palliative surgery for unresectable gastric cancer yields poor results overall [4], although for antral tumours, a proximal anterior gastroenterostomy does benefit patients with gastric outlet obstruction. The same considerations apply to patients with cancer of the head of the pancreas involving the duodenum and pyloric region. In these patients, the gastroenterostomy is combined with a bilioenteric bypass (Chap. 9, this volume).

Percutaneous gastrostomy is undertaken for patients with bulbar palsy and is most commonly performed endoscopically − percutaneous endoscopic gastrostomy (PEG) [5, 6]. The procedure can be carried out expeditiously by the laparoscopic approach, as can feeding jejunostomy in nutritionally compromised patients.

Preoperative Work-up and Preparation

All the operations are conducted under antibiotic prophylaxis with cephuroxime administered at the time of induction. Chemoprophylaxis against deep vein thrombosis by heparin administered subcutaneously is used in elderly patients and in those suffering from cancer. In addition, these patients should wear graduated antithrombosis stockings. Complete deflation of the stomach by a 16-F Salem sump nasogastric tube attached to a continuous low suction is essential for all gastric laparoscopic procedures.

Anaesthesia

All the gastric operations described in this chapter are performed under general anaesthesia with endotracheal intubation. The exact details and premedication vary with the practice of the anaesthetist.

Patient Positioning and Skin Preparation

For gastric procedures, the anaesthetized patient is placed in the supine position with a head-up tilt. The skin of the entire abdomen is washed with medicated soap (Hibiscrub; ICI, UK) and then disinfected with the disinfectant of choice. The operating field left exposed by the sterile drapes extends from the costal margins to the suprapubic region.

Layout of Ancillary Instruments and Positioning of Staff

During laparoscopic gastric surgery, the surgeon operates mainly from the left side of the operating table with the camera person by his side and the first assistant and the scrub nurse on the right side. A two-monitor visual display is essential. The electrosurgical unit, preferably of the microprocessor controlled type (Erbe; Tübingen, Germany), suction irrigation, insufflator, light source and camera unit are placed on a stack behind the surgeon.

Laparoscopic Witzel Gastrostomy

Instrumentation and Consumables

In addition to the ordinary straight laparoscopic instrumentation, a pair of 5-mm needle holders, rubber-shod suture holder, a 10-mm plastic retraction rod and a straight Duval or Babcock's grasping forceps are needed. A silicon balloon-tipped gastrostomy tube (14–16 F) is used and suturing is performed with 3/0 Polysorb mounted on endoski needles (USSC; Norwalk, USA).

Sites of Trocar and Cannulae

The sites of the access cannulae are shown in Fig. 12.1. The optic is introduced through a subumbilical port (11-mm; p1) to the left of the midline. The two working cannulae (5.5-mm1 p2, p3) are placed along the linea semilunaris, low down at umbilical level. The retracting cannula (10.5-mm; p4) is inserted in the right subcostal region along the anterior axillary line and the assistant's cannula (5.5-mm; p5), used to hold the suture tension, is placed in the left subxiphoid region.

Operative Steps

After the quadrate and left lobe of the liver together with the falciform – round ligament complex are lifted up by the plastic rod, the stomach is grasped along the greater curvature and pulled

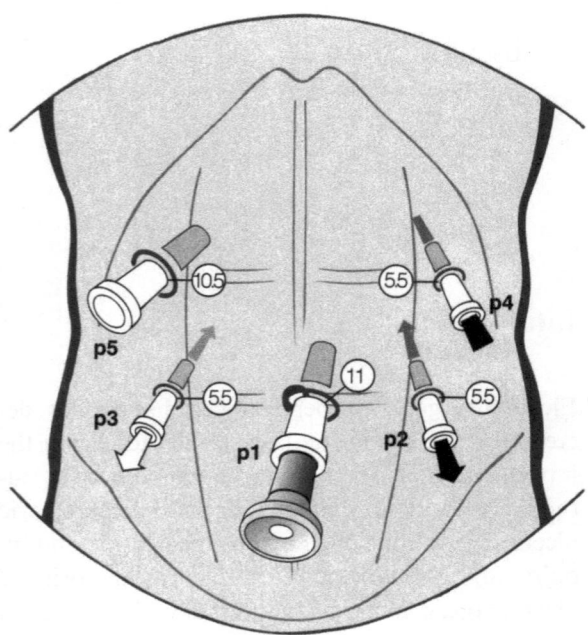

Fig. 12.1. Sites of access port for laparoscopic Witzel gastrostomy

down. Any overlying portion of the greater omentum is displaced to expose the anterior surface of the middle third of the stomach. A longitudinal incision is made halfway between the lesser and greater curvatures using the electrosurgical knife and cutting current until the gastric mucosa is reached. As the upper edge of the cut muscle coat is grasped and tented upwards, the mucosa is opened with electrocutting. Despite this, the cut mucosal edges often bleed. This requires soft coagulation after the bleeding submucosal vessels are grasped with an insulated forceps. The suction device is then inserted inside the lumen and the stomach aspirated. The gastrostomy catheter is inserted through a stab wound in the left hypochondrium, the exact site being determined by the finger depression test. Once inside the peritoneal cavity, it is grasped and pulled further in. The integrity of its balloon is tested before the catheter is inserted through the gastrotomy. A sufficient length of the catheter (at least 7 cm) must be threaded inside the stomach so that its tip lies in the pyloric region and, preferably, in the first part of the duodenum. The position of the catheter tip inside the stomach is easily determined by inflation of the balloon.

The first suture is placed in a purse-string fashion around the entrance of the catheter into the stomach, taking deep seromuscular bites and starting above and behind the tube. Once in position, the suture is tied securely around the tube using a standard internal microsurgical knot. The long limb of the suture is then wound around the tube before being tied again to the tail of the first knot. The inversion of the gastrostomy catheter within the gastric walls is carried out by a continuous suture. Taking deep seromuscular bites, the adjacent gastric wall is picked up on either side of the catheter some 2.5 cm proximal to its entrance into the stomach and the starter knot tied. The stomach walls are then approximated over the tube with continuous suturing towards and 1 cm beyond the gastrostomy site, with tension being held on the suture line by the assistant using a rubber-shod suture holder. Once the catheter and the gastrostomy site have been oversewn completely, the end of the suture is tied using an Aberdeen knot. Alternatively, the suture is tied to the long limb of an anchoring knot introduced and tied by the surgeon as the assistant maintains tension on the suture line. At the end of this stage of the operation, the gastrostomy site and the adjacent section of the catheter are buried within the gastric walls (Fig. 12.2).

Traction applied to the external section of the tube should approximate the "gastric tube" to the anterior abdominal wall without tension. At the stage of the operation, it may be necessary to reduce the intra-abdominal pressure to facilitate this approximation.

Fixation of the Witzel's gastrostomy tube to the anterior abdominal wall around the exit site of the catheter can be performed either by internal or external suturing.

Internal Technique

In the internal technique the preformed Dundee jamming loop starter knot tied at the end of the atraumatic sutures is employed. After fashioning the starter jamming loop knot, the suture is introduced through a reducer tube and then passed through the anterior abdominal wall behind the exit site of the catheter. It is then inserted through the corresponding side of the gastric tube, taking a

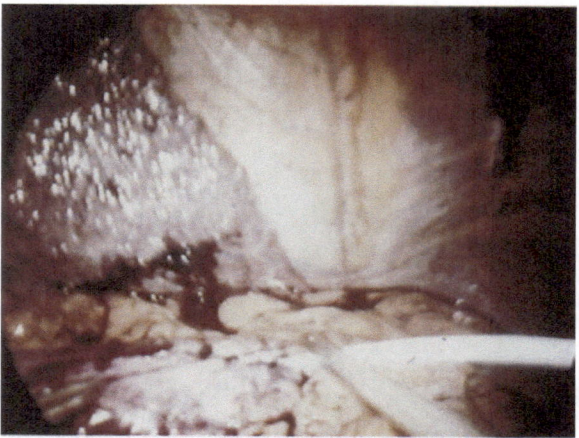

Fig. 12.2. Completed oversewing of the gastrostomy catheter

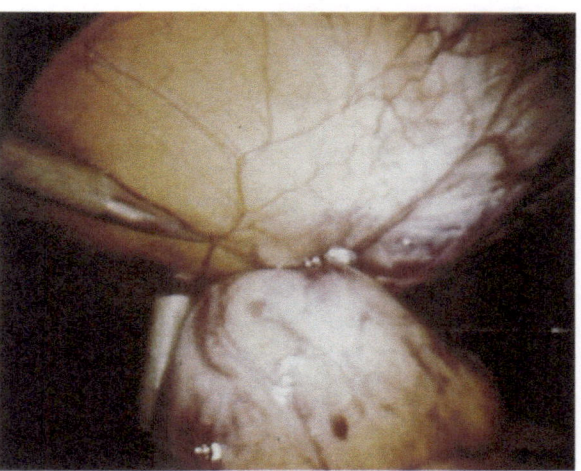

Fig. 12.3. Completed approximation of the gastric tube behind the catheter

deep seromuscular bite. After the needle holder is passed through the loop, it is used to grab the standing part of the suture which is withdrawn through the loop before the loop is slipped and locked from the tail. After completion of the approximation of the stomach tube behind the catheter (Fig. 12.3), an identical suture is inserted to approximate the stomach tube in front of the gastrostomy catheter.

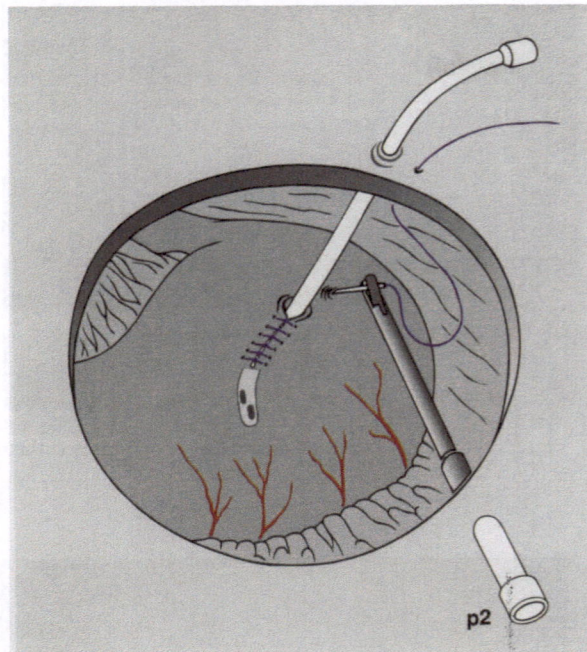

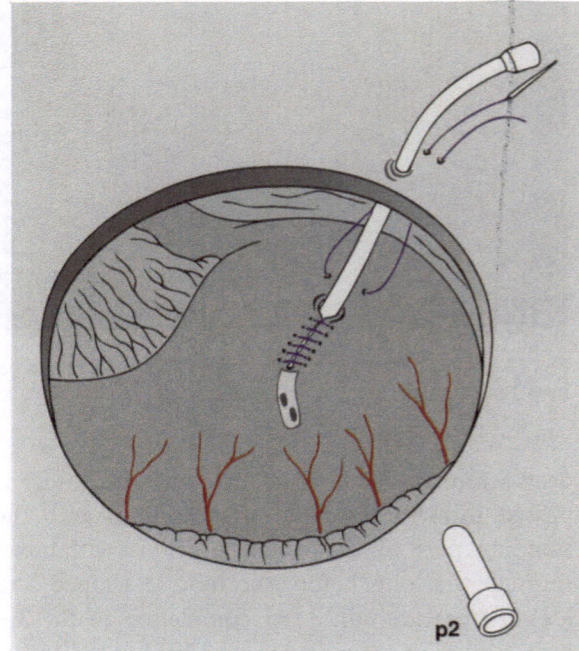

Fig. 12.4 a, b. External fixation of the gastric tube to the anterior abdominal wall. **a** The straight 60-mm needle is passed through the abdominal wall behind the catheter into the peritoneal cavity. **b** The suture is inserted through the stomach tube behind the catheter and then exteriorized

External Technique

Two atraumatic sutures mounted on a straight 60-mm needle are used. After the skin incision admitting the gastrostomy catheter is enlarged (2 cm), the needle is passed through the subcutaneous and muscular layers behind the catheter into the peritoneal cavity where it is grasped by the needle holder. The needle is then passed through the stomach tube behind the catheter (Fig. 12.4a) before its direction is changed such that the tip impinges on the abdominal wall close to the initial entrance site (Fig. 12.4b). The needle is then passed through the abdominal wall, from inside out, using the following technique: as one needle holder is placed halfway along the needle to maintain its direction, the second holder is applied further distally and is used to drive the needle through the parieties. Once the needle has been exteriorized, the two ends of the suture are held in a Spencer Wells forceps. An equivalent suture is placed in front of the catheter after which the two sutures are tied, thereby approximating the stomach tube to the entry site. The edges of the skin wound are then approximated by absorbable sutures.

Feeding Jejunostomy

There are two techniques which can be used for the laparoscopic construction of a feeding jejunostomy. One approach consits of nontunnelled intubation of an upper jejunal loop with fixation of the loop to the abdominal wall by external sutures [7] or by a kit employing the use of four T fasteners around the jejunostomy catheter. The alternative, favoured by the author, is a tunneled Witzel-type feeding jejunostomy. There are no published comparative studies between the two methods. The externally fixed nontunnelled techniques are quicker but the tunnelled jejunostomy provides a greater safety margin against catheter dislodgement.

Laparoscopic Nontunnelled Externally Fixed Jejunostomy

Sites of Trocar and Cannulae

The three cannulae (one 10.5-mm for the optic; p1 and two 5.5-mm for atrumatic gasping forceps and needle holders; p2, p3) are placed as shown in Fig. 12.5.

Operative Steps

With the patient in the reversed Trendlenburg position, the upper jejunum is exposed by lifting the left half of the transverse colon. The jejunum is grasped and followed proximally until the ligament of Trietz is identified. The loop is selected (usually some 50 cm from the duodenojejunal flexure). The appropriate external site of the jejunostomy is then selected by finger depression. The position of this should ensure that the jejunal loop can be brought to the anterior abdominal wall without any tension. The site is marked by a small skin stab wound. At this stage, air is insufflated through a nasogastric tube to distend the upper jejunal loops. This facili-

tates the subsequent steps, including the insertion of the jejunostomy catheter.

Fixation of the selected loop can be effected in two ways:

1. The simplest is the use of three external atraumatic monofilament stay sutures mounted on a 60-mm straight needle. The needle is introduced through the abdominal wall. It is then grasped by a needle holder and passed through the seromuscular wall of the bowel before it is reversed and exteriorized. Three such sutures are placed equidistant from each other and from the site of the proposed jejunostomy on the antimesenteric border of the selected jejunal loop. Each stay suture is held by small artery forceps until the jejunostomy tube is in place.
2. The other method employs the use of four Brown/Mueller T fasteners. Each of these is preloaded inside a slotted needle which is inserted through the parieties into the jejunal lumen. At this point, the T fastener is advanced and the needle withdrawn. Traction on the T fastener approximates the bowel lumen to the anterior abdominal wall (Fig. 12.6). Four such T fasteners are placed in a rectangular configuration around the proposed jejunostomy site.

The next step consists of the insertion of the jejunostomy catheter using commercially available needle jejunostomy kits (e. g. Vivonex). These have three components: (1) 18-gauge needle and J-guide wire, (2) introducer peel-away sheath with an internal dilator and (3) J-jejunostomy tube (8 – 12 F). The 18-gauge needle attached to an air-filled syringe is inserted percutaneously (through the previously created stab wound) into the bowel in the selected area of the antimesenteric aspect of the jejunal loop (at the centre of the area marked by the three external sutures or the four T fasteners). Air is injected into the jejunal loop to confirm the intralumenal position of the needle tip. The guidewire is then passed through the needle into the jejunum when the needle is removed. The introducer/dilator is then passed over the guidewire well into the jejunal lumen. Thereafter, the guidewire and the dilator are removed, leaving the peel-away introducer sheath. The jejunostomy catheter is then passed into the distal limb of the jejunum for at

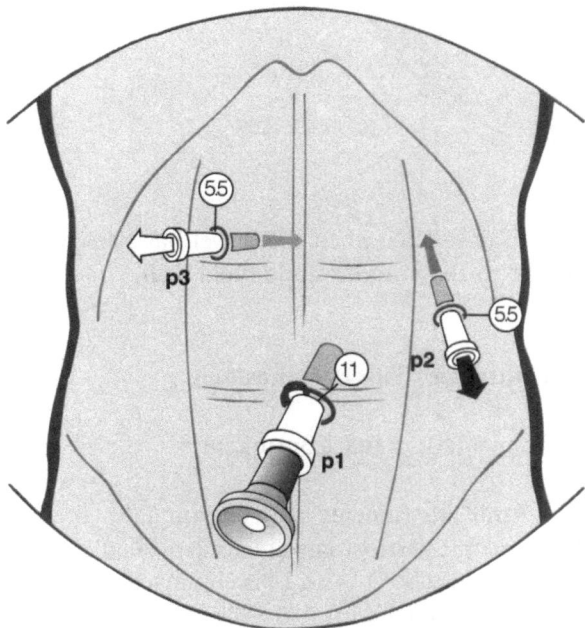

Fig. 12.5. Sites of trocar and cannulae for nontunnelled jejunostomy

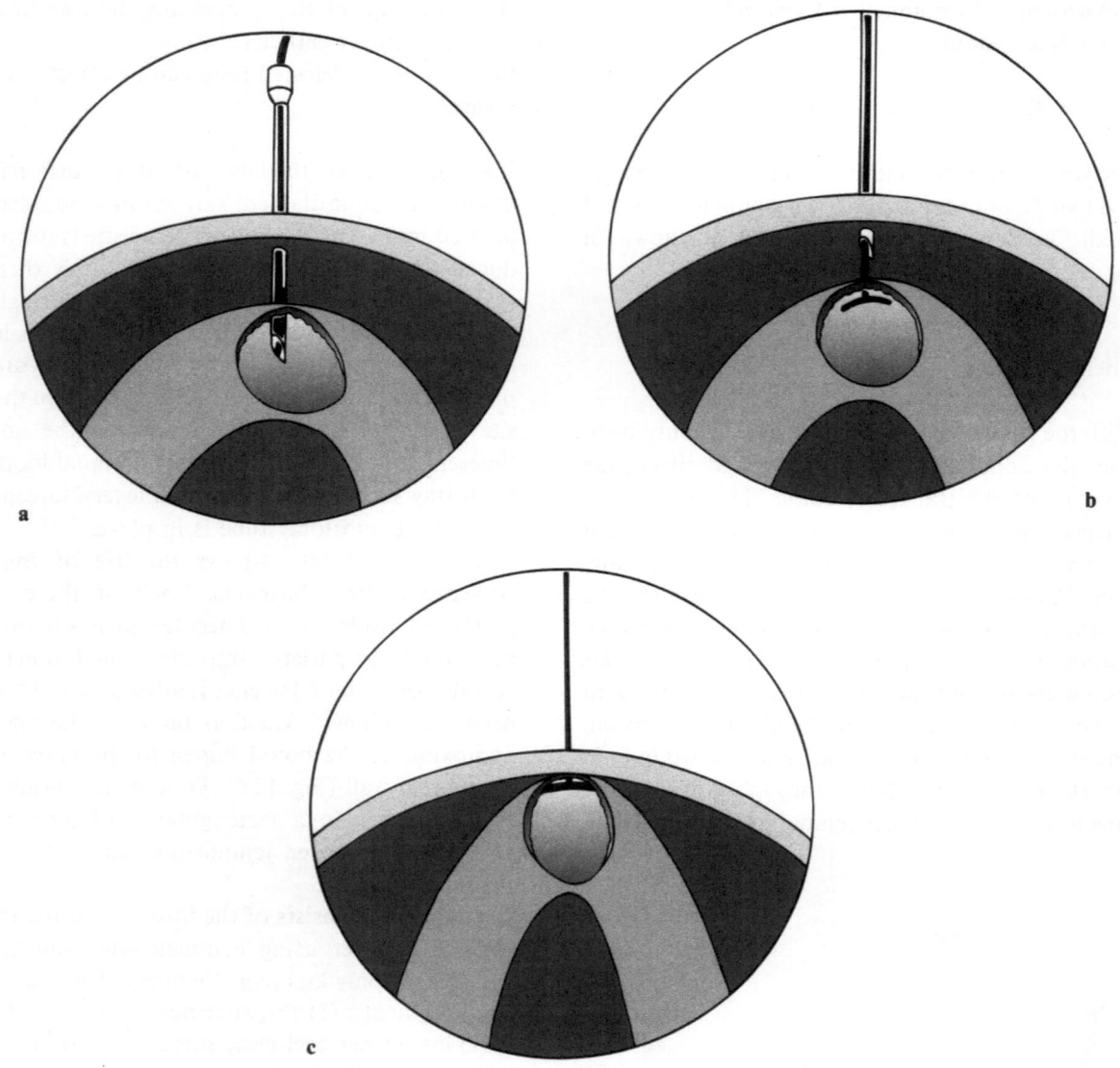

Fig. 12.6a–c. The mechanism of T fasteners. Once inside the lumen of the bowel, the T fastener is advanced as the needle is withdrawn. Traction on the T fastener approximates the bowel lumen to the anterior abdominal wall

10–14 days later when the bowel has become adherent to the anterior abdominal wall.

least 10 cm and the jejunostomy sheath peeled away.

The next step consists in the approximation of the bowel around the jejunostomy site either by tying the three external sutures or by sliding the nylon washer and then crimping the aluminium ring to hold the T fasteners in position. The jejunostomy catheter is then sutured to the adjacent skin. The jejunal fixation sutures or the T fasteners are cut

Laparoscopic Witzel Jejunostomy

Instrumentation and Consumables

The same instruments and consumables used in laparoscopic gastrostomy are needed. A silicon balloon-tipped tube (14–16 F) is employed and suturing is performed with 3/0 Polysorb (USSC; Norwalk, USA) or Vicryl (Ethicon; Edinburgh, UK) mounted on endoski needles.

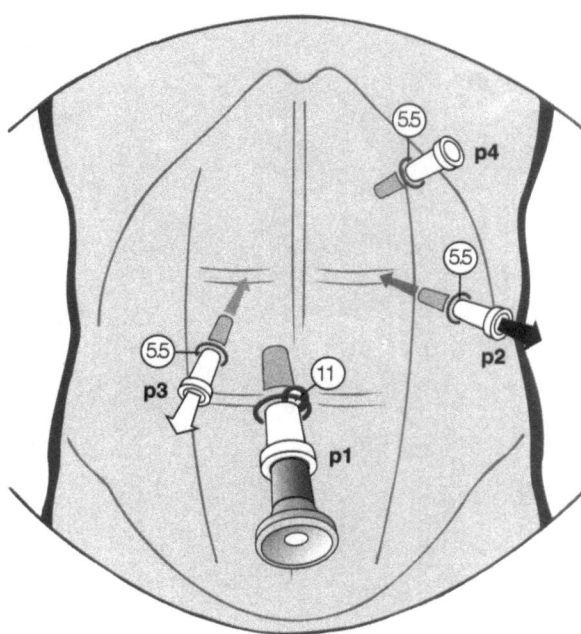

Fig. 12.7. Sites of access ports for laparoscopic Witzel feeding jejunostomy

Sites of Trocar and Cannulae

The sites of the four access cannulae are shown in Fig. 12.7. The optic is introduced through a subumbilical port (11-mm; p1) to the right of the midline. The two working cannulae (5.5-mm; p2, p3) are placed along the linea semilunaris, low down at umbilical level. The assistant's cannula (5.5-mm; p5) is positioned in the left subxiphoid region.

Operative Steps

The initial step consists in the selection of the appropriate loop of upper jejunum. For this purpose, the left half of the transverse colon is grasped and lifted up by the assistant, whilst the upper jejunal loops are followed up by the surgeon using two atraumatic graspers to the ligament of Trietz. A loop some 60–80 cm from the duodenojejunal flexure is selected and its easy approximation to the anterior abdominal wall of the left upper quadrant ascertained. After selection of the appropriate site, determined by the finger depression test, a full-thickness incision is made with a pointed scalpel and the jejunostomy catheter introduced into the

peritoneal cavity by means of a Spencer Wells forceps. A purse-string seromuscular suture (circle diameter of 1–1.5 cm) is placed on the antimesenteric aspect of the jejunal loop using 2/0 Polysorb or Vicryl mounted on an endoski needle. The bowel is then opened inside the purse-string by the electrosurgical hook knife and the catheter introduced into the jejunal lumen for a distance of 10–12 cm), after which the purse-string suture is tied securely using an internal microsurgical knot with two 5-mm needle holders. The long limb of the suture is then wound around the tube before being tied again. The extraluminal section of the jejunostomy tube over a distance of 3 cm and the enterostomy site are then buried underneath adjacent jejunal walls using a continuous suturing technique as previously described in the section on gastrostomy.

Fixation of the jejunostomy to the anterior abdominal wall around the exit site of the catheter is performed either by internal or external suturing, also as described in the gastrostomy section.

Vagotomy and Antrectomy for Prepyloric Ulcer Disease

The advent of laparoscopic surgery has resulted in a confused situation with regard to the elective surgical management of patients with intractable duodenal ulcer disease. Aside from the exact indications for surgical treatment, various procedures are being advocated, sometimes disregarding the results of past, well-conducted clinical trials on the efficacy and adverse sequelae of some of the procedures [7]. In this respect, there is no doubt that the operation of bilateral truncal vagotomy with pyloric dilatation is an untested procedure whether it is performed laparoscopically, thoracoscopically or by the open approach.

Previous reported surgical studies indicate that the best overall clinical outcome of patients with uncomplicated duodenal ulceration is obtained by the operation of parietal cell vagotomy with preservation of the nerve supply to the antrum. This can be performed either by the classical highly selective vagotomy (HSV) technique [8, 9] or by posterior truncal vagotomy and anterior seromyotomy [10–12]. Both these operations, which give equivalent results [13], can now be conducted expeditiously by the laparoscopic approach [14]. The operation of posterior truncal vagotomy and anterior HSV first described by Hill et al. [15] can also be performed laparoscopically [16] although there are no large long-term studies of the efficacy of this procedure.

All the above operations are accompanied by unacceptably high nonhealing and recurrence rates in patients with prepyloric ulcers [3] for which the only effective surgical management is bilateral truncal vagotomy and antrectomy.

Instrumentation and Consumables

The operation of bilateral truncal vagotomy and antrectomy is both tedious and protracted if straight laparoscopic instruments are employed. The use of the curved coaxial instruments greatly expedites the procedure. Other requirements include: plastic retraction rod, a pair of 5-mm needle holders, rubber-shod or diamond-coated suture grasper and atraumatic 3/0 sutures (absorbable or nonabsorbable) mounted on endoski needles. The author's preference is for Polysorb (USSC), although coated Vicryl also handles well. If nonabsorbable sutures are used, silk is much easier to use laparoscopically than polyamide. Other consumables include, Foley catheter, endoloops (Surgitie, USSC, or Ethibinder, Ethicon) and the EndoGIA* (USSC). Both blue and white cartridges are needed.

The stomach is kept decompressed by low suction attached to a 16-F Salem sump nasogastric tube.

Sites of Trocar and Cannulae

The sites and types of access ports are shown in Fig. 12.8. The optical (11-mm; p1) cannula is placed in the immediate subumbilical region and the two operating cannulae (flexible metal 8-mm; p2, p3) along the linea semilunaris at the level of the umbilicus. One 15-mm cannulae is inserted in each subcostal region. They are used for the introduction of the EndoGIA stapler. The right subcostal cannula is also employed to retract the left lobe of

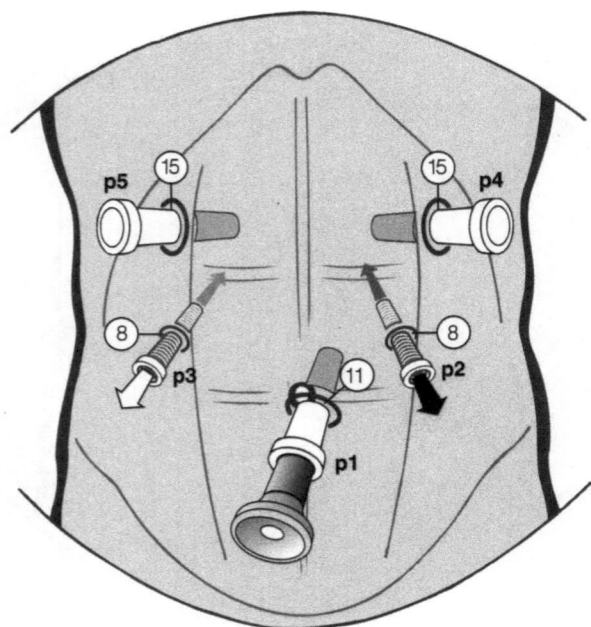

Fig. 12.8. Sites of access ports for bilateral truncal vagotomy and antrectomy

the liver and as the assistant's grasping/holding cannula (with 5.5-mm reducer).

Operative Steps

Exposure of the Hiatus and Truncal Vagotomy

A falciform – round ligament sling is inserted to elevate the central portion of the liver. The black plastic rod is then introduced through the right subcostal port and used to elevate the left lobe of the liver and thus expose the oesophageal hiatus. The bilateral truncal vagotomy is carried out first using the technique described in Vol. 1, Chap. 20. Complete dissection of the oesophagus and division of all accessory vagal branches including the nerves of Grassi is important to ensure a complete vagotomy.

Indentification and Marking of the Pylorus

The identification of the pylorus is essential and should be the next step. It is marked by a suture on its anterior surface. If the surgeon overlooks this measure, he will encounter problems during the antrectomy, when as a result of oozing, determination of the distal limit of the resection becomes difficult and he then incurs a real risk of either leaving antral tissue behind or resecting an excessive segment of the first part of the duodenum, rendering the anastomosis difficult.

Antral Mobilization

The mobilization of the stomach is commenced at the junction of the upper with the lower third of the organ by ligature and division of one or two vessels supplying the greater curvature from the gastroepiploic arcade. These vessels are surrounded by fat and therefore cannot be secured safely by clips. The author's technique for securing these vessels before their division entails ligation of the distal end in continuity with chromic catgut using a Roeder or Melzer knot. A curved grasper is then passed inside a preformed chromic catgut endoloop and applied to the vessel close to its origin from the gastro-epiploic arcade (Fig. 12.9). The vessel is then divided between the grasper and the proximal tie. The endoloop is positioned and tightened on the vessel behind the grasper before this is released.

The stomach is then elevated with the curved coaxial grasper and any adhesions between its posterior surface and the pancreas are divided by the curved coaxial scissors. As the stomach is held tented upwards, the EndoGIA* (loaded with white cartridge) is introduced through the left subcostal cannula; the open limbs of the stapler are placed on either side of the greater omentum and then approximated close to the greater curvature before the device is fired. The process is repeated until the right gastroepiploic artery its accompanying vein are reached. The proximal ends of these vessels (Fig. 12.10) are best ligated in continuity with silk or Dacron using an external slip knot of the Tayside or Melzer type. The distal end is secured by an endoloop inside a curved grasper as described above.

The curved duck-bill forceps is then passed behind the stomach and used to push and tent the lesser omentum forwards (Fig. 12.11). This is divided with scissors through its avascular section from the duodenum to the O-G junction. An anomalous hepatic artery arising from the left gastric may be encountered in some patients. This should be pre-

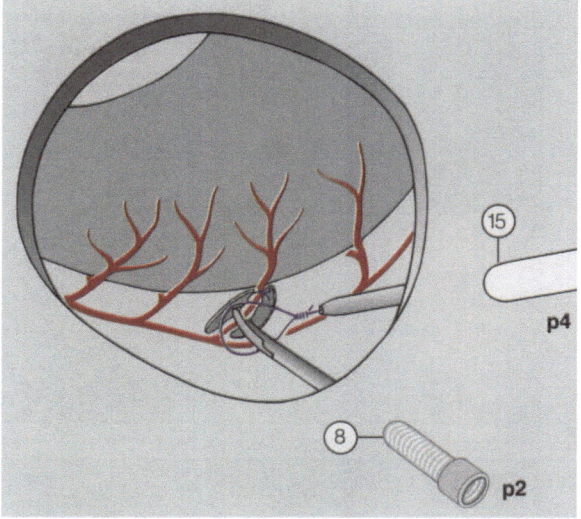

Fig. 12.9. Technique for securing vessels to the greater curvature of the stomach

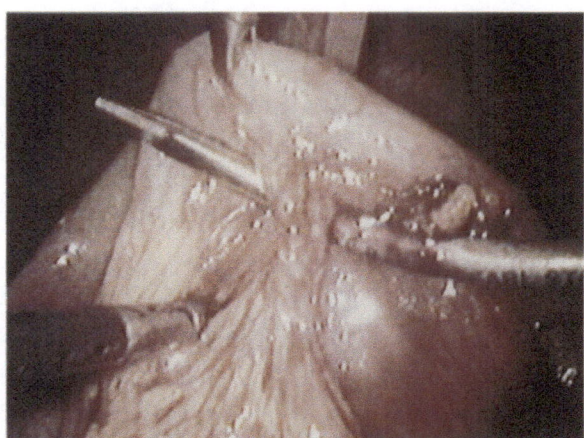

Fig. 12.10. Curved coaxial duckbill grasper around the right gastroepiploic artery and vein prior to their ligation

served if at all possible. The left gastric vessels are suture ligated close to the mobilized lesser curvature 1 cm proximal to the proposed transection line. For this purpose, a 3/0 silk suture mounted on an endoski needle is passed through the serosa of the lesser curvature and then tied over the vessels using a standard microsurgical knot. The right gastric artery is also suture ligated in continuity with 3/0 black silk at the proximal end using a similar technique. A clip is placed on the vessel close to the antrum before the artery is divided. This completes the mobilization of the distal stomach (Fig. 12.12).

Transection and Stapling

The extent of stapling of the proximal end depends on the type of reconstruction intended. For Billroth I procedures, the EndoGIA* stapler 3.0 cm or powered 6.0 cm type (with blue cartridges) introduced through the left subcostal cannula is applied from the lesser curve side slightly obliquely and with the ends of the stapler limbs some 2.5–3 cm from the lesser curve, the exact distance depending on the width of the first part of the duodenum (Fig. 12.13a). The stapler is then fired (Fig. 12.13b). With the 3.0 cm stapler two overlapping applications are needed to reach the appropriate distance. If a Polya-type reconstruction is intended, the proximal stapling is continued until the stomach is stapled and transected in a slightly oblique fashion from the lesser to the greater curvature. Usually two stapler applications suffice but sometimes three are needed. Thereafter, the left lobe of the liver is allowed to drop down on the proximal stomach and the plastic rod used to elevate the right lobe of the liver to expose the antroduodenal segment.

The technique of duodenal transection also varies with the type of anastomosis which is intended. For a Polya or end-to-side Billroth I anastomosis, the duodenum is completely stapled and transected with the EndoGIA* (with blue cartridges) just distal to the pylorus.

For gastroduodenal reconstructions (end-to-end or end-to-side), the proximal gastric resection line extends from the stapled proximal part of the stomach vertically down to the greater curvature. This division of the stomach walls is performed with the L-shaped electrosurgical hook-knife using cutting current. Often, submucosal vessels bleed. These are grasped by an insulated duck-bill forceps and electrocoagulated. If an end-to-end gastroduodenal anastomosis is intended, both distal and proximal resection lines are effected with electrosurgical cutting.

A laparobag is introduced through the left 12-mm subcostal cannula and the detached antrum placed inside the bag. Extraction of the antrum is best delayed until the continuity of the gastrointestinal tract has been restored.

12.11a

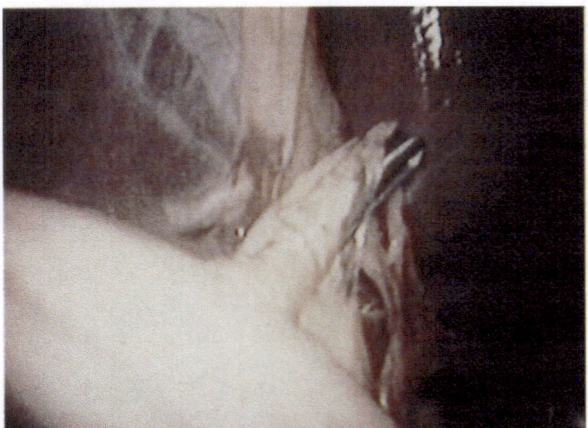

b

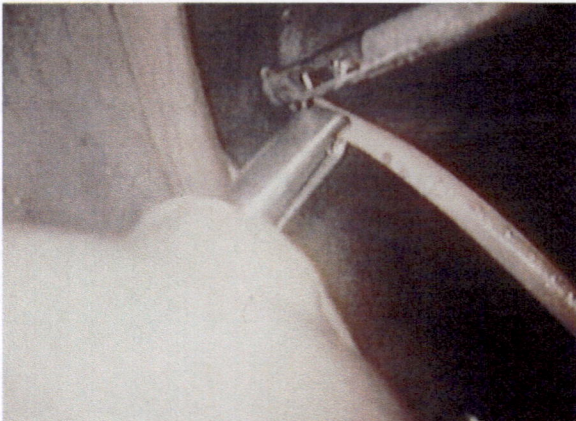

12.12

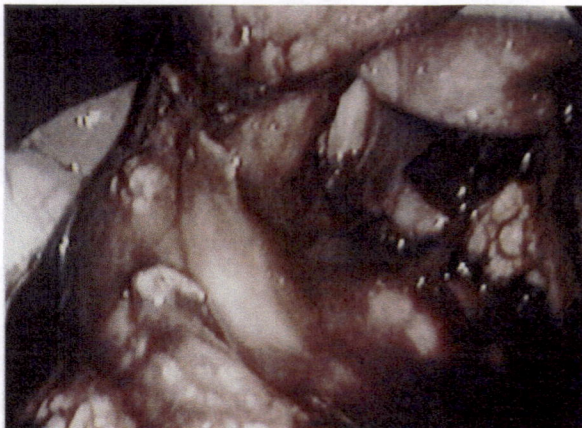

Fig. 12.11a, b. Curved duck-bill grasper passed behind the stomach and used to tent the lesser omentum

Fig. 12.12. Completed mobilization of the antrum

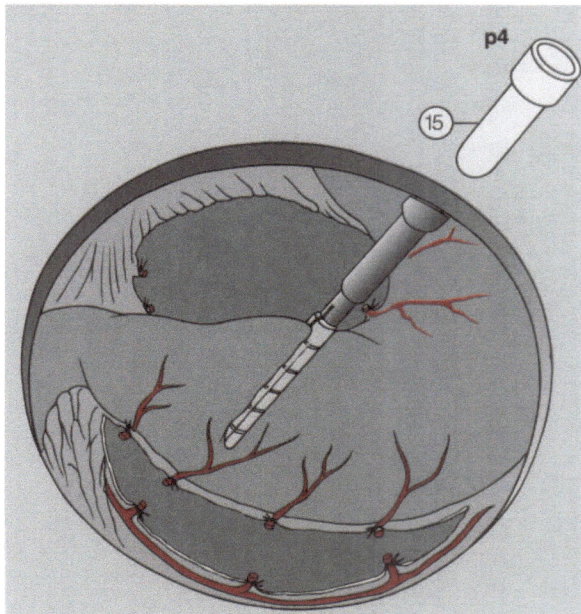

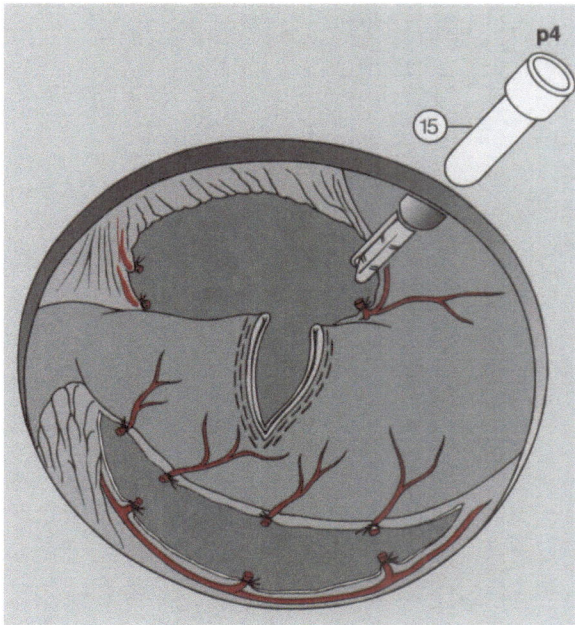

Fig. 12.13 a, b. Proximal partial transection for Billroth I procedures. **a** The EndoGIA* 60 mm stapler is applied from the lesser curve side in an oblique fashion across the stomach some 2.5 – 3 cm from the lesser curve. **b** When the stapler is fired, the stomach is stapled and transected for part of the distance between the lesser and greater curvatures

Anastomosis

Polya antecolic anastomosis. Polya antecolic anastomosis is the easiest type and is performed using the EndoGIA* (with blue cartridges). An upper jejunal loop some 40 – 50 cm from the ligament of Trietz is selected and brought up by the assistant with an atraumatic grasper to the stapled body of the stomach such that the efferent loop lies near the lesser curvature. A 3/0 deep seromuscular suture is passed through the upper antimesenteric corner of the jejunum and then through the anterior wall of the stomach just proximal to the stapled line and close to the lesser curve. The suture is tied, using an internal microsurgical knot, and cut. A corresponding suture is placed at the opposite end close to the greater curvature. After tying, this suture is left uncut (Fig.12.14a). As traction is maintained on the tail of lower corner suture, an opening is made with the electrosurgical hook knife in the lower end of the aligned jejunal loop and in the adjacent stomach proximal to the corner knot (Fig. 12.14b). The stapler limbs of the 6.0 cm powered stapler are introduced into the jejunal and gastric lumens, respectively, their ends lifted anteriorly and then approximated. If the position of the opposed limbs of the stapler is judged to be correct, the instrument is fired and then released. If a 3.0 cm stapler is used the second application of the stapler overlaps the first by about 1 cm. Again after ensuring correct application, the instrument is fired and then released. On completion, the anterior wall of the anastomosis is lifted up to inspect the interior and exclude mucosal bridges, which are cut with scissors if present. The defect at the lower end is closed with a running deep seromuscular suture using the lower corner suture, which is carried upwards until the stapler line is reached. The suturing is terminated by an Aberdeen knot or tied to a separate anchor knot.

End-to-Side Billroth I Gastroduodenal Anastomosis. The end-to-side Billroth I anastomosis is fashioned along an oblique line running from the top stapled corner of the duodenal stump to the upper aspect of the anterior wall of the second part of this organ. A hand suturing technique is used. The upper corner seromuscular suture is passed through the stomach and then the duodenum medi-

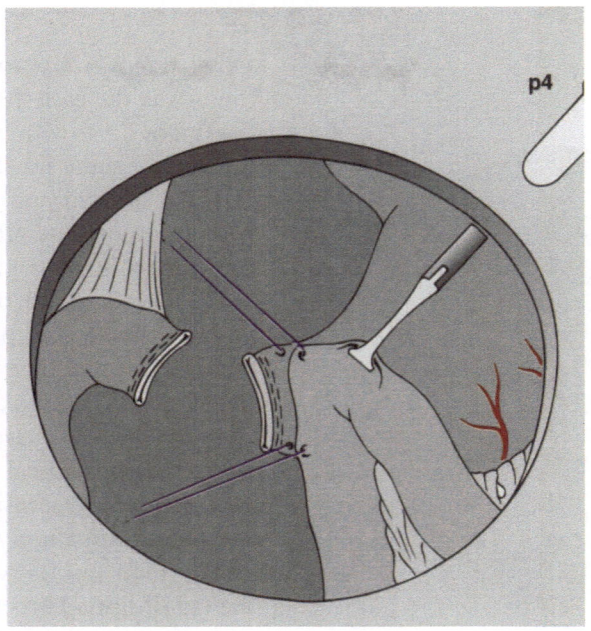

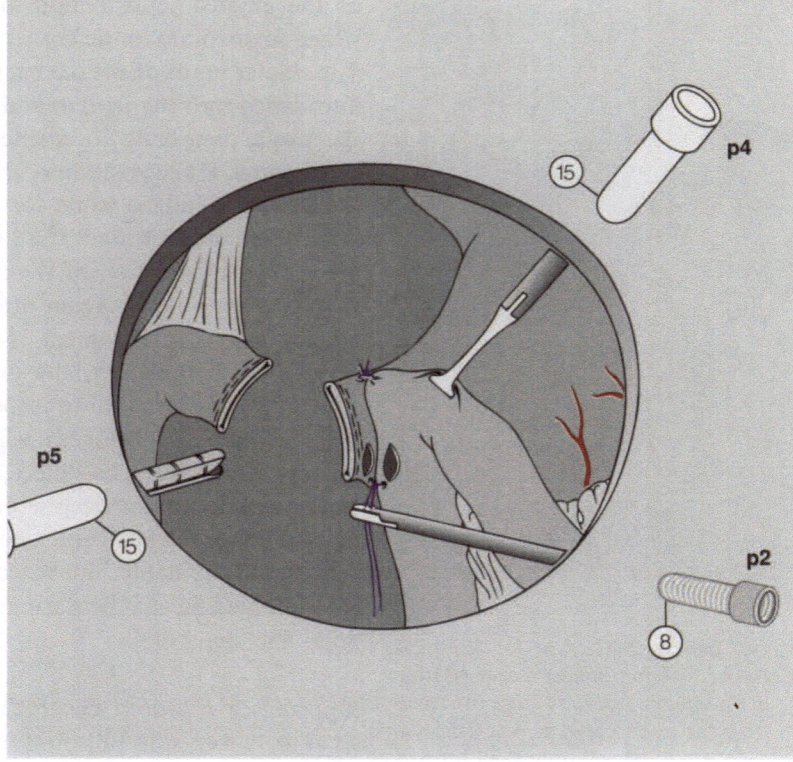

Fig. 12.14a, b. Polya antecolic reconstruction. **a** The selected jejunal loop is aligned along the stapled body of the stomach by two stay sutures, which are tied. **b** Openings are made in the lower end of the aligned jejunal loop and in the adjacent stomach

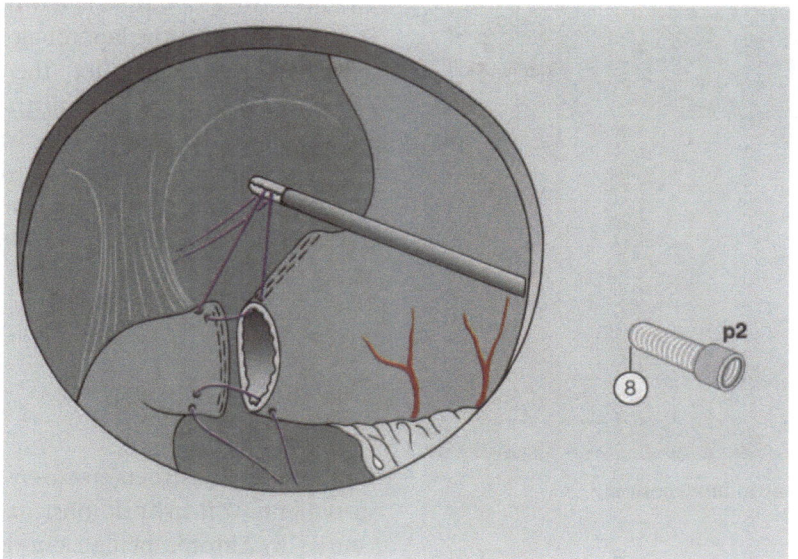

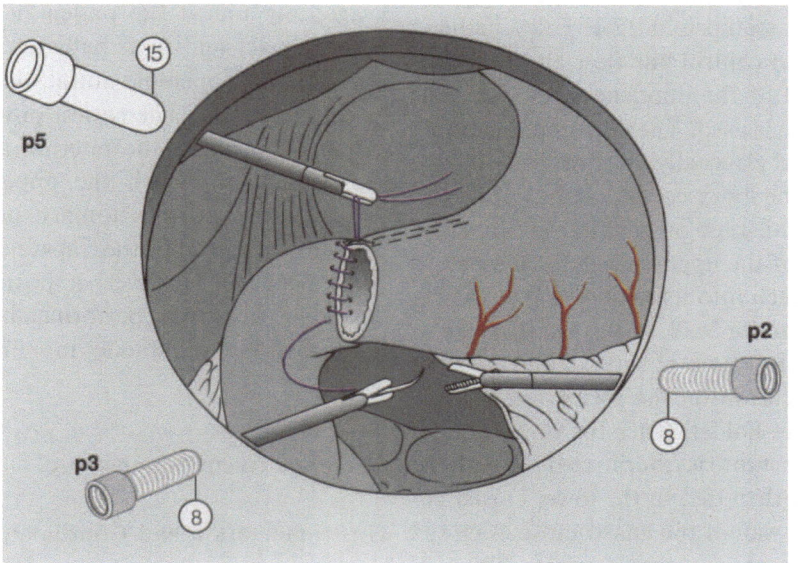

Fig. 12.15 a, b. End-to-side Billroth I gastroduodenal anasto-mosis. **a** Proximal and distal corner seromuscular sutures. **b** Running posterior suture line using deep seromuscular bites

al to the upper end of the stapled line and tied (Fig. 13.15 a). A corresponding corner suture is placed at the lower end and after it is tied, the tail is grasped by the assistant to align and steady the anastomosis (Fig. 12.15 a). The posterior suture line is effected in a continuous fashion using deep seromuscular bites (Fig. 12.15 b) until the lower cor-

ner is reached, at which time the suture is tied to the tail held by the assistant. The duodenum and the stomach are then opened on either side of the com-pleted posterior suture line using the electrosurgical hook knife. Often bile flow from the second part of the duodenum obscures the field. In this situation, a 12-F Foley catheter is introduced through a stab wound in the right hypochondrium and placed in-side the second part of the duodenum before the balloon is inflated with air. The anterior wall of the anastomosis is sutured either with a continuous or interrupted technique using inverting sutures.

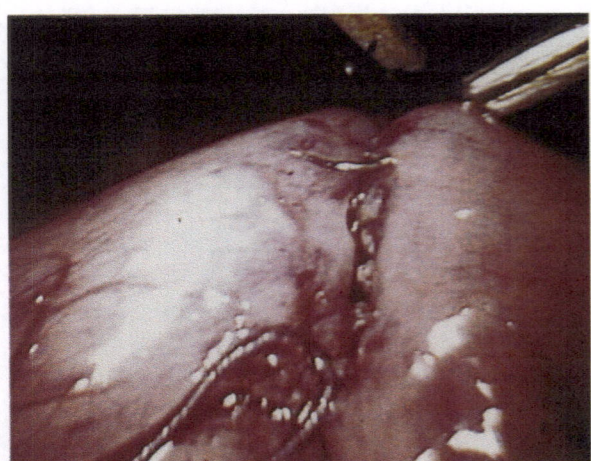

Fig. 12.16. Sutured gastroduodenostomy

End-to-End Billroth I Anastomosis. For end-to-end Billroth I anastomosis a 12-F Foley catheter must be inserted to control bile flow and to stretch the posterior wall of the duodenum. An all-coats suturing technique is used. The upper corner suture is inserted and tied externally. A corresponding suture is placed at the lower corner of the anastomosis, tied and the tail kept on traction by the assistant. The needle of the upper suture is then passed through the stomach into its lumen so that the suturing of the posterior wall of the anastomosis is performed from the mucosal aspect. The assistant must keep even tension on the suture line using a rubber-shod suture holder. Once the opposite corner is reached, the suture is exteriorized through the stomach side and then tied to the lower corner suture. The anterior wall of the anastomosis is closed with a continuous or interrupted suture. The balloon catheter is deflated and removed as the approximation of the anterior walls of the gastroduodenostomy is nearing completion (Fig. 12.16).

Extraction of the Antrum and Toilet of the Peritoneal Gutters

Irrespective of the restoration of continuity which is performed, on completion, air is injected through the nasogastric tube to test the integrity of the anastomosis. Thereafter, the stomach is deflated and nasogastric tube is left in situ. The antrum is extracted inside the laparobag through one of the subcostal cannulae after the placement of a speculum-type retractor to distract the wound edges. The gutters are thoroughly irrigated with saline and aspirated dry. Any clots or tissue debris are removed, the cannulae withdrawn under vision and the pneumoperitoneum desufflated. No drain is inserted.

Gastroenterostomy

Laparoscopic gastroenterostomy may be performed in patients with pyloric obstruction from stenosis caused by chronic benign duodenal ulcer disease, where it is usually accompanied by truncal vagotomy unless the patient is elderly or hypochlorhydric; and as a palliative procedure in patients with inoperable antral, duodenal or pancreatic cancer [18]. The easiest procedure to perform laparoscopically is the anterior (antecolic) gastrojejunostomy, in which the upper jejunal loop is anastomosed to the stomach near to the greater curvature in front of the transverse colon and greater omentum. However, a posterior anastomosis (retrogastric) can be performed laparoscopically although it is undoubtedly more difficult.

Anterior Gastrojejunostomy

Instrumentation and Consumables

Although anterior gastrojejunostomy can be performed with straight laparoscopic instruments, its execution is facilitated by the use of the curved co-axial scissors and duck-bill forceps. Other requirements include a pair of 5-mm needle holders and rubber-shod suture grasper. Suturing is done with atraumatic 3/0 sutures mounted on endoski needles and either absorbable (Polysorb or coated Vicryl) or nonabsorbable (Sofsilk, USSC, or polyamide) can be used. Other consumables include endoloops (Surgitie or Ethibinder) and the EndoGIA* with the blue cartridge.

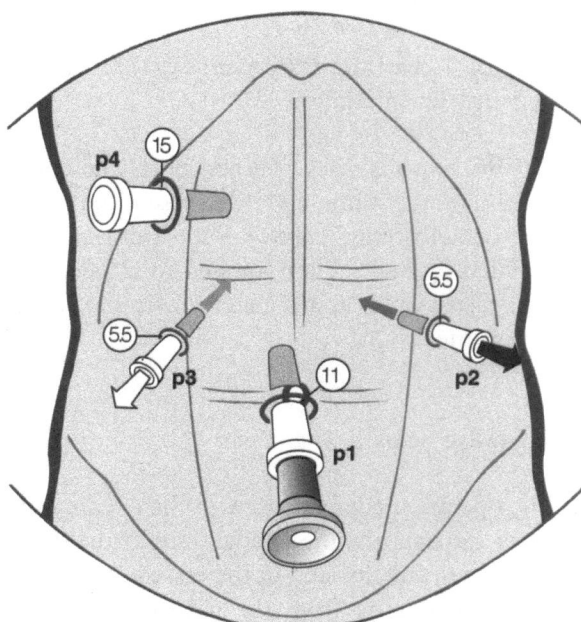

Fig. 12.17. Sites of access ports for gastroenterostomy

Sites of Trocar and Cannulae

The positioning of trocar and cannulae are shown in Fig. 12.17. The optical (11-mm; p1) cannula is placed in the immediate subumbilical region and the two operating cannulae (5.5-mm; p1, p2) along the linea semilunaris at the level of the umbilicus. A 15-mm cannula (p4), used to introduce the EndoGIA* stapler, is inserted in the right subcostal region in the anterior axillary line along the plane of the greater curvature of the stomach (determined visually by the finger depression test). This cannula (with the appropriate reducer) is also used by the assistant for retraction and for holding tension on the suture line during suturing.

Operative Steps

The first step of the operation consists in the insertion of the falciform − round ligament lift to elevate the central portion of the liver and expose the anterior aspect of the antrum of the stomach. In the absence of malignancy, the ideal site of the anastomosis of the jejunal loop is with the antrum along its greater curvature. If the procedure is being performed for obstructing cancer, the gastroje-

junostomy is fashioned 5 cm proximal to the tumour. A loop of upper jejunum some 40−50 cm from the duodenojeunal junction is selected. This step requires elevation of the left half of the transverse colon by the assistant as the surgeon follows the upper jejunal loops to the ligament of Trietz. The selected loop is marked by a serosal suture, which is tied loosely.

Next, attention is paid to the stomach. One or more vessels supplying the greater curvature from the gastroepiploic arcade at the proposed site of the anastomosis are ligated and divided as described in the antrectomy section (see above). The next step consists in the alignment of the stomach and the selected jejunal loop by the insertion of two-corner deep-seromuscular sutures which are approximately 5 cm apart. The left extremity suture is inserted first. The needle picks the jejunum on the medial side of the antimesenteric border and then the adjacent stomach. The suture is tied internally using a standard microsurgical knot and then cut long. Traction is kept on this suture by the assistant as the right corner suture is inserted though the two organs, tied and left uncut). This suture is subsequently used to close the defect created for the insertion of the stapler (see below). As traction is held on the tail of the right extremity suture, appropriately sized openings are made in the jejunum and stomach (medial to the suture) for the insertion of the limbs of the EndoGIA* stapler. The two limbs of the opened EndoGIA* stapler are introduced into the stomach and the jejunum, respectively. Once inside the lumen of the stomach and jejunum, the stapler limbs are elevated to tent the two organs and then closed before the instrument is fired. Thereafter, the instrument is released and withdrawn from the anastomosis. After the 3-cm stapler is reloaded with a new cartridge, it is reintroduced and a second application made beyond but overlapping (by 0.5 to 1 cm) the left extremity of the first stapled anastomotic line. If a 6-cm stapler is available, only one application is used to effect the anastomosis. The anterior wall of the gastrojejunostomy is then lifted up to inspect the stapled anastomotic line (Fig. 12.18) and to ensure that there are no mucosal bridges (encountered in 10% of cases in our experience). If present, these mucosal bridges are cut with scissors.

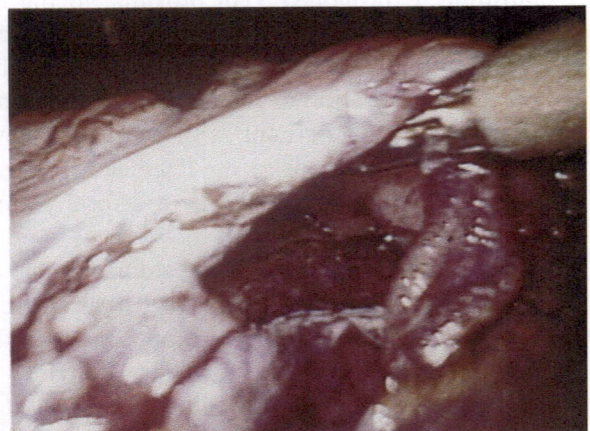

12.18

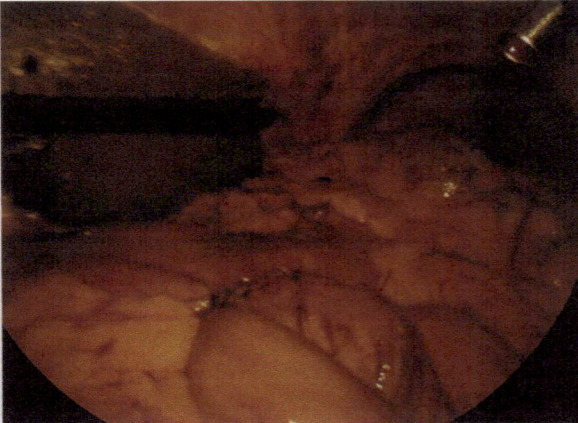

12.19

Fig. 12.18. Close-up of the interior view of an anterior stapled gastrojejunostomy

Fig. 12.19. Completed anterior gastroenterostomy

The final stage of the procedure consists in the suture closure of the defect. The right corner suture is used to approximate the two edges with a continuous seromuscular technique. The suturing is carried to the left until the anterior staple line is reached (Fig. 12.19). The suture is ended either by an Aberdeen knot or by being tied to a separate anchor knot. At the end of the procedure, air is injected through the nasogastric tube to distend the stomach and test the integrity of the anastomosis, after which the stomach is deflated and the nasogastric tube left in situ.

Posterior Gastrojejunostomy

Sites of Trocar and Cannulae and Instrumentation

The instruments, sites of access ports and consumables are the same as those used for anterior gastroenterostomy. Likewise, the stomach is kept deflated by low suction applied to a Salem sump nasogastric tube and a falciform/round ligament lift inserted.

Operative Steps

The operation commences with the opening of the lesser sac opposite the middle third of the stomach by ligature and division of the vessels supplying the greater curvature from the gastroepiploic arcade using the technique previously described.

The left half of the transverse colon is lifted up by the assistant and the middle colic vessels identified. A 3-cm opening is cut by scissors in the transverse mesocolon just to the left of the middle colic vessels. An upper jejunal loop some 20 cm from the ligament of Trietz is grasped by an atraumatic forceps and inserted through the defect into the lesser sac. At this stage, the transverse colon and greater omentum are released and allowed to drop over the grasper holding the bowel. A curved Duval grasper is applied to the anterior wall of the mobilized greater curvature, which is then pulled up to expose the lesser sac, the posterior surface of the stomach and the transposed jejunal loop being held by the infracolic grasper. After the assistant grasps the jejunal loop by an atraumatic forceps inserted into the lesser sac between the transverse colon and the stomach, the infracolic grasper is released. The transposed jejunal loop is secured to the posterior surface of the stomach by the right corner suture, which is left uncut after it is tied. The assistant then releases hold on the jejunal loop. The left corner suture is then inserted some 5 cm proximally, tied and cut. The anastomosis is fashioned using the EndoGIA* stapler as described previously and the defect closed using a running suture. On completion, the edges of the mesocolic defect are attached to the stomach by a few interrupted sutures above the anastomosis.

Pyloroplasty

A Heineke-Mikculicz pyloroplasty can be performed laparoscopically without much difficulty, provided the surgeon has mastered the technique of interrupted suturing with internal knotting. The procedure is carried out either as a component of bilateral truncal vagotomy for duodenal ulcer disease or as drainage operation in patients with gastroparesis from any cause. Gastroparesis is encountered in a few patients with reflux disease (before and after fundoplication) and in diabetic patients. In addition to the appropriate symptoms, the diagnosis of gastroparesis must be confirmed by emptying studies after the ingestion of isotope-labelled standardized meals. In patients with confirmed delayed emptying, a truncal vagotomy is not performed, but if the patient is not hypochlorhydric, the procedure is followed by long-term therapy with H_2 receptor antagonists. In patients with associated symptomatic gastro-oesophageal reflux, the pyloroplasty is performed at the same time as the laparoscopic antireflux operation.

A Finney pyloroplasty is difficult to perform laparoscopically as it requires complete mobilization of the second and proximal part of the third portion of the duodenum. This procedure is seldom performed in open surgery nowadays and to the author's knowledge has not been attempted by the laparoscopic route.

Heineke-Mikculicz Pyloroplasty

Instrumentation and Consumables

In addition to the ordinary straight laparoscopic instrumentation, the following are required: a pair of 5-mm needle holders, rubber-shod suture holder, a straight Babcock's grasping forceps and a Foley balloon catheter. Suturing is performed with 3/0 silk or polyamide mounted on endoski needles.

Sites of Trocar and Cannulae

The sites of the access cannulae are shown in Fig. 12.20. The optic is introduced through a subumbilical port (11-mm; p1) to the left of the

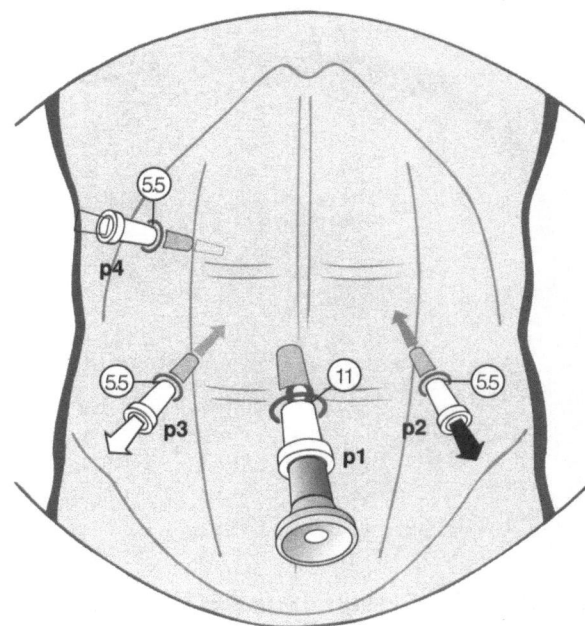

Fig. 12.20. Sites of access ports for pyloroplasty

midline. The two working cannulae (5.5-mm; p2, p3) are placed along the linea semilunaris at the level of the umbilicus. The assistant's cannula (5.5-mm; p5) is inserted in the right subcostal region along the anterior axillary line. The quadrate lobe and segment five of the right lobe of the liver is elevated by the insertion of the falciform – round ligament lift (see below). Excessive leakage of bile through the antroduodenotomy, which can obscure the field during the suturing of the pyloroplasty, can be controlled by the temporary insertion of a Foley balloon catheter into the second portion of the duodenum.

Operative Steps

Throughout the entire procedure, it is essential that the stomach be kept empty and collapsed by the continuous low suction to a size 16-F Salem sump nasogastric tube. The first step of the procedure consists of the insertion of the round ligament – falciform lift to elevate the central portion of the liver from the antropyloroduodenal segment. The exact position of the pylorus is then identified by reference to the prepyloric veins of Mayo and a stay suture is inserted on its lower border, tied internally

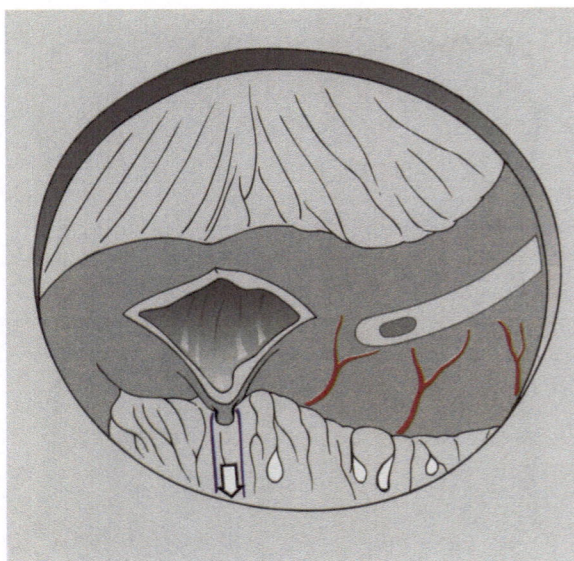

Fig. 12.21. Traction applied to the bottom corner suture converts the horizontal incision to a vertically disposed rhomboid defect

Fig. 12.22. The first stitch, which approximates the margins of the proximal end of the rhomboid, is cut long so that the assistant can hold it under tension, thereby facilitating the insertion of the second suture

and then cut some 3 cm from the knot. The proposed pyloroplasty incision is then mapped with soft electrocoagulation using either the Berci spatula or the L-shaped electrosurgical hook knife. The coagulated line runs horizontally in the centre of the antropyloroduodenal segment and extends from the duodenal bulb across the pyloric sphincter to the adjacent antrum over a distance of 4 cm. The incision is deepened, preferably using microprocessor – controlled electrocutting (Erbe ACC unit; Tübingen, Germany) with the cutting panel on the generator set at mark 3. During this step, an insulated forceps is held in the left hand and used to grasp and coagulate bleeding submucosal vessels as and when they are encountered. On completion, traction is applied to the suture previously applied to the lower border of the pylorus, converting the horizontal incision to a vertically disposed rhomboid defect (Fig. 12.21). Leakage from the stomach should be minimal, but large quantities of bile often escape from the defect and aspiration is required. If bile flow continues at a rate which obscures the operative field, a 12-F Foley catheter is used to deal with this problem as outlined in the section on antrectomy.

Interrupted all-coats inverting sutures are used to fashion the pyloroplasty. As traction is maintained on the stay suture, the first stitch approxi-

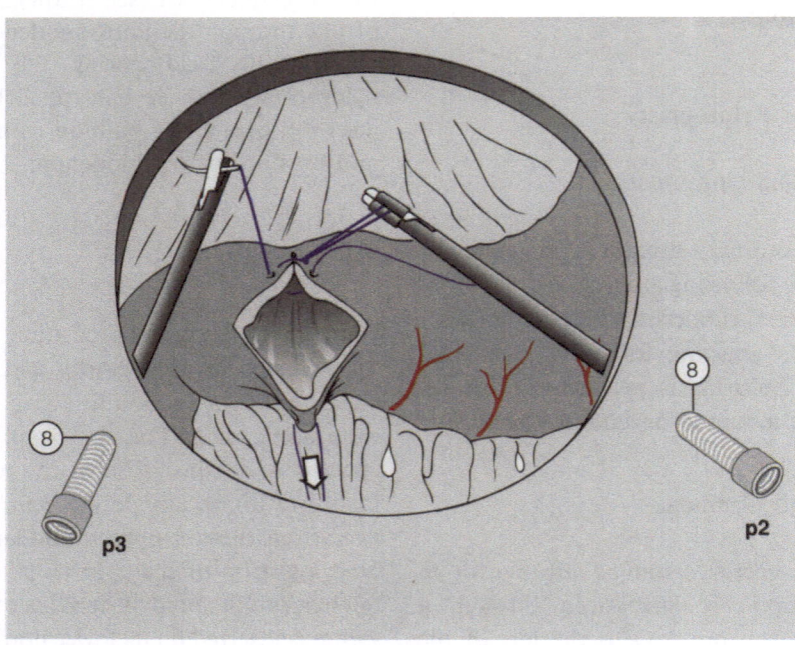

mating the margins of the proximal end of the rhomboid is inserted, tied internally and cut long. The assistant then grasps the long ends of the tied first suture to facilitate the insertion of the second suture (Fig. 12.22); the process is repeated until the lower 1 cm of the defect is reached. It is important that the last two sutures are inserted first before being tied. If a Foley balloon catheter has been placed in the second part of the duodenum, the balloon is deflated and the catheter removed before the last two sutures are tied. Once the suturing of the pyloroplasty has been completed, the suction on the nasogastric tube is disconnected and air injected using a 50-ml syringe to test the integrity of the suture line. The Salem sump nasogastric tube is left in situ at the end of the procedure.

Postoperative Care

It is our practice to remove the nasogastric tube early, after recovery of consciousness. A second dose of antibiotic is administered 12 h after the operation. Analgesia with opiates is usually required during the first 24 h. All patients in whom a gastroenterostomy, gastroduodenal anastomosis or pyloroplasty has been performed are investigated with a gastrografin swallow on the third to fourth postoperative day to establish that there is no anastomotic leakage. During this period, the patients do not receive anything by mouth except for hourly sips of water. A tube contrast study is performed before enteral feeding is commenced in patients who have had a laparoscopic gastrostomy or jejunostomy. This is usually conducted 24 h after the operation.

References

1. Alexandre-Williams J (1991) A requiem for vagotomy. BMJ 302:547–548
2. Strom M, Berstad A, Bodemar G, Walan A (1986) Results of short and long-term cimetidine treatment in patients with juxtapyloric ulcers, with special reference to gastric acid and pepsin secretion. Scand J Gastroenterol 21:521–530
3. Andersen D (1985) Prevention of ulcer recurrence – medical versus surgical treatment. The surgeon's view. Scand J Gastroenterol 20[Suppl 110]:89–92
4. Srivastava A, Hughes LE (1986) Role of palliative surgery in gastric cancer. In: Preece PE, Cuschieri A, Wellwood JM (eds) Cancer of the stomach. Grune and Stratton, London, pp 189–207
5. Miller RE, Winkler WP, Kotler DP (1988) The Russell percutaneous endoscopic gastrostomy: key technical steps. Gastrointest Endosc 34:339–341
6. Deitel M, Bendago M, Spratt EH, Burul CJ, To TB (1988) Percutaneous endoscopic gastrostomy by the pull and introducer methods. Can J Surg 31:102–104
7. Albrink MH, Foster J, Rosemurgy AS, Carey LC (1992) Laparoscopic feeding jejunostomy: also a simple technique. Surg Endosc 6:259–260
8. Cuschieri A (1992) Laparoscopic vagotomy. Surg Clin N Am 72:357–367
9. Amdrup E, Andersen D, Hostrup H (1978) The Aarhus county vagotomy trial. An interim report on primary results and incidence of sequelae following parietal cell vagotomy and selective gastric vagotomy in 748 patients. World J Surg 2:85
10. Stoddard CJ, Vassilakis JS, Duthie HL (1978) Highly selective vagotomy or truncal vagotomy and pyloroplasty for chronic duodenal ulceration; a randomized, prospective clinical study. Br J Surg 65:793
11. Taylor TV, Gunn AA, MacLeod DAD (1982) Anterior lesser curve seromyotomy and posterior truncal vagotomy in the treatment of chronic duodenal ulcer. Lancet ii:846–848
12. Taylor TV, Holt S, Heading RC (1985) Gastric emptying after lesser curve myotomy and posterior truncal vagotomy. Br J Surg 72:620–622
13. Taylor TV, Lythgoe JP, McFarland JB, Gilmore IT, Thomas PE, Ferguson GH (1990) Anterior lesser curve seromyotomy and posterior truncal vagotomy versus truncal vagotomy and pyloroplasty in the treatment of chronic duodenal ulcer disease. Br J Surg 77:1007–1009
14. Oostvogel HJM, van Vroonhoven TJMV (1988) Anterior lesser curve seromyotomy with posterior truncal vagotomy versus proximal gastric vagotomy. Br J Surg 75:121–124
15. Katkhouda N, Mouiel J (1991) A new surgical technique of treatment of chronic duodenal ulcer without laparotomy by videocoelioscopy. Am J Surg 161:361–364
16. Hill GL, Barker CJ (1978) Anterior highly selective vagotomy with posterior truncal vagotomy: a simple technique for denervating the parietal cell mass. Br J Surg 65:702–705
17. Bailey RW, Flowers JL, Graham SM (1991) Combined laparoscopic cholecystectomy and selective vagotomy. Surg Laparosc Endosc
18. Wilson RG, Varma JS (1992) Laparoscopic gastroenterostomy for malignant duodenal obstruction. Br J Surg 79:1348

13 Laparoscopy and Laparoscopic Contact Ultrasound Scanning in Disorders of the Liver, Biliary Tract and Pancreas

A. CUSCHIERI

Diagnostic laparoscopy can provide clinically useful information which influences management in patients suffering from both acute and chronic intra-abdominal disorders but is especially useful in hepatic, biliary and pancreatic disease. Diagnostic and staging laparoscopy provides clear benefit to patients suffering from intra-abdominal malignancy [1−9], and it is indeed surprising that the procedure has been overlooked in the routine work-up of these patients, although the situation has changed drastically in the last few years. Instead of repeated, expensive imaging tests such as computed tomography (CT) and magnetic resonance imaging (MRI) scannning with or without percutaneous guided biopsy, a laparoscopic examination will, in most instances, provide direct visualization of the lesion, a more reliable tissue sample and often yields accurate information on staging of the disease, establishing dissemination and resectability of the primary lesion. These advantages are certainly true for pancreatic, hepatic, gastric, oesophageal and colorectal cancer. There is no radiological imaging technique which can detect peritoneal seedlings or small metastatic deposits in the liver with the same reliability as laparoscopy [5, 6].

Diagnostic laparoscopy should be an integral part of general surgical practice. The technique of diagnostic laparoscopy and the common indications for the procedure are outlined in Vol. 1, Chap. 14. The present chapter deals specifically with laparoscopy in the evaluation of patients with hepatic, biliary and pancreatic disease.

Laparoscopic Evaluation of Liver Disease

There are many reports [10−12], monographs [9] and colour atlases [13] which document the usefulness of diagnostic laparoscopy in the evaluation of both benign and malignant liver disease.

Chronic Liver Disease

The benefits of laparoscopy in the assessment of patients with chronic liver disease include visual information of the macroscopic appearance and size of the liver, the nature of surface nodularity and the presence of portal hypertension and splenomegaly. At the same time, it provides increased scope for multiple biopsies of both the diseased hepatic parenchyma and any suspect lesions. Aside from the targeted nature of the biopsy, bleeding which may complicate the procedure, particularly in patients with advanced chronic liver disease with impaired clotting function and thrombocytopoenia, is easily dealt with by compression and use of electrocoagulation whenever necessary. In this respect, there is no doubt that laparoscopic biopsy is safer and has a higher diagnostic yield than the blind percutaneous procedure. The combined visual appearance of the liver together with histological examination of the liver biopsies result in a firm diagnosis in virtually all patients.

Laparoscopy is of particular value in patients with ascites. The nature of the ascitic fluid − serous, bile-stained, chylous or haemorrhagic − its cellular composition, and the state of the peritoneal lining − inflammation or nodular deposits − can be assessed by laparoscopy, and this helps to establish the exact cause in the individual patient. Special care is needed in performing diagnostic laparoscopy for ascites as the air-filled small bowel loops float on the surface of the ascitic fluid and are therefore closely opposed to the anterior abdominal wall. This enhances the risk of bowel injury by the Veress needle during the creation of the pneumoperitoneum unless special precautions are taken. One approach which obviates this problem is the use of open laparoscopy. The alternative is the careful insertion of the Veress needle unconnected to any tubing and with the tap opened. In this way, ascitic fluid will spurt out as soon as the tip of the Veress needle enters the peritoneal cavity. Sufficient ascitic fluid (1–2 l) should be withdrawn to reduce the intra-abdominal pressure and fluid volume, before insufflation is started and the trocar/cannula inserted. During laparoscopic inspection, more fluid may need to be aspirated to ensure a thorough examination of the peritoneal cavity and its contents.

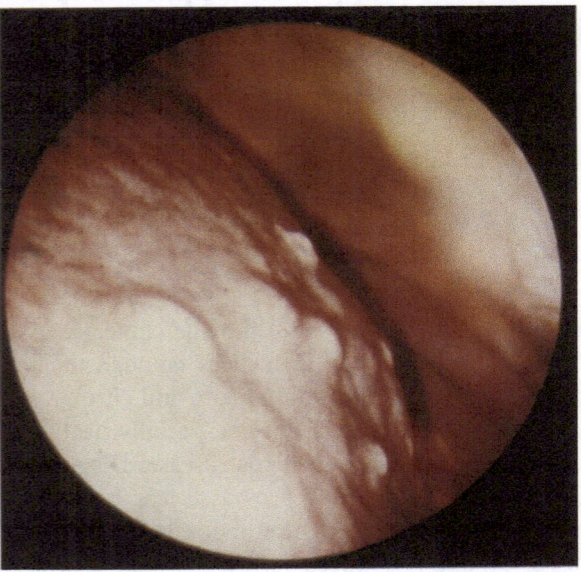

Fig. 13.1. Secondary deposits in the liver from a primary carcinoma of the sigmoid colon

Hepatic Malignancy

The laparoscopic assessment of hepatic malignancy consists of inspection of the liver surface, contact ultrasound scanning of the hepatic parenchyma and targeted biopsy. These combined techniques allow accurate diagnosis with histological confirmation of both primary and secondary hepatic tumours, an assessment of the extent of the tumour burden and a realistic appraisal of resectability.

In patients with secondary tumour deposits (Fig. 13.1), the size, number, extent and bilateral involvement of the liver will determine whether treatment is indicated and, if so, its nature.

In primary hepatomas, information is gained on the state of the hepatic parenchyma (normal or cirrhotic), the exact location, size, sectorial involvement, invasion of the diaphragm and the presence or absence of satellite lesions. The operability by liver resection is ascertained from this information.

Laparoscopy is also useful in the assessment of hilar cholangiocarcinoma. These tumours are visualized by retraction of the right lobe and gallbladder from the hepatoduodenal ligament. Extent and precise location of tumour, local infiltration, nodal disease and hepatic involvement are ascertained by the use of laparoscopic ultrasound scanning.

Laparoscopic Examination of the Pancreas

In the author's opinion, laparoscopy is essential in the management of patients with pancreatic disease, benign or malignant. It provides essential information on the nature and extent of the disease and, in the case of pancreatic cancer, it is the only consistently reliable means of establishing dissemination and inoperability [5–8]. Diagnostic laparoscopy should be regarded as an integral part of routine management of these patients. Its use will spare a substantial number of patients with advanced disease an unnecessary laparotomy. In patients with incurable cancer, palliation of jaundice and duodenal obstruction can also be conducted laparoscopically (Chap. 10). In the author's reported experience of a series of patients with pancreatic cancer in whom laparotomy was immediately preceded by laparoscopy, no instance of laparoscopically assessed inoperability was found to be incorrect at operation [6]. However, some 20% of patients who were judged to be operable by laparoscopy were found to be unresectable at laparotomy due to invasion of the portal vein. This study was, however, conducted before the advent of laparoscopic ultrasound examination, which can reliably detect vascular invasion.

Examination for Lesions of the Head of the Pancreas

These patients present with cholestatic jaundice and the diagnosis is usually confirmed by abdominal ultrasonography followed by endoscopic retrograde cholangiopancreaticographic study (ERCP). Preparation for laparoscopy includes administration of intramuscular vitamin K analogue and catheterization of the urinary bladder to measure the urine output. As the procedure is performed under general anaesthesia, adequate intravenous hydration with crystalloid solutions is necessary and an osmotic or loop diuretic is given at the time of induction of anaesthesia. A size 16-F Salem sump nasogastric tube is inserted and attached to continuous low suction, as total gastric and duodenal decompression is essential for laparoscopic examination of the head of the pancreas.

Sites of Trocar and Cannulae and Instrumentation

The basic procedure is performed through four ports (Fig. 13.2). The 30° forward oblique optic is introduced through a subumbilical 11-mm cannula and the two operating (5.5-mm) ports are placed along each linea semilunaris at the level of the umbilicus. The left 10.5-mm subxiphoid port is needed for elevation of the quadrate and right lobe of the liver (together with the round ligament − falciform complex) by the assistant, using the black 10-mm plastic rod. An extra 10.5-mm port is needed for laparoscopic ultrasound examination of the head of the pancreas and the hepatoduodenal ligament with the structures it contains. This is placed on the right side along the anterior axillary line.

The instruments needed include dissecting scissors, electrosurgical hook and a variety of insulated graspers (traumatic and atraumatic). The cholecystocholangiogram, which must be regarded as an integral part of the laparoscopic examination of jaundiced patients with mass lesions in the pancre-

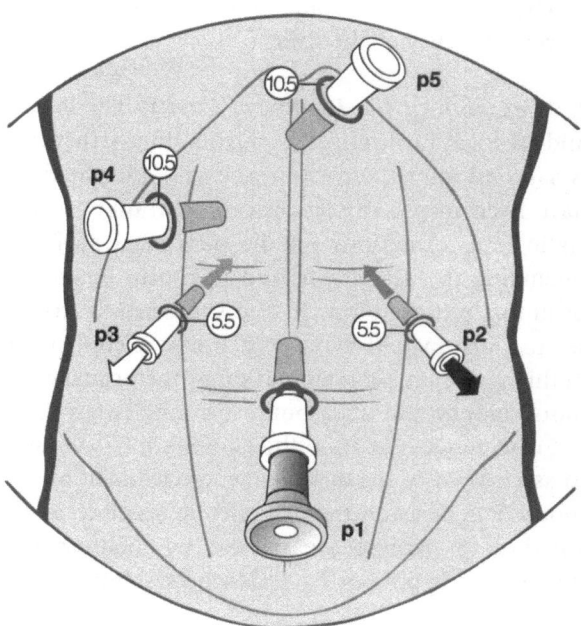

Fig. 13.2. Sites of trocar and cannulae for laparoscopic examination of the head of the pancreas

atic head, is best performed using the Veress needle. A modern portal C-arm image intensifier with image processing system is essential for efficient and complete radiological visualization of the biliary tract in these patients. Finally, biopsy (Trucut; Bioptit) and cytological equipment (fine needle aspiration system) should be available. A pair of 5-mm needle holders and atraumatic sutures mounted on endoski needle should also be included in the sterile instrument tray.

Laparoscopic Diagnosis and Staging

Laparoscopic diagnosis and staging consists of six steps, in the following order:

1. Inspection of the peritoneal cavity, omentum, serosal surfaces of the small intestine and liver with biopsy of suspect lesions
2. Inspection and palpation of the gallbladder, duodenum and hepatoduodenal ligament
3. Biopsy and cytology of primary lesion
4. Cholecystocholangiography
5. Mobilization of the head of the pancreas and duodenal curve

6. Ultrasonographic examination of the pancreas, portal vein and the liver

1. Inspection of the Peritoneal Cavity. The lesion and its local infiltration to surrounding structures is assessed after the peritoneal cavity and the liver have been inspected. Suspicious or frankly metastatic transformations on the peritoneal surfaces (including the diaphragm and falciform ligament) or in the liver are biopsied and subjected to frozen section histology. If metastatic disease is confirmed in this way, detailed examination of the primary tumour, biopsy and ultrasound scanning (steps 2, 3, 5, 6) are unnecessary and the examination is limited to assessment of the duodenal encroachment by tumour. The decision then should be made to as to whether to palliate the patient by laparoscopic bilioenteric bypass or by endoscopic stenting.

2. Inspection and Palpation. The round ligament – falciform complex, the quadrate and the right lobe of the liver are held up by the assistant by placement of the plastic rod obliquely across the neck of the gallbladder (Fig. 13.3). The antrum of the stomach is grasped near the greater curvature

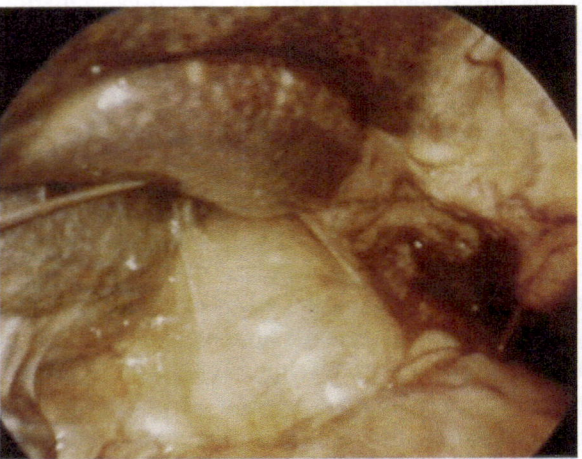

Fig. 13.4. Dilated common bile duct in a patient with inoperable carcinoma of the head of the pancreas

by an atraumatic forceps and pulled down. This manoeuvre results in anterior bulging of the "mass lesion" which compresses the duodenum from behind. The mobility of the mass in the coronal plane is assessed by pushing it from the side by a closed atraumatic grasper. The hepatoduodenal area is then inspected. Usually the dilated common bile duct is obvious (Fig. 13.4) and in some cases, the upward extension of the tumour beyond the duodenal bulb can be detected. Enlarged lymph nodes in the porta hepatis and to the right of the bile duct, low down, can be visualized as well.

After the grasper on the antrum of the stomach has been released, the involvement of the duodenum by the tumour is assessed by picking its anterior wall and lifting it from the mass. The degree of lift, pliability or induration of the walls of the duodenum are determined, starting at the level of the pylorus and proceeding along the duodenal bulb and the second part of the duodenum.

3. Biopsy and Cytology of Primary Lesion. If a mass lesion in the pancreatic head is palpated when the stomach is pulled down, then the best and safest technique is transduodenal biopsy. This is ideally performed by use of the Biopty spring-loaded core needle system (Fig. 13.5) although a disposable long Trucut needle is adequate for the purpose. In either case, the optimal side of entry of the needle through the anterior abdominal wall is determined by the finger depression test. A small stab wound

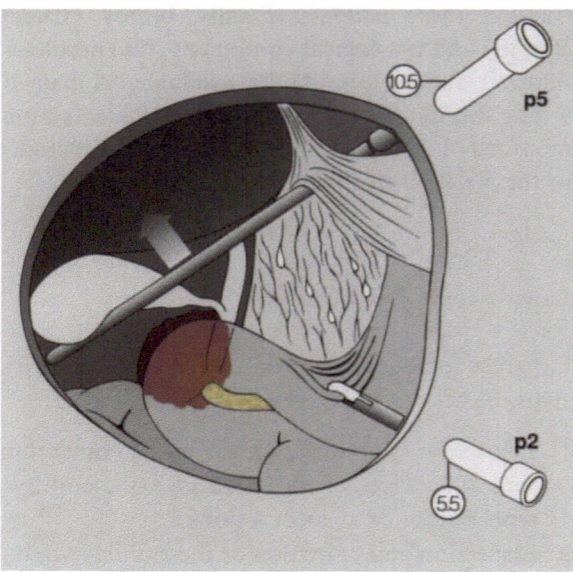

Fig. 13.3. The round ligament – falciform complex, the quadrate and the right lobe of the liver are held up by placement of the plastic rod obliquely across the neck of the gallbladder and the antrum of the stomach is grasped near the greater curvature and pulled down

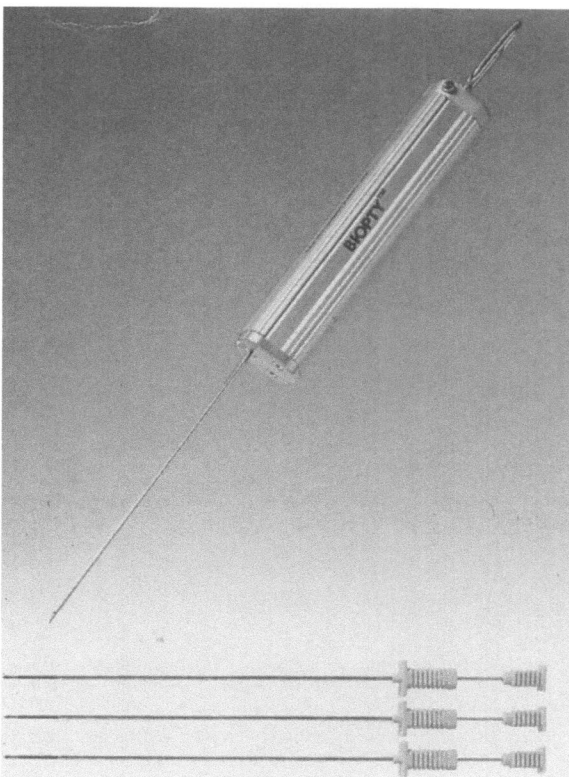

Fig. 13.5. Biopty spring-loaded core needle system used for transduodenal biopsy

is made by a pointed scalpel in this site and the biopsy needle introduced and guided to the proximal end of the second part of the duodenum (Fig. 13.6a). The needle is then advanced through the duodenal walls until the lesion is felt by the tip of the needle, which is advanced for a further 1 cm, fired and then removed (Fig. 13.6b). If an adequate specimen is obtained, the hole in the anterior duodenal wall is closed by a single interrupted black silk or polyamide suture tied internally with two 5-mm needle holders (Fig. 13.6c).

Fine needle aspiration cytology can be used instead but the yield is lower than obtained by the needle core biopsy technique. The advantage of the fine needle aspiration is that the small needle puncture in the anterior duodenal wall does not require suturing.

4. Cholecystocholangiography Cholecystocholangiography is indicated: (a) When the ERCP demonstrates complete or near total occlusion of the bile

duct such that the proximal biliary tree is not outlined by this investigation [14–16] and (b) before laparoscopic bilioenteric bypass, when it is essential in the selection of the appropriate bypass: cholecystojejunostomy or a choledochojejunostomy, depending on the proximity of the upper extension of the tumour to the entry of the cystic duct into the common bile duct [17].

The essential requirement for laparoscopic cholecystocholangiography is the availability of a modern portal C-arm image intensifier with the necessary software for rapid imaging processing and storage, such as the Diasonics (Utah, USA) machine (Fig. 13.7).

The best instrument for cholecystocholangiography is the Veress needle. This is attached via a three-way tap to a line leading to two 50-ml syringes (one containing isotonic saline and the other sodium diatrizoate, 20% – 30%) and to a suction line. The site of entry of the Veress needle (opposite the central fundus and in line with the long axis of the organ) is determined by finger depression of the anterior abdominal wall. After a small stab wound is made in the skin, the Veress needle is introduced into the peritoneal cavity. When the gallbladder is reached, the spring-loaded inner blunt stylet is held retracted so that the bevelled cutting tip is exposed (Fig. 13.8a). This is then advanced through the gallbladder fundus into the lumen, at which time the inner blunt component is released. Confirmation of the intraluminal position of the needle is achieved by injection of a few millilitres of saline followed by aspiration. The Veress needle is then advanced further in and the position of its blunt, rounded tip determined by needle deflection such that the tip tents the medial wall of the gallbladder (Fig. 13.8b). The optimum position is near the neck of the organ. Once this position has been reached, the gallbladder is aspirated of bile until it becomes nearly empty. Before fluorocholangiography is commenced, the operating table is tilted head-down (30°) and slightly to the right and the C-arm is brought in place with the usual precautions to ensure against contamination of the operating area. If metal cannulae are used, those that are in the area of the intended exposure are removed temporarily over a plastic radiolucent rod and reinserted once the cholangiography has been completed.

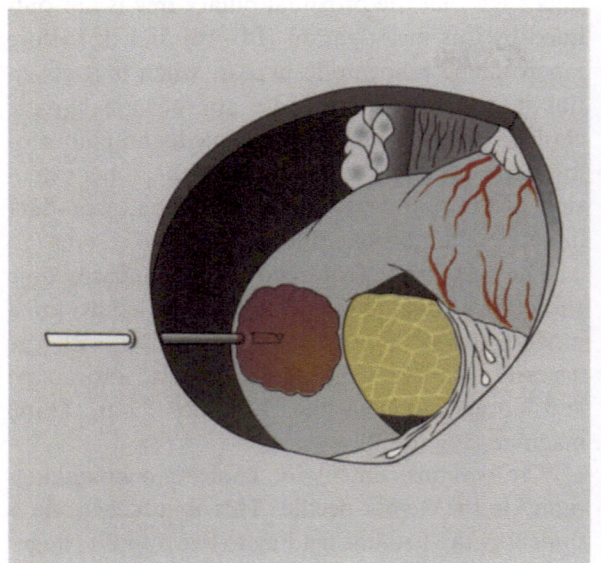

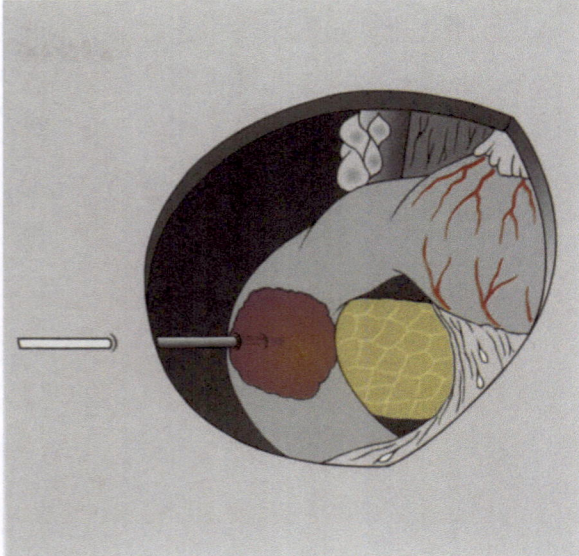

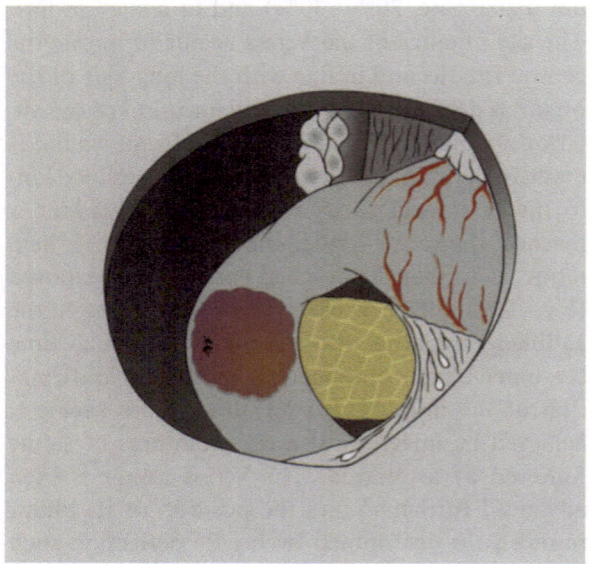

Fig. 13.6a – c. Transduodenal biopsy of a lesion in the head of the pancreas. **a** Guiding biopsy needle. **b** Advancing, firing, and removing the needle. **c** Sutured hole in the anterior duodenal wall

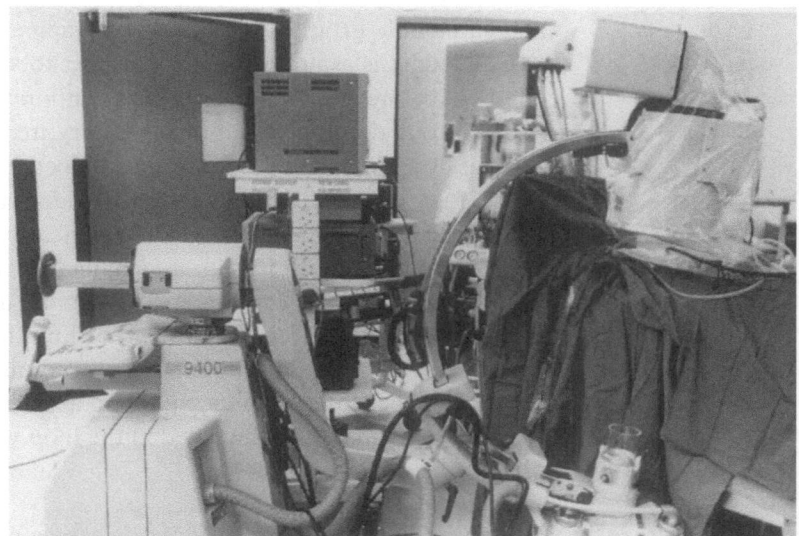

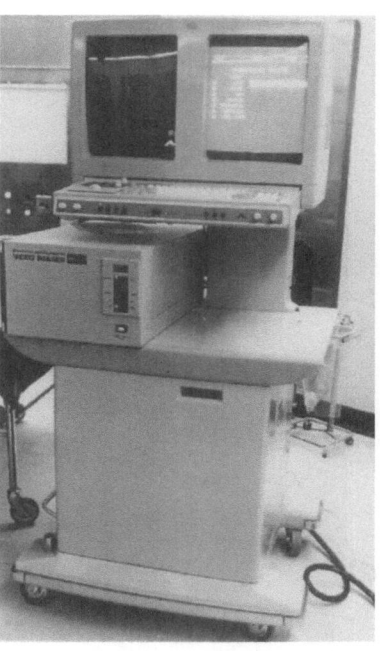

Fig. 13.7 a, b. Modern portable C-arm image intensifier with advanced imaging processing software

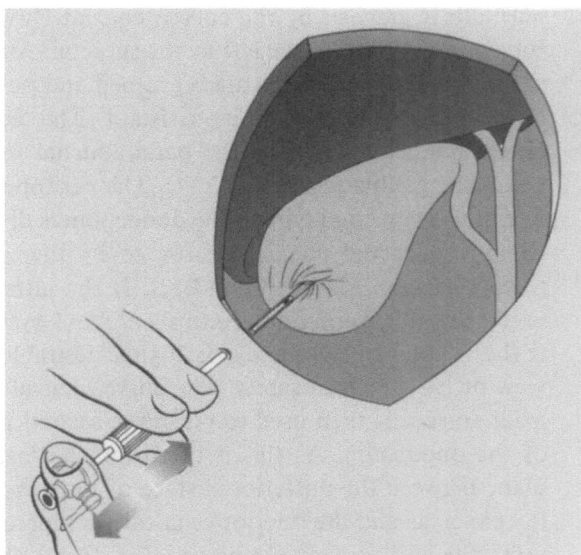

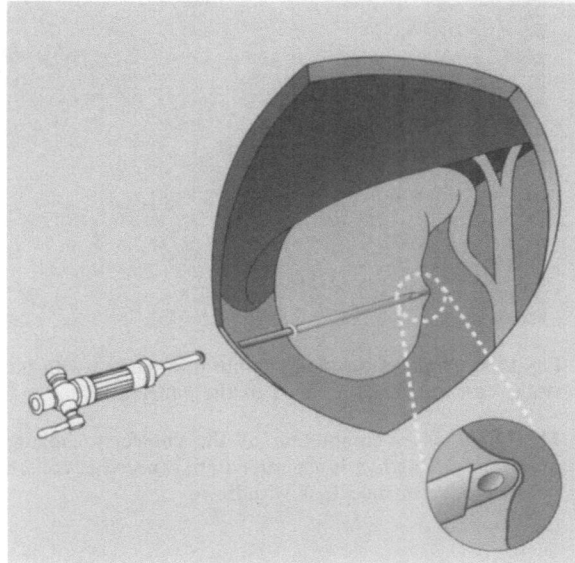

Fig. 13.8 a, b. Transcystic cholecystocholangiography. **a** Advancing the bevelled cutting tip of the Veress needle through the gallbladder fundus into the lumen, when the glallbladder lumen is entered the stylet is released. **b** Determining the position of the Veress needle by needle deflection such that the rounded tip tents the medial wall of the gallbladder

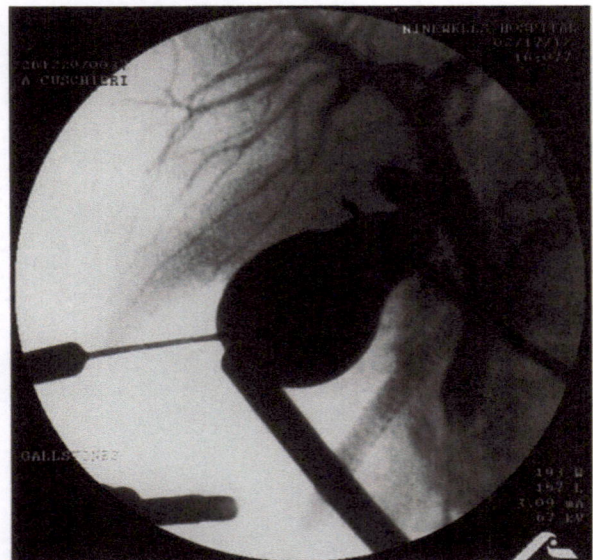

13.9

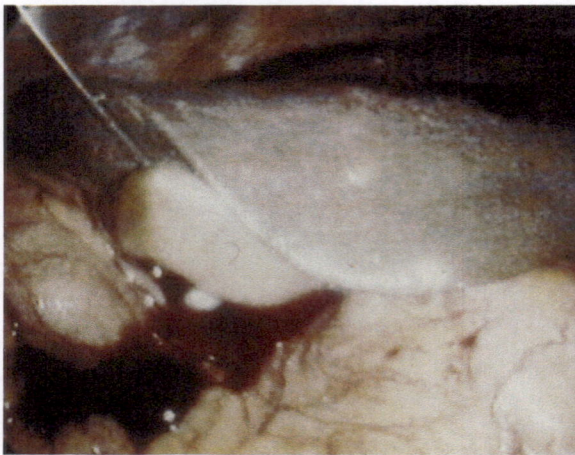

13.10

Fig. 13.9. Cholecystocholangiogram in a patient with inoperable carcinoma of the head of the pancreas

Fig. 13.10. After completion of the cholecystocholangiogram, the gallbladder is aspirated until it becomes collapsed before the Veress needle is withdrawn

Fluoroscopy is started with contrast medium injection. On average, some 40–50 ml contrast medium are needed to fill the gallbladder before it starts to opacify the cystic duct and then the biliary tract. Exposures are stored throughout by pressing on the appropriate foot switch (Fig. 13.9). The important information needed from the cholecystocholangiogram includes the distance between the cystic duct insertion and the upper limit of the tumour and the state of the proximal biliary tree: extent of dilata-

tion, secondary stones, other lesions or strictures. On completion of the cholecystocholangiogram, the gallbladder is aspirated until it becomes totally collapsed before the Veress needle is withdrawn (Fig. 13.10). If decompression of the biliary tree is intended by an immediate laparoscopic bilioenteric bypass, then the small hole in the gallbladder can be ignored. Closure of the gallbladder puncture is necessary if decompression is not contemplated. This is carried out by a single interrupted suture using 3/0 Polysorb or Vicryl with internal knotting using two 5-mm needle holders. On no account may the hole be closed with an endoloop as necrosis of the gallbladder wall included in the loop will ensue.

5. Mobilization of the Head of the Pancreas and Duodenal Curve. Mobilization of the head of pancreas and duodenum requires experience and can be difficult with straight laparoscopic instruments, but is easier using coaxial curved instruments introduced through flexible metal cannulae. The duodenal bulb is grasped by the curved coaxial Duval's forceps and pulled to the left by the surgeon. At the same time the hepatic flexure is grasped and pulled down and to the left by the assistant. This combined manoeuvre exposes the paraduodenal fossa below the gallbladder (Fig. 13.11). The peritoneum lateral to the second part of the duodenum is divided by the curved coaxial scissor or by the electrosurgical hook knife (Fig. 13.12). If the latter is used, the microprocessor-controlled ACC system (Erbe, Tübingen, Germany) is highly desirable in view of its enhanced safety. The curved Duval coaxial grasper is then used to grasp the second part of the duodenum. As this is lifted up, the fascial plane between the posterior surface of the head of the pancreas and the inferior vena cava is separated using the curved coaxial scissors (Fig. 13.13). This plane is obliterated if there is posterior extension of the tumour; under these circumstances attempts to dissect it should be resisted as the lesion will prove to be inoperable and dissection would likely lead to major bleeding from damage to the vena cava, the right adrenal or the left renal vein.

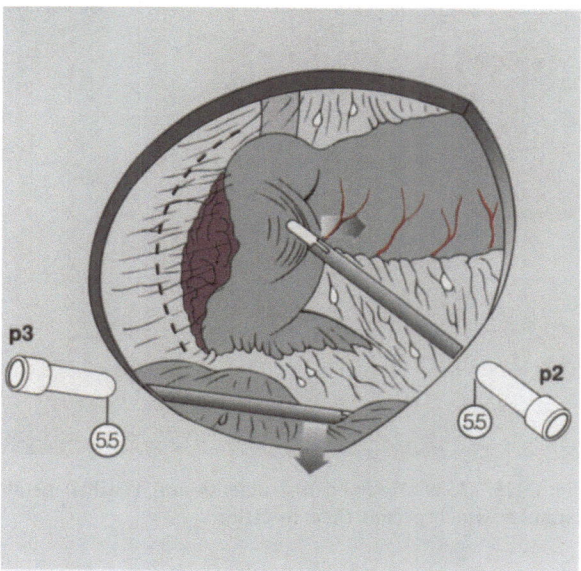

Fig. 13.11. Grasping the duodenal bulb and pulling it to the left and the hepatic flexure down to expose the paraduodenal fossa below the gallbladder

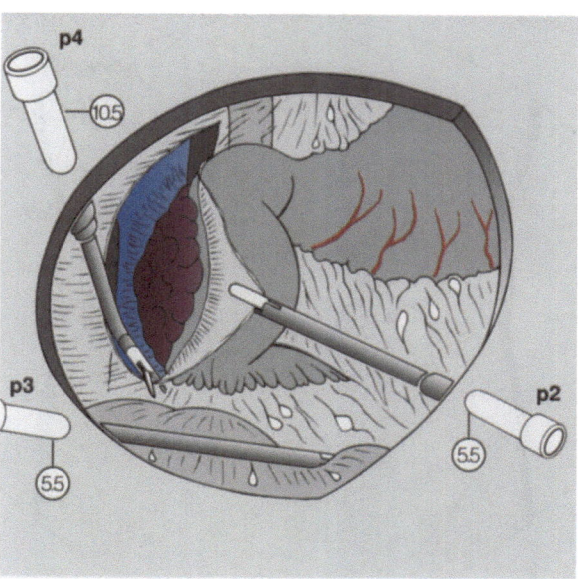

Fig. 13.13. Separating the fascial plane between the posterior surface of the head of the pancreas and the inferior vena cava using the curved coaxial scissors as the second part of the duodenum is lifted up

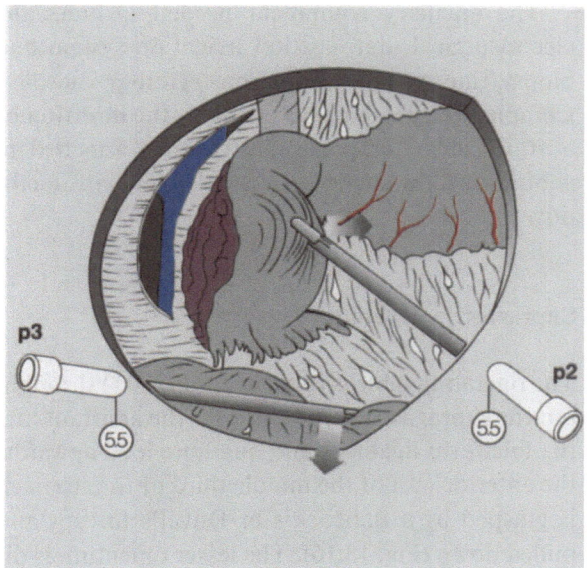

Fig. 13.12. Dividing the peritoneum lateral to the second part of the duodenum by the curved coaxial scissor or by the electrosurgical hook knife

Examination of the Body and Tail of the Pancreas

Two approaches are available: the supragastric and the infragastric techniques [4, 18, 19]. To some extent they are complementary in that both can be used in the same patient and the number and sites of the access ports necessary are the same. The supragastric technique provides a good exposure of the central portion of the pancreas in thin patients. The method is difficult in obese individuals and is impossible if there are adhesions binding the pancreas to the lesser sac. In addition, the neck of the pancreas (region close to the gastroduodenal artery) and the tail of the organ cannot be inspected adequately by this technique. By contrast, the infragastric approach is almost always technically feasible as adhesions can be divided and the entire region from the gastroduodenal artery on the right side to the tail of the gland and the splenic hilium on the left can be visualized.

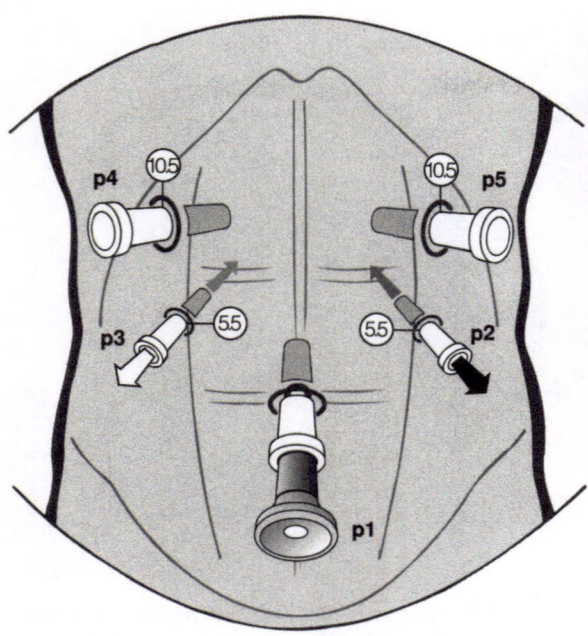

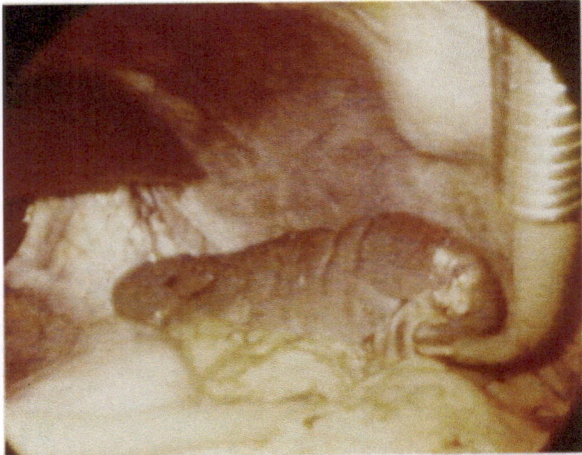

Fig. 13.15. Coaxial curved instruments and flexible metal cannulae which permit their insertion

Fig. 13.14. Sites of trocar cannulae for examination of the body and tail of the pancreas

Sites of Trocar and Cannula and Instrumentation

Four trocar cannulae are needed for either the supragastric or infragastric technique of laparoscopic inspection of the pancreas. These are shown in Fig. 13.14. The optic is introduced through a subumbilical 11-mm cannula. Two operating cannulae (5.5-mm for straight instruments, 8-mm metal flexible for curved coaxial instruments) are placed one on each side along the linea semilunaris at the level of the umbilicus. A 10.5-mm cannula is placed in the right upper quadrant along the anteriorly axillary line. This is the assistant's cannula and is also used for introduction of the ultrasound probe. Usually another cannula placed in the corresponding position on the left side is required for complete ultrasound examination of the pancreas (see below).

Although both infra- and supragastric methods of laparoscopic exposure of the pancreas can be performed using standard straight laparoscopic instrumentation, there is no doubt that both techniques are considerably facilitated by the use of coaxial curved instruments introduced through metal flexible cannulae (Fig. 13.15). Both the ease

of execution and the time taken to perform the procedures are influenced by the type of instruments used. A 30° forward oblique telescope is essential for both the supra- and infragastric techniques.

The ancillary equipment needed includes the electrosurgical unit, suction irrigation system and biopsy/fine needle aspiration cytology needles. Complete gastric decompression by the insertion of a 16-F Salem sump nasogastric tube attached to continuous low suction is essential for both methods.

Supragastric Technique

The operating table is tilted head-up (30°) throughout the supragastric procedure. As the assistant lifts the falciform ligament and quadrate lobe upwards, the anterior wall of the middle third of the stomach is grasped by a Babcock's or Duval's forceps and pulled down (Fig. 13.16). The lesser omentum is divided by scissors in an oblique transverse direction some distance from the lesser curve to avoid the left gastric vascular arcade and the incision extended from the region of the antrum to the transparent section (pars flaccida) close to the oesophagogastric junction (Fig. 13.17) provided an anomalous left hepatic artery arising from the left gastric is not encountered. In such a case, the left extension of the lesser omental window is stopped short of

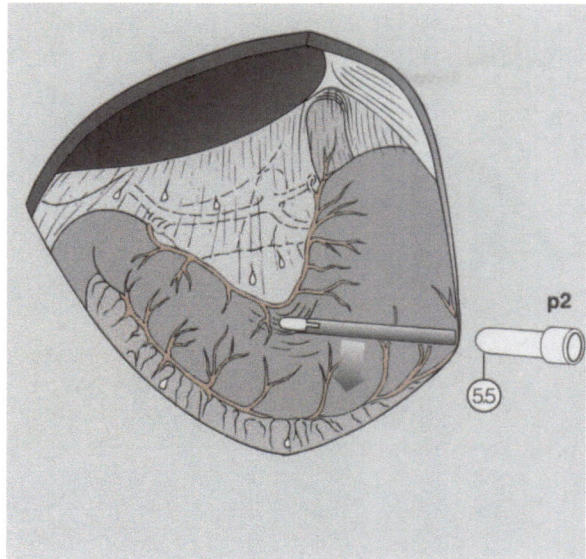

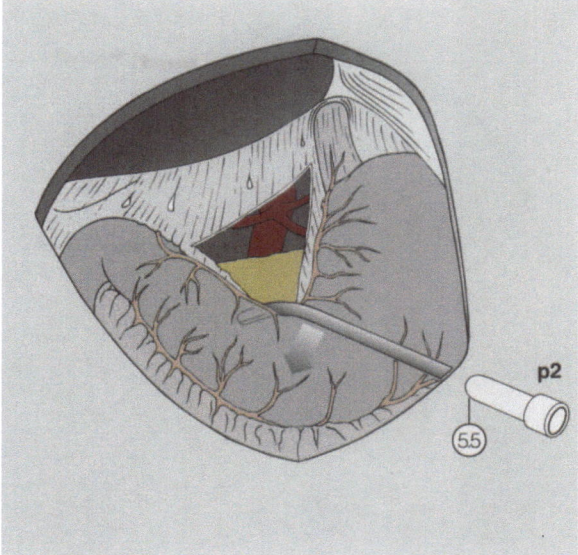

Fig. 13.16. Grasping and pulling the anterior wall of the middle third of the stomach

Fig. 13.17. Dividing the lesser omentum in an oblique transverse direction some distance from the lesser curve to avoid the left gastric vascular arcade and extending the incision from the region of the antrum to the transparent section close to the oesophagogastric junction. In examination of the pancreas by the supragastric approach the curved coaxial grasper is used as a hook to lift the stomach upwards and in a distal direction thereby exposing the body of the pancreas. The curved grasper is slid along the lesser curvature to the right to expose the proximal part of the body of the pancreas and then to the left for visualization of the left hemipancreas

this vessel because it must be preserved. The curved coaxial grasper is then placed behind the stomach with the tip pointing downwards used as a hook to lift the stomach upwards and in a distal direction, thereby exposing the body of the pancreas. The curved grasper is slid along the lesser curvature to the right to expose the proximal part of the body of the pancreas and then to the left for visualization of the left hemipancreas (Fig. 13.17). The exposed pancreas is palpated with a closed atraumatic forceps and any suspicious lesion biopsied. A good exposure of the distal splenic artery in its tortuous course along the upper border of the pancreas is obtained.

Infragastric Technique

The infragastric technique undoubtedly provides better exposure of the pancreas and is feasible even in the presence of adhesions binding the posterior wall of the stomach and lesser omentum to the pancreas. It, however, takes longer and is more technically demanding.

The first step of the procedure consists of creation of an infragastric window in the greater omentum near the greater curvature. For this pur-

pose, the stomach is grasped at the junction of its middle with the upper third by a coaxial curved grasper which is used to lift the greater curvature upwards to identify an avascular window between vessels running from the gastroepiploic arcade to the stomach. Usually two to three such vessels require to be secured and divided to create a sufficient window. As these gastric vessels are soft and surrounded by fat, they do not hold clips well and often continue to bleed despite correct clip application. Furthermore, clips applied to these gastric vessels can be brushed off easily during the manipulations. For these reasons, ligature of these greater curvature vessels is necessary. This is achieved as follows: The peritoneum is divided on either side of the selected vessel (Fig. 13.18), which is then tied in continuity at its origin from the arcade using an external slip knot of 1/0 chromic catgut (Fig. 13.18). A preformed chromic catgut en-

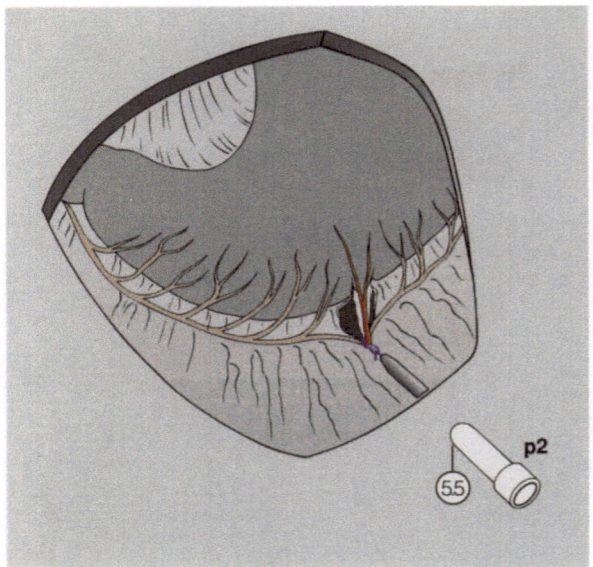

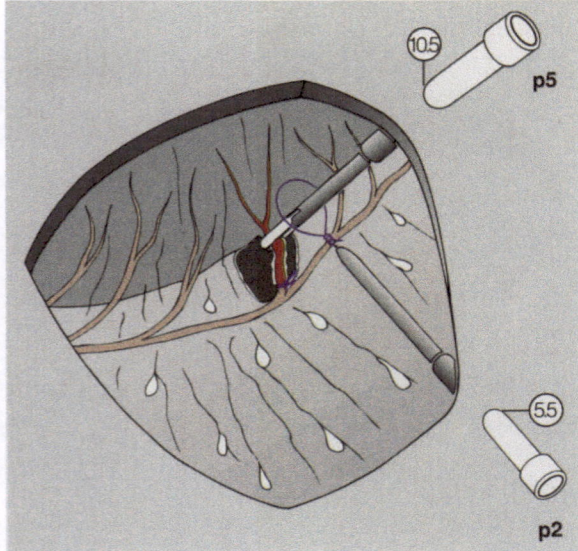

Fig. 13.18. Ligature and division of the greater curve vessels to create the infragastric window. Dividing the peritoneum on either side of the selected vessel, using an external slip knot of 1/0 chromic catgut to tied the vessel in continuity at its origin from the arcade

Fig. 13.19. A curved grasper is passed through the endoloop before being applied to the vessel close to the stomach wall

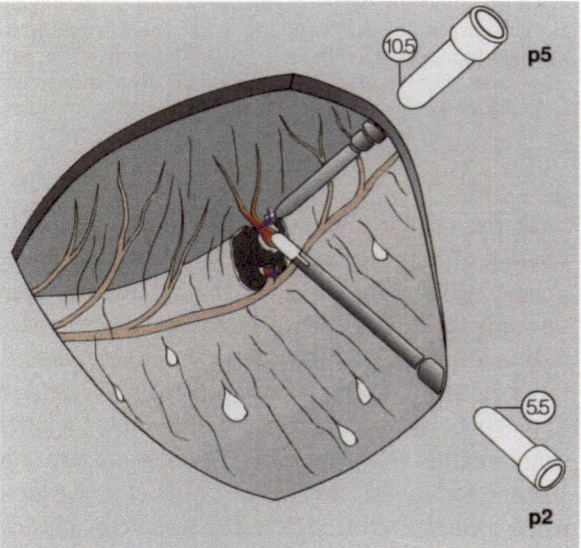

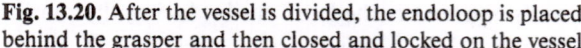

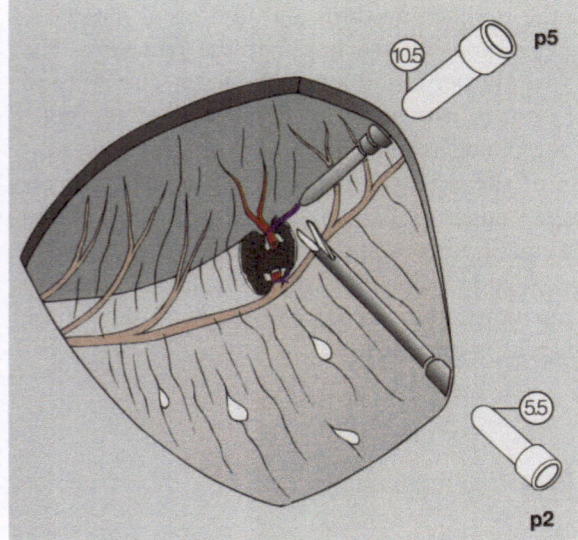

Fig. 13.20. After the vessel is divided, the endoloop is placed behind the grasper and then closed and locked on the vessel

Fig. 13.21. The grasper is released and the ligated vessel divided by scissors

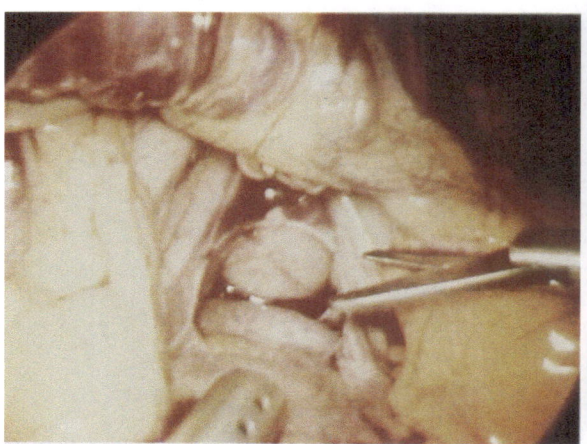

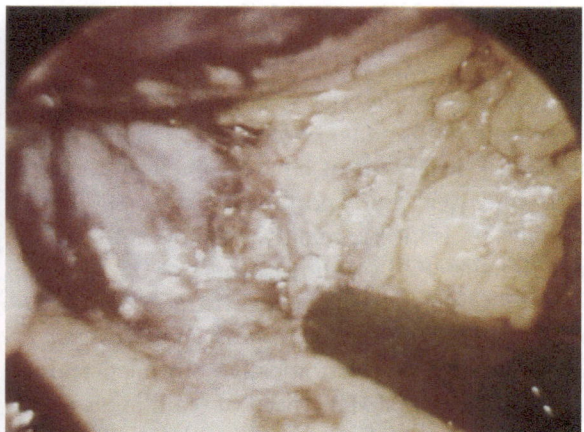

a

Fig. 13.22. Division of adhesions between the posterior surface of the stomach and the pancreas

doloop is then inserted and a curved grasper is passed through the loop before grasping the vessel close to the stomach wall (Fig. 13.19). After the vessel is divided by scissors, the endoloop is placed behind the grasper (Fig. 13.20) and then closed and locked on the vessel (Fig. 13.20) before the grasper is released (Fig. 13.21). The long limb of the endoloop is then cut. The entire process is repeated to ligate and divide adjacent vessels until a suficient window is achieved. The posterior wall of the stomach is then lifted by the coaxial curved grasper when the central portion of the pancreas is exposed. In the vast majority of patients adhesions are present between the posterior surface of the stomach and the pancreas. These are divided by the coaxial curved scissors (Fig. 13.22). Eventually, the entire surface of the pancreas from the gastroduodenal artery on the right to the tail and splenic artery and hilium on the left can be inspected and palpated (Fig. 13.23 a–c). Lesions can be biopsied or subjected to fine needle aspiration cytology.

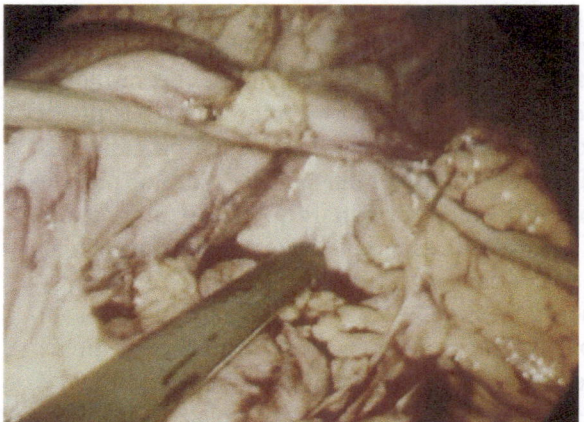

b

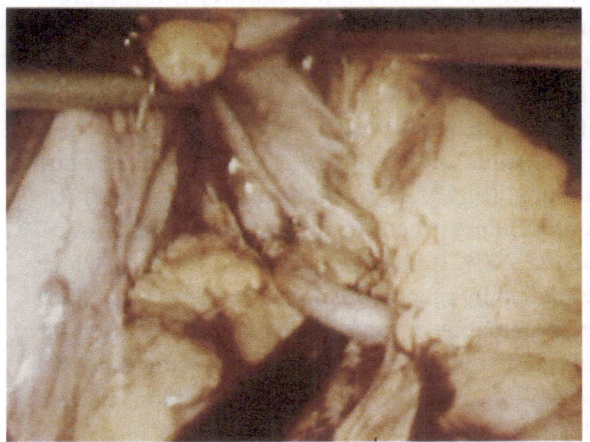

c

Fig. 13.23 a–c. Infragastric exposure of the lesser sac. **a** Gastroduodenal artery, neck and proximal body of pancreas. **b** Left hemi-pancreas. **c** Splenic artery

Laparoscopic Ultrasound Scanning

There is littledoubt that the scope of diagnostic and staging laparoscopy has been considerably enhanced with the advent of laparoscopic transducer probes and real-time portable units. Modern ultrasonic transducers mainly employ lead zirconate titanate (PZT), although some of the newer probes utilize vinylidene fluoride trifluoroethylene copolymer (P (VDF-TrPE)). In most modern scanners, mechanical or electronically controlled real-time systems are used. The speed of scanning is determined by the speed of sound and the resolution is dependent on the wavelength and thus on the attenuation in the tissue [20]. Wavelength frequency (MHz) aside, the improvement in the resolution provided by modern ultrasonic scanners is due to more sophisticated electronic signal processing of reflected sound providing a wider range of registration of the received signals on video storage tubes.

Contact ultrasonography employed during open and laparoscopic surgery allows the use of high frequency probes (5–7.5 MHz) for maximum resolution. As the probe is in direct contact with the tissue, the sacrifice in depth of field (far field = 5–6 cm at these frequencies) which is inevitable with increased wavelength frequency is not a problem. If the organ's depth exceeds this range (e. g. right lobe of liver), contact scanning from the relevant two opposite surfaces ensures imaging of the entire parenchymal depth.

The value of intraoperative contact ultrasound scanning (IOCUS) in open surgery for liver tumours, biliary tract and pancreas is beyond question [21–27]. It detects deposits in the liver which are missed by preoperative imaging tests and which are impalpable or invisible at operation, permits scan-guided biopsy and assists in defining both inoperability and the extent of resection needed [21–25]. In the cases of pancreatic insulinomas, palpation of the pancreas together with IOCUS. permits localization of these tumours in 100% of cases [26]. The reports on the use of the technique for the detection of ductal calculi during open cholecystectomy have been favourable [27], although whether IOCUS is an effective substitute to intraoperative cholangiography (IOC) remains unsettled.

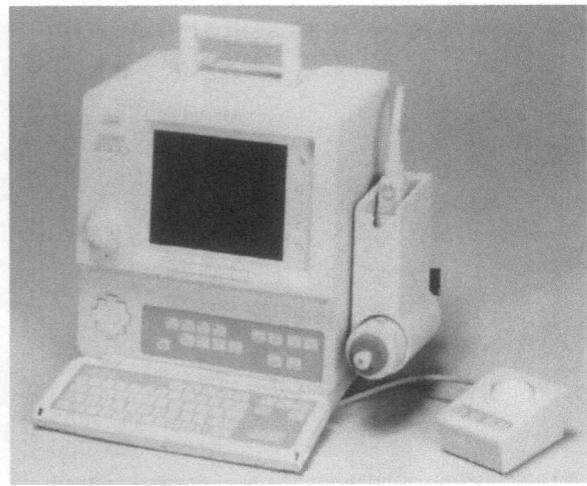

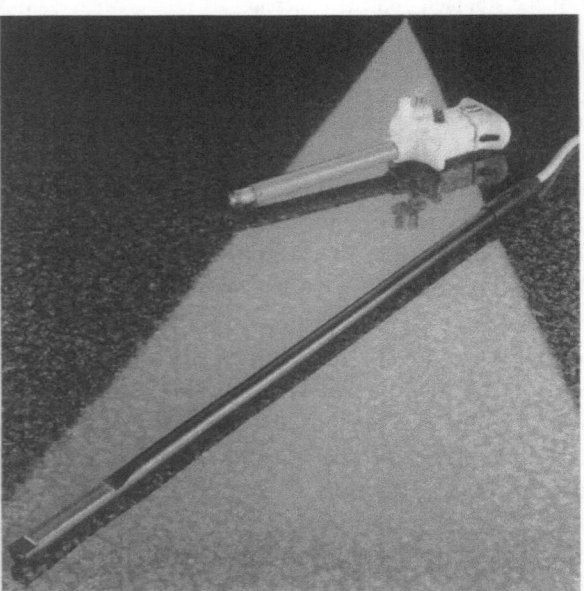

Fig. 13.24a, b. Aloka laparoscopic ultrasound scanning system and probe

The reported experience to date with laparoscopic contact ultrasonography is limited [28–30], but the results are encouraging and the benefit should be equivalent to that which has been accrued by IOCUS during open surgery. Laparoscopic ultrasound scanning has been used in the diagnosis of hepatic and gallbladder disease, ductal calculi, staging of cancer of the head of the pancreas and liver tumours, and examination of the hepatic parenchyma for secondary deposits. More recently we have extended the scope of laparoscopic ultrasound scanning to include examination of the neck and body of the pancreas [31].

In our institution, we have evaluated and used two systems in laparoscopic diagnosis and staging: the Aloka SSD 500 system (Tokyo, Japan), which uses a high density linear array 7.5-MHz probe (Fig. 13.24) and the Laparoscan (Endomedix, Irvine, California, USA) which has end- or sideviewing 5-MHz sector probes. Both the Aloka and the Laparoscan probes are introduced through standard 10.5-mm cannulae. In general, linear array probes outline the anatomy better and provide higher resolution in both the near and far fields. More than any other imaging modality, ultrasonography requires a skilled operator who is also an experienced interpreter. There is little doubt that with training, surgeons, by virtue of their knowledge of the structural and topographical anatomy, can become experienced reliable ultrasound operators within a relatively short period of time. The utility of laparoscopic ultrasound scanning is as much dependent on the acquisition of the necessary skills in manipulation of the probe and in the interpretation of the scanned images as it is on the quality of the equipment and probes used. The best advice that can be given to surgeons who have no previous experience is to enlist the services of a trained ultrasonographist (usually a radiologist colleague) to guide them through as many cases as is necessary to achieve full proficiency in both the execution of the technique and in its interpretation.

Laparoscopic Ultrasound Scanning of the Liver

Laparoscopic ultrasound examination of the liver is invaluable in the evaluation of cirrhosis, detection of focal lesions and secondary deposits and in the assessment of the resectability of primary tumours [29, 30]. The contact ultrasound scanning permits the detection of deep lesions within the hepatic parenchyma which do not reach the liver capsule and cannot therefore be visualized by inspection of the liver surface during diagnostic laparoscopy.

The technique is similar to the that used in open surgery. The ultrasound scanning using the sector Aloka probe starts on the anterosuperior surface by identification of the vena cava at the back of the liver and subsequently the three hepatic veins which form the boundaries of the four sectors of the liver. The hepatic parenchyma of each sector is scanned from the vena cava downwards to the free margin of the liver. On completion of the examination through the anterosuperior surface, the probe is placed underneath the liver lobes for scanning of the hepatic parenchyma from below. The examination of the entire depth of the hepatic parenchyma (especially on the right side) is assured by this combined approach.

Cystic structures within the liver parenchyma are readily identified as they contain few or no internal echoes, exhibit good transmission and have sharply defined walls. Solid lesions (tumours) are more difficult to delineate and exhibit three sonographic patterns: hypoechoic or sonolucent, hyperechoic or complex. The hypoechoic lesions can usually be differentiated from cysts because they have a different sound attenuation and indefinite margins. Hypoechoic lesions are usually composed of solid tumours without necrosis [32]. Hyperechoic lesions exhibit intense and uniform echo reflectivity, which is indicative of a prominent vascular component consisting of dilated vessels [32]. Hyperechoicity can also be caused by fatty change. Complex lesions have both hyper- und hypoechoic regions which reflect viable and necrotic areas within a lesion, respectively. In some malignant tumours alternating rings of hypo and hyperechoic regions give rise to a "bull's eye" appearance. However, it must be stressed that there are no reliable ultrasonographic findings which differentiate benign from malignant tumours or between primary and metastatic liver disease.

The most hyperechoic lesion encountered in the liver is the haemangioma. This is, however, readily identified by its macroscopic appearance during laparoscopy and is, of course, compressible. Haemangiomas should never be biopsied.

If a solid lesion is detected, an ultrasonically guided biopsy using the Bioptit or Trucut needle is performed.

Laparoscopic Ultrasound Scanning of the Gallbladder and Extrahepatic Biliary Tract

Laparoscopic ultrasound examination is useful in the evaluation of gallbladder disease. Direct contact scanning of the gallbladder is indicated in those patients with symptoms attributable to disease in this organ where the usual preoperative work-up is normal or equivocal or raises suspicion of serious disease. The most common indication is the patient who presents with symptoms of biliary colic but has negative investigations. Small calculi or biliary sludge can be detected in some of these patients with laparoscopic contact ultrasonography. Other lesions which are best confirmed by scanning of the gallbladder during laparoscopy include adenomyomatosis, cholesterolosis and polyps. In cancer of the gallbladder, contact ultrasonography of this organ provides information on the extent of mural involvement and presence and sectorial location of invasion of the hepatic parenchyma.

Laparoscopic scanning of the extrahepatic bile ducts for the detection of ductal calculi is currently under investigation in a number of centres [28]. Although early results are encouraging, it is doubtful whether it has the potential for providing the detailed anatomical information which is elicited by IOC and for this reason, it is unlikely to replace this contrast examination. Laparoscopic biliary ultrasonography may be used as a substitute for IOC in easy, uncomplicated cases without a previous history of jaundice or acute pancreatitis as a quick screen for unsuspected ductal calculi. When positive or suggestive, it requires confirmation by IOC. Another potentially useful role for laparoscopic ultrasonography with colour Doppler (when this becomes available) is in the course of a difficult laparoscopic cholecystectomy. Where it would ideal for the identification of vascular structures, including the common hepatic artery and its branches.

More detailed information can be obtained by intraluminal biliary ultrasound. The system which is introduced percutaneously is used to image the interior of the gallbladder and bile ducts [33], thereby documenting the presence of biliary sludge, stones, ductal strictures and tumours. This technique provides useful information on the nature of intraluminal filling defects, intramural pathology of the gallbladder and bile ducts and allows the examination of inaccessible duct territories.

Ultrasound Scanning of the Pancreatic Head

The mobilization of the head of the pancreas described above permits excellent ultrasound scanning of the pancreas by placement of the linear array Aloka probe behind the head of the pancreas with the transducer facing forwards. Detailed examination of the pancreatic parenchyma, the intrapancreatic segment of the bile duct, the common channel and ampullary region, the lesion and its encroachment on the pancreatic duct and portal vein can be determined.

Contact Scanning of the Body and Tail of the Pancreas Through the Infragastric Approach

This provides the best technique for outlining the detailed anatomy of the pancreas and has been used successfully for the location of occult insulinoma [31]. The Aloka system is employed. As the current sector probe is straight, contact with the surface of the pancreas requires two ports: a right subcostal for scanning the distal hemipancreas and an ipsilateral port for scanning the neck and proximal body of the organ (Fig. 13.25). Each half of the

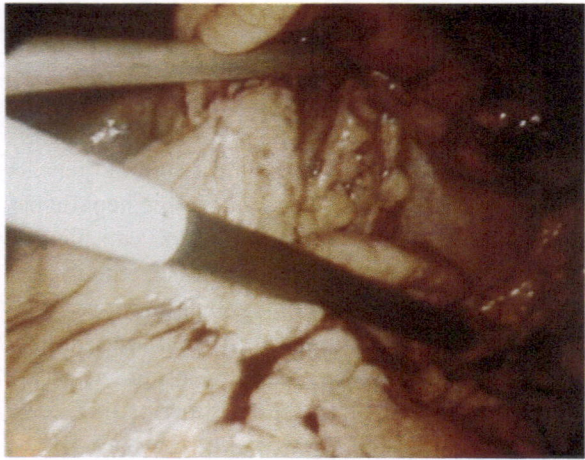

Fig. 13.25. Probe scanning the distal hemipancreas

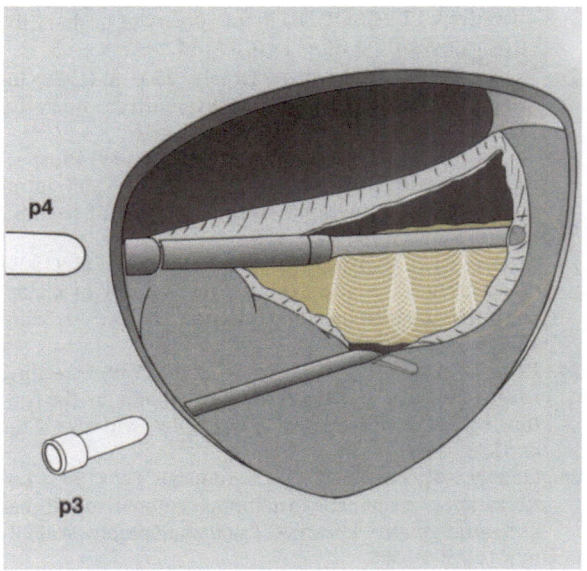

Fig. 13.26. Scanning each half of the pancreas with the probe lying along the longitudinal axis of the organ, starting at the upper border and sweeping down the anterior surface to the lower border of the pancreas

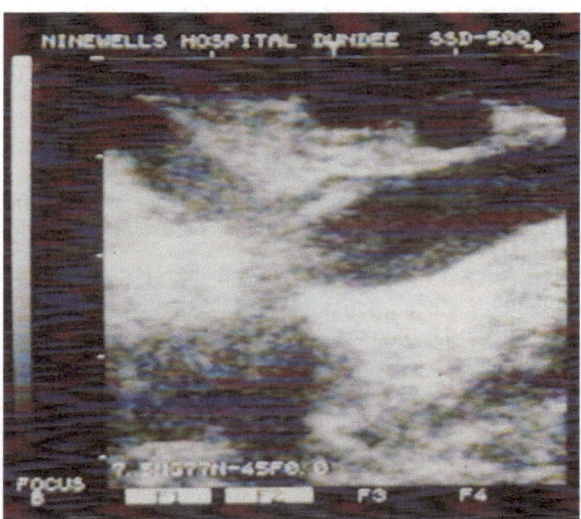

Fig. 13.28. The portal vein and its junction with the splenic vein, the proximal pancreatic duct and the central pancreatic artery in the proximal pancreas

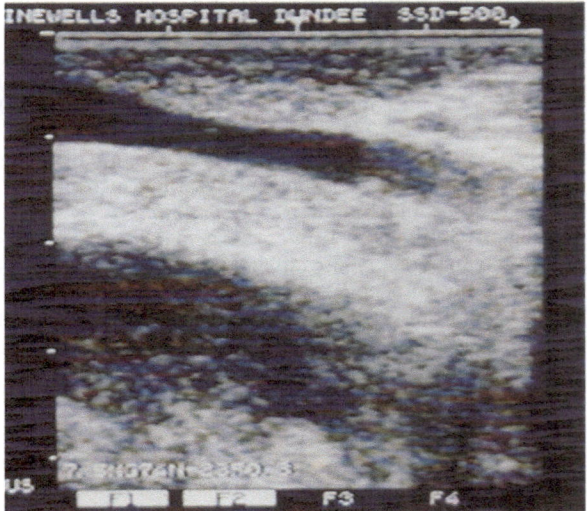

Fig. 13.27. The pancreatic duct in the distal hemipancreas just above the splenic vein, separated from it by the central artery of the pancreas

pancreas is scanned with the probe lying along the longitudinal axis of the organ, starting at the upper border and sweeping down the anterior surface to the lower border of the pancreas (Fig. 13.26). In this sweep of the left hemipancreas, the pancreatic duct appears just above the splenic vein and is sepa-

rated from it by the central artery of the pancreas (Fig. 13.27). In the proximal pancreas, the portal vein and its junction with the splenic vein, the proximal pancreatic duct, and the central pancreatic artery are clearly visible (Fig. 13.28). Having completed the contact scanning on the anterior surface, the probe is transferred to the lower border of the pancreas with the transducer facing upwards and is used to lift the organ and any mass (see Figure 13.25). This manoeuvre provides excellent imaging of the deeper portion of the pancreas and the retropancreatic nodes.

References

1. Lightdale CJ (1982) Clinical application of laparoscopy in patients with malignant neoplasms. Gastrointest Endosc 28:99–102
2. Shandall A, Johnson C (1985) Laparoscopy or scanning in oesophageal and gastric carcinoma? Br J Surg 22:449–451
3. Possik RA, Franco EL, Pires DR et al (1986) Sensitivity, specificity and predictive value of laparoscopy for the staging of gastric cancer and for the detection of liver metastases. Cancer 58:1–6
4. Cuschieri A, Hall AW, Clark J (1978) Value of laparoscopy in the diagnosis and management of pancreatic cancer. Gut 19:672–677

5. Warshaw AL, Tepper JE, Shipley WU (1986) Laparoscopy in the staging and planning of therapy for pancreatic cancer. Am J Surg 158:76–80
6. Cuschieri A (1988) Laparoscopy for pancreatic cancer: does it benefit the patient? Eur J Surg Oncol 14:41–44
7. Ishida H, Furukawa Y, Kuroda H et al (1981) Laparoscopic observation and biopsy of the pancreas. Endoscopy 13:68–73
8. Ishida H (1983) Peritoneoscopy and pancreas biopsy in the diagnosis of pancreatic disease. Gastrointest Endosc 29:211–218
9. Berci G, Cuschieri A (1984) Practical laparoscopy. Baillière Tindall, London
10. Henning H, Look K (1985) Laparoskopie. Thieme, Stuttgart
11. Fornari F, Rapaccini L, Cavanna L et al (1988) Diagnosis of hepatic lesions: ultrasonically guided fine needle biopsy or laparoscopy? Gastrointest Endosc 34:231–234
12. Jensen DM, Berci G (1981) Laparoscopy: advances in biopsy and recording techniques. Gastrointest Endosc 27:150–153
13. Beck K (1984) Colour atlas of laparoscopy. Saunders, Philadelphia
14. Berci G, Morgenstern L, Shore JM, Shapiro S (1973) A direct approach to the differential diagnosis of jaundice. Laparoscopy with transhepatic cholecystocholangiography. Am J Surg 126:372–378
15. Cuschieri A (1975) Value of laparoscopy in hepatobiliary disease. Ann Coll Surg Engl 57:33–38
16. Irving AD, Cuschieri A (1978) Laparoscopic assessment of the jaundiced patient. Br J Surg 65:678–680
17. Shimi S, Banting S, Cuschieri A (1991) Laparoscopy in the management of pancreatic cancer: endoscopic cholecystojejunostomy for advanced disease. Br J Surg 79:317–319
18. Meyer-Burg J, Ziegler U, Palma C (1969) Zur supragastralen pankeaskopie. Ergebnisse aus 125 laparoskopien. Dtsch Med Wochenschr 97:1969–1971
19. Strauch M, Lux G, Ottenjann R (1973) Infragastric pancreascopy. Endoscopy 5:30–32
20. Wells PN (1988) Ultrasound imaging. J Biomed Eng 10:548–554
21. Bismuth H, Castaing D, Garden OJ (1987) The use of operative ULTRASOUND in the surgery of primary liver cancer. World J Surg 11:610–614
22. Parker GA, Lawrence W Jr, Horsley JS et al (1989) Intraoperative ultrasound of the liver affects operative decision making. Ann Surg 209:569–576
23. Clarke MP, Kane RA, Steele G Jr et al (1989) Prospective comparison of preoperative imaging and intraoperative ultrasonography in the detection of liver tumours. Surgery 106:849–855
24. Brower ST, Dumitrescu O, Rubinoff S et al (1989) Operative ultrasound establishes resectability of metastases by major hepatic resection. World J Surg 13:649–657
25. Russo A, La Rosa C, Cajozzo M et al (1989) Screening for liver metastases of colorectal carcinoma by the routine use of intraoperative echography. Minerva Chir 44:1893–1900
26. Galiber AK, Reading CC, Charboneau JW (1988) Localization of pancreatic insulinoma: comparison of pre- and intraoperative US and CT and angiography. Radiology 166:504–508
27. Mosnier H, Audy JC, Boche O, Guivarc'h M (1992) Intraoperative sonography during cholecystectomy for gallstones. Surg Gynec Obstet 174:469–473
28. Rothlin M, Schlumpf R, Largiader F (1991) The technique of intraoperative ultrasonography in laparoscopic cholecystectomy. Chirurg 62:899–901
29. Fornari F, Civardi G, Cavanna L et al (1989) Laparoscopic ultrasonography in the study of liver disease. Preliminary results. Surg Endsc 3:33–37
30. Miles WFA, Paterson-Brown, Garden OJ (1992) Laparoscopic contact hepatic ultrasonography. Br J Surg 79:419–420
31. Pietrabissa A, Shimi S, Cuschieri A Detection of occult insulinoma by laparoscopic infragastric pancreatic contact ultrasound scanning
32. Tanaka S, Kitamura T, Imaoka S et al (1983) Hepatocellular carcinoma: sonographic and histological correlation. Am J Roentgenol 140:701–707
33. van Sonnenberg E, D'Agostino HB, Sanchez RL et al (1992) Percutaneous intraluminal US in the gallbladder and bile ducts. Radiology 182:693–696

Subject Index

Springer-Verlag
and the Environment

We at Springer-Verlag firmly believe that an international science publisher has a special obligation to the environment, and our corporate policies consistently reflect this conviction.

We also expect our business partners – paper mills, printers, packaging manufacturers, etc. – to commit themselves to using environmentally friendly materials and production processes.

The paper in this book is made from low- or no-chlorine pulp and is acid free, in conformance with international standards for paper permanency.